W9-CYY-745

Osteoarthritis

Osteoarthritis

Public Health Implications for an Aging Population

EDITED BY

David Hamerman, M.D.

Distinguished University Professor of Medicine, Professor of
Orthopedic Surgery, and Director, Resnick Gerontology Center,
Albert Einstein College of Medicine and Montefiore Medical Center,
Bronx, New York

THE JOHNS HOPKINS UNIVERSITY PRESS
BALTIMORE AND LONDON

© 1997 The Johns Hopkins University Press
All rights reserved. Published 1997
Printed in the United States of America on acid-free paper
05 04 03 02 01 00 99 98 97   5 4 3 2 1

The Johns Hopkins University Press
2715 North Charles Street
Baltimore, Maryland 21218-4319
The Johns Hopkins Press Ltd., London

Library of Congress Cataloging-in-Publication Data will be found at the end of this book.
A catalog record for this book is available from the British Library.

ISBN 0-8018-5561-6

Contents

Contributors

John P. Allegrante, Ph.D., Professor and Director, Division of Health Services, Sciences and Education, Columbia University, New York, New York; and Adjunct Professor of Behavioral Science and Health Education in Medicine and Associate Director, Education, Epidemiology and Health Services Research, Cornell Arthritis and Musculoskeletal Disease Center, New York, New York

Philip W. Brickner, M.D., Professor of Clinical Medicine, New York Medical College, Valhalla, New York; Chair, Department of Community Medicine, St. Vincent's Hospital, New York, New York

Emmanuelle Cambois, Institut National de la Santé et de la Recherche Médicale, Equipe "Démographie et Santé," Montpellier, France

Christine K. Cassel, M.D., Professor and Director, Department of Geriatrics, Mt. Sinai School of Medicine, New York, New York

Flavia M. Cicuttini, M.B., Ph.D., Senior Lecturer, Department of Epidemiology and Preventive Medicine, Monash University, Australia

Helmut Fenner, Ph.D., Lecturer in Pharmaceutical Science, Swiss Federal Institute of Technology, Hofgut Siegmatt, Gelterkinden, Switzerland

William F. Forbes, Ph.D., D.Sc., Distinguished Professor Emeritus, Elizabeth Bruyere Health Center, University of Ottawa, Ottawa, Ontario, Canada

Andrew A. Guccione, Ph.D., P.T., Lecturer, Department of Orthopedics, Harvard Medical School, and Director of Physical Therapy Services, Massachusetts General Hospital, Boston, Massachusetts

Laurance D. Hall, Ph.D., Professor, Herchel Smith Laboratory for Medicinal Chemistry, University of Cambridge School of Clinical Medicine, Cambridge, United Kingdom

Marc C. Hochberg, M.D., M.P.H., Professor of Medicine and Epidemiology and Preventive Medicine, and Head, Division of Rheumatology and Clinical Immunology, University of Maryland School of Medicine, Baltimore, Maryland

James Oat Judge, M.D., Assistant Professor, Department of Medicine, Travelers Center on Aging, University of Connecticut School of Medicine, Farmington, Connecticut

Margaret Lethbridge-Cejku, M.Sc., Research Associate, Division of Rheumatology and Clinical Immunology, Department of Medicine, University of Maryland School of Medicine, Baltimore, Maryland

Marian A. Minor, P.T., Ph.D., Associate Professor, Physical Therapy Program, School of Health Related Professions, University of Missouri, Columbia, Missouri

S. Jay Olshansky, Ph.D., Associate Professor, Center on Aging, Health and Society, University of Chicago, Chicago, Illinois

A. Robin Poole, Ph.D., D.Sc., Director, Joint Diseases Laboratory, Shriner's Hospital for Children, Montreal, Quebec, Canada; and Professor, Department of Surgery, McGill University, Montreal, Quebec, Canada

Jean-François Ravaud, M.D., Institut National de la Santé et de la Recherche Médicale, Equipe "Handicap et Société," Institut Fédératif de Recherche sur le Handicap, Paris, France

Jean-Marie Robine, Institut National de la Santé et de la Recherche Médicale, Equipe "Démographie et Santé," Montpellier, France

Tim D. Spector, M.D., Consultant Rheumatologist and Honorary Senior Lecturer, Department of Rheumatology, St. Thomas' Hospital, London, United Kingdom

Jenny A. Tyler, D.Phil., Head, Matrix Biochemistry Department, Strangeways Research Laboratory, Cambridge, United Kingdom

Paul J. Watson, Ph.D., Herchel Smith Laboratory for Medicinal Chemistry, University of Cambridge School of Clinical Medicine, Cambridge, United Kingdom

Foreword

Osteoarthritis affects the lives of a large percentage of older people. Although much has been written about osteoarthritis, the attention it has gotten in the research community is still relatively small in proportion to its tremendous impact on functional abilities and quality of life in the older population. In this context, this book is a major addition to the field, and will be welcomed by those interested in issues both of aging and of osteoarthritis itself. Its contribution to our understanding of osteoarthritis goes well beyond that of standard texts on pathology and clinical management. Additionally, readers of this book will find that some of the most intriguing issues in aging can be approached through the study of different aspects of osteoarthritis.

Dr. David Hamerman should be congratulated for bringing together a diverse group of distinguished investigators whose contributions complement each other so well. The result is a volume that characterizes osteoarthritis and aging from a variety of perspectives, with the overall effect being a clear elucidation of the major themes of the book.

One provocative theme is the relationship of the aging process to age-associated diseases and the question of where osteoarthritis fits into this framework. While improving our knowledge of the development of osteoarthritis is important in its own right, studying osteoarthritis can provide a more general understanding of basic aging processes. From a population perspective, considering the relative impact of osteoarthritis also leads to important questions that are addressed here. How does this nonlethal disease's impact on disability and quality of life differ from that of the diseases that are the leading causes of death? How will the relative impacts of lethal and nonlethal diseases change as mortality rates continue to decline, especially in the oldest segment of the population? How does the overall impact of osteoarthritis change in the presence of other comorbidities?

The themes of prevention and intervention also receive a great deal of attention in this book. Review of the risk factors for osteoarthritis makes it clear that the disorder is not an inevitable part of growing old. It is true that there are not a large number of established risk factors for osteoarthritis, and only a few are modifiable. However, these risk factors are common and have a strong relationship to osteoarthritis, and therefore account for a substantial proportion of this condition in the older population. The book is particularly innovative in its approach to interventions. Its chapters on early diagnosis, research methodologies to monitor new therapeutic approaches, and potentials for new pharmaceuticals are very useful. Other new, nonpharmacologic interventions, particularly exercise, receive a gratifying amount of attention, and the chapters on those topics are an especially important contribution.

Osteoarthritis is beginning to receive the attention it is due as an important condition in older people. This book describes how public health aspects of osteoarthritis are being actively investigated and provides us with a conceptual framework that considers the relationship between aging and disease. It presents a vision of the way in which understanding this framework can give direction to the search for ways to prevent and treat osteoarthritis, exciting prospects for our aging population.

—Jack M. Guralnik, M.D., Ph.D.
Chief, Epidemiology and Demography Office
Epidemiology, Demography, and Biometry Program
National Institute on Aging

Introduction

Human aging, the overarching theme of this book, is an increasingly important concern of society. At the start of the twentieth century, "elderly" persons, or those aged 65 and over, constituted about 4 percent of the U.S. population. The factors that have contributed to longer life, and to the growth of the number of elderly persons to about 13 percent of the population at present, are well known: improved methods of sanitation, antibiotic therapy, advances in medical and surgical care, and widespread promotion of personal health practices. This trend favoring the growth of the elderly cohort will continue: according to demographic projections for the early decades of the twenty-first century, the proportion of the population that is aged 65 and over will approach 20 percent (McGinnis, 1988).

The most significant aspect of these projections relates to those members of the elderly population who are aged 85 and over, sometimes referred to as the "oldest old" or the "extreme aged," to distinguish them from a cohort a decade or so younger, termed the "young old" (Taeuber and Rosenwaike, 1992). The oldest old are the fastest-growing segment of the elderly population, and conservative projections indicate that by the early decades of the twenty-first century they will constitute more than 5 million people, while other projections double that number. The impressive growth of this group has profound implications for every segment of society, reflecting what is undeniable and inevitable about living a very long life: morbidities, or diseases associated with advancing age, become a dominant feature in the health profile and affect well-being and the quality of life. Thus, there are implications for those aged individuals and their caregivers, generational issues facing younger cohorts, concerns among planners who must define how health needs will be met and financed, and responsibilities on the part of health professionals who must provide for those needs.

Osteoarthritis (OA) is of great public health importance because it often imposes a *chronic* disability that is additive to other morbidities that are also highly age associated but are generally more *lethal.* Some years ago, Paul Dieppe commented, "Osteoarthritis remains an enigma; everyone recognizes it when they see it, but no one can define it" (Dieppe, 1984, p. 161). The difficulty in providing a unifying definition, even today, reflects the variable clinical and radiographic manifestations of OA in single or multiple joints, in which findings upon patient presentation may be minimal or far advanced. There is no specific diagnostic test, the course is not predictable, and the effects of medical therapies are uncertain. However, joint pain, limited range of motion, and instability, combined with radiographic evidence of joint space narrowing secondary to cartilage loss, sclerosis of the subchondral bone, and osteophytes (spurs) at the articular margins, are accepted as classical manifestations of disease (Hamerman, 1993). While OA may involve the diarthrodial joints of the extremities and the facet joints of the spine, this book will focus exclusively on the former, as this orientation makes for a more coherent and unifying presentation of the related subjects under consideration.

The four parts of this book survey the links between aging and the consequences of OA. Part One explores the association of aging and disease. Aging provides a setting for the expression of many conditions seen especially in elderly persons, such as OA, osteoporosis, cardiovascular diseases, stroke, late-onset diabetes, and dementia; their ultimate expression—the time when clinical manifestations appear, their severity, and their duration—are likely to depend on the interplay of environmental and genetic factors (chapter 1). A number of epidemiologists and gerontologists are engaged in a debate about the impact of emerging morbidities as the population ages: the issue is whether, with medical advances and health practices, those morbidities that become expressed with age will be "compressed" or "postponed" to the very last year or so of a long life of good quality, or whether they will "expand" or "extend" over the years of late life, with cumulative disabilities impairing the quality of life until death. Personal health practices have delayed the expression of diabetes, cardiovascular diseases, osteoporosis, and stroke, and therapeutic advances have limited their impact, but these conditions have not been eliminated; for other conditions, such as cancer, OA, and the so-called degenerative diseases that impair vision, hearing, and cognitive function, neither amelioration nor remedies are on the scene (chapter 2). The provision of health care for those persons achieving advanced age must meet the needs of ever-increasing numbers who are homebound due to disability. This will create challenges for health planners and for the medical profession in particular, which until now has been only peripherally involved in such efforts to care for very old people at home (chapter 3).

Part Two focuses on OA of the peripheral joints as the prototype of a chronic condition in the aging population which is unlike the disorders that are associated with mortality. Thus, in looking at OA in depth, we can seek to understand its association with aging itself (chapter 4), and consider aspects of disablement in general (chapter 5) and the impact of OA specifically in the presence of other morbidities that impair functional status (chapter 6). One dreaded event that occurs in very elderly persons is hip fracture, which is usually associated with osteoporosis, in which bone density is at least 2.5 standard deviations (SD) below the young normal mean. The evidence, presented in some studies, that hip fracture in older persons may occur less frequently in those with OA than in those with osteoporosis has been attributed to increased bone density in the former group. The contrasting states of bone density in OA and osteoporosis are examined in chapter 7. The public health implications of these conditions of the aging skeleton bear on virtually every other chapter in this book.

Joint restoration is the tertiary "preventive" measure now widely practiced for the management of advanced osteoarthritic joint disease. In Part Three, rather than discuss these surgical procedures or the use of anti-inflammatory and analgesic medications, subjects that are presented in depth in other reviews and do not lend themselves to the theme of aging, we focus on exercise as an intervention to promote the health of very old persons in general (chapter 8) and to improve outcomes for those with OA in particular (chapter 9).

Finally, in Part Four we look at the prospects for a future in which our knowledge of aging and OA may permit advances in health practices, diagnosis, and therapies that make secondary or even primary prevention of OA a reality. Even now, there are suggestions that some health practices, such as the maintenance of an ideal body weight, the use of exercises to strengthen lower-limb muscles, and the avoidance of joint trauma, may ameliorate OA or reduce its incidence (chapter 10). If aging is separable from the pathologic expression of OA as a disease, then it may be possible to detect OA early by biochemical analyses of "markers" derived from cartilage matrix or bone and present in synovial fluid and serum, and/or by the use of genetic tests to detect altered components of connective tissue (chapter 11); for example, type II collagen gene mutations have been demonstrated in a small subset of younger individuals with generalized OA and heritable forms of chondrodysplasias (Jiminez and Dharmavaram, 1994). Highly sophisticated computer-based imaging of joints is emerging as a potential means of identifying articular cartilage that appears free of OA and differentiating it from articular cartilage that shows changes that seem to coincide with the early stages of OA (chapter 12). Perhaps these newer imaging techniques and their potential for application to population studies will help to unravel the relationship between OA as a continuum of aging, on the one hand, and, on the other hand, OA as the additive expression of disease, albeit associated with the aging process. More precise visualization of joint structures in prospective clinical studies could encourage the pharmaceutical industry in the next decade to design new therapeutic modalities aimed at arresting the progression of OA at an early stage (chapter 13).

In this book, professionals representing a range of disciplines consider the implications of a potentially disabling chronic disease of peripheral joints which occurs almost exclusively in elderly persons. We believe that the multidisciplinary perspectives presented in these chapters and the need to respond to the imperatives that aging will increasingly impose on our society make this book timely and of interest to those concerned with epidemiology, social demography, rheumatology, orthopedic surgery, gerontology, public health, rehabilitation, and newer diagnostic and therapeutic measures for the identification and management of osteoarthritis.

REFERENCES

Dieppe P. 1984. Osteoarthritis: Are we asking the wrong questions? *Br J Rheumatol* 23:161–165.
Hamerman D. 1993. Aging and osteoarthritis: Basic mechanisms. *J Am Geriatr Soc* 41:760–770.
Jiminez SA, Dharmavaram RM. 1994. Genetic aspects of familial osteoarthritis. *Ann Rheum Dis* 53:789–797.
McGinnis JM. 1988. The Tithonus syndrome: Health and aging in America. In: *Health promotion and disease prevention in the elderly,* edited by R Chernoff, DA Lipschitz. Vol. 35, *Aging.* Pp. 1–16. New York: Raven Press.
Taeuber CM, Rosenwaike I. 1992. A demographic portrait of America's oldest old. In: *The oldest old,* edited by RM Suzman, DP Willis, KG Manton. Pp. 3–14. New York: Oxford University Pp. 3–14. New York: Oxford University Press.

PART I

The Association of Aging and Disease

1

General Concepts of the Association of Aging and Disease

William F. Forbes, Ph.D., D.Sc.

This chapter reviews our knowledge of the relationship between aging and disease. The first section of the chapter deals with population aging, providing a summary of the various demographic factors that contribute to the formation of a more elderly population. The elderly population is of special interest from the point of view of this chapter, since it is this cohort that is mainly affected by chronic diseases (Fried and Bush, 1988) that accrue as part of various aging processes.

The next section discusses aging processes and disease. Although work on aging has proceeded for many years, there is still no agreement on what constitutes a quantitative definition of aging. Moreover, there is considerable discussion about what aging processes represent in terms of biological entities and which measurements can be used to differentiate aging from disease.

These difficulties are illustrated in the section devoted to osteoarthritis (OA), a condition that afflicts many elderly persons. The question is whether OA should be regarded as a disease or as a consequence of an underlying aging process, and this illustrates the difficulty of disentangling the two. This is not entirely a theoretical issue: if OA can be shown to be the consequence of a basic aging process, and if this process (or these processes) can be identified and reduced (as considered in chapter 10), the prevalence of OA could be diminished and there would be an impact on a number of other chronic, age-related diseases. A reduction in OA would not have such an impact if OA were a disease with its own underlying characteristics and possibly its own unique set of risk factors.

Demographic Trends toward an Older Population

The term *population aging* is used to describe how our population now and in the immediate future contains a greater proportion of older individuals than has been the case in the past (Davies, 1985). In fact, individuals in the oldest age groups, namely, those more than 85 years old, represent the fastest-growing segment of the elderly population. Moreover, the proportion of older persons will increase, not only because people are living longer but also because with relatively low fertility rates there are fewer young persons. It is also known that the oldest population contains a majority of women (because males die younger) and a disproportionate number of widows and widowers.

Because of the increasing number of people living longer and hence the increasing incidence of advanced age in the population, there is little doubt that a variety of chronic diseases which are generally associated with age will assume an increasing importance. There has been discussion about whether many of these diseases represent aging processes (e.g., Bierman, 1978; Berg, 1985). Some of these diseases are important as causes of death. Of particular importance in this respect are the clinical manifestations of arteriosclerosis, namely, heart attacks and strokes—for which, incidentally, the mortality rates have been decreasing markedly during the last few decades (Brody, 1985; Davies, 1985). In addition to diseases that contribute to mortality, there are those that affect the quality of life; of particular importance in this regard are the various dementias. However, the most common disability associated with old age results from diseases of the joints, among which OA plays the most prominent part. Thus the question arises—and it is the focus of this chapter—should OA be regarded as a disease or as part of a normal aging process? This has important implications for society as a whole, particularly with respect to the future of health care.

Aging, Disease, and the Relationship between Them

Disease is defined relatively easily as a condition in which various functions of the organism are disturbed by comparison with a "normal" reference condition. But what is normal? If, for example, bone strength at the age of 20 is used as the normal reference, then age-related changes in bone-strength may be regarded as disease. This brings us to the definition of aging, for which there is not complete agreement. One generally accepted definition of aging is that it represents a normal biological process (one that is not necessarily understood) that occurs to a varying extent in everyone following maturation, and that it causes irreversible changes in cells and organs which permanently increase the probability that an individual will be afflicted by harmful consequences, namely, disease or death (Forbes and Thompson, 1990; Thompson and Forbes, 1990; Forbes and Hirdes, 1993). Although this definition seems straightforward, it does not address a number of issues. For example, this definition assumes that aging occurs after maturation, but it may be argued that aging begins at birth, or even at conception, since as soon as we are born, or conceived, aging processes occur. However, we believe (following Kohn, 1978, 1982) that it is preferable to think of maturation and aging as distinct processes, since their outcomes differ markedly.

A second issue arises from the above definition—namely, the inevitability of the aging that occurs in everyone. That aging is inevitable seems reasonable and intuitively correct, but when we consider OA, it is not clear whether the *clinical* manifestations of OA are an expression of disease, or an aging process that occurs in every member of the population who lives long enough. If OA met the criterion of universality (that is, if it occurred in everyone), it could be regarded as an aging process. If only a subset of the population is affected by OA, however, OA could be considered a disease, because its clinical characteristics will not occur in everyone. In fact, it seems possible that everyone would eventually be affected by OA if death did not occur before the clinical manifestations of OA became apparent. That is, we lean toward the view that OA represents an aging process, yet this discussion indicates why it is not easy to decide whether a particular condition, such as OA, should be regarded as a disease or an aging process (Evans, 1993; Hamerman, 1993, 1995).

To expand on this matter: we know that, on average, the degree of impairment (i.e., adverse changes that may lead to clinical symptoms) increases with chronological age, and at some "threshold level" at the higher end of the distribution of the degree of impairment, disability or a handicap occurs, as reflected by severe symptoms (see fig. 1.1). The concept of disablement is discussed comprehensively in chapter 5. Representations similar to that in figure 1.1 have been described previously (Brown and Forbes, 1974; Fries, 1988; Hamerman, 1993; Perls, 1995).

It is reasonable to assume that the degree of impairment is distributed differently at different ages. That is, the degree of impairment will vary for different individuals, and figure 1.1 shows that, in older cohorts, the greater average extent of impairment, together with the greater variability in the degree of impairment, will lead to an increased risk of symptoms. Figure 1.1 also shows that there is a progression of the disease with age, and that certain manifestations of this disease, as determined by a threshold level, can be tolerated; below this level no disability is apparent. However, as individuals grow older, the prob-

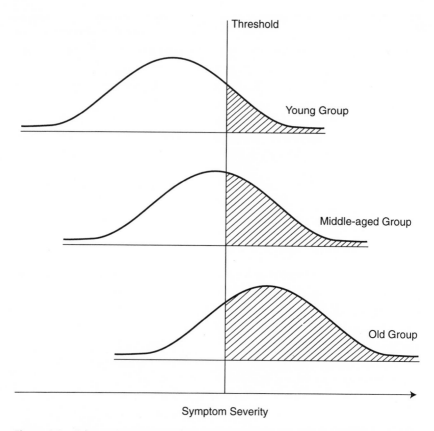

Figure 1.1.   Schematic presentation of the development of osteoarthritis and other chronic diseases. This representation shows a number of aspects relating to population aging and the incidence of the severity of clinical symptoms. The distribution of symptoms is displayed in populations at three arbitrarily selected ages—early adulthood (about 30 years), middle age (about 50 years), and old age (75 years and older). Assuming the distribution of symptom severity is normal for each population, the proportion of subjects in the youngest group exceeding the threshold is lowest, while the proportion in the eldest group is highest. The *cross-hatched areas* under the curve show this relationship. The figure also demonstrates what the text discusses more fully, that within each age group there will be variability (low and high) in the prevalence of symptoms.

ability that the clinical manifestations will rise above the threshold level of the disease will increase dramatically.

The representation shown in figure 1.1 is, of course, not confined to OA; it applies to most of the chronic diseases (Brown and Forbes, 1974). Most diseases show a similar pattern with age; that is, with time, the probability of being affected by a disability or disease, and by disease leading to death, increases in an approximately exponential manner (Forbes et al., 1993). In addition, in older cohorts many chronic diseases tend to occur together, and it is often a matter of chance whether a person will die from one particular disease or from another. These age-related patterns, and the fact that chronic diseases often occur together, have been said to show the synchronous nature of disease processes.

Following Kohn (1978, 1982), one can assume that aging processes account for this synchronous nature of disease processes. According to this view, aging is regarded as an inevitably fatal disease that afflicts everyone, and other diseases, such as OA, are seen as complications caused by these more basic aging processes. This model is statistically consistent with the known relationship between a variety of diseases, since if a number of variables (a variety of diseases) are strongly associated with respect to their prevalence as a function of age, this association can be explained by the presence of a third variable, namely, basic aging processes. This explanation is attractive because the alternative explanation—namely, that one disease, such as OA, causes another disease, such as a malignancy—seems most unlikely. This model can also explain why diseases tend to occur together in older individuals, since basic aging processes would have progressed, thus increasing the risk of a variety of chronic diseases. This, in turn implies that if OA could be prevented, or reduced, a basic aging process would also be reduced. Since this basic aging process is assumed to cause other chronic diseases as well, these would be reduced at the same time, with important public health implications.

There is a substantial amount of knowledge about the factors that affect life expectancy (see also chapter 2); for example, those individuals with higher income have a relatively longer life expectancy, and those who smoke cigarettes have a considerably shorter life expectancy than those who do not (Branch and Jette, 1984; Adams, 1990). Numerous other factors are also relevant to projections of life expectancy. These include exercise, diet, levels of serum glucose and lipids, and extent of obesity and stress. There are also relationships between these factors (e.g., between diet and serum lipids), some of which are not completely understood. We also do not know the importance of these risk factors or aspects of these risk factors (e.g., different components of the diet) for chronic diseases and for aging processes.

There is also an alternative way of explaining the synchronous nature of disease processes. This is to assume that different diseases, possibly caused by a variety of aging processes, show a similar age-related pattern of incidence and mortality because of evolution: any genetic change that delayed the onset of a disease would be favored by selection, and individuals who had incorporated this genetic change would become dominant in the population over time. In this way, natural selection would tend to synchronize different disease processes, and they would all tend to occur at the more advanced ages, even if they were physiologically independent. However, there are difficulties with this hypothesis. For example, there have been different historical patterns of mortality, and it is doubtful whether even 100 years ago the chronic diseases, the present main causes of mortality, played an important role in determining reproductive ability and mortality and thus were susceptible to natural selection. Hence, it is not clear how evolution would have given rise to similar age-related patterns of chronic diseases. In spite of these and other reservations, natural selection probably has some relevance, and there may be no need to hypothesize the existence of basic aging processes.

In the evolutionary model of chronic disease, the conquest of OA might have little effect on survival to a disease-free old age, since other chronic diseases would tend to replace OA because they develop in synchrony as a result of natural selection. Aging processes and natural selection are not mutually exclusive, however, since some important molecular changes (e.g., changes with respect to specific collagen cross-links) brought about by natural selection could contribute to more than one disease process. Hence, there may be a continuum in the sense that some chronic diseases are caused by aging processes, whereas at the other end of the continuum, some disabilities and diseases are not related to aging processes.

The use of the plural, *aging processes*, is deliberate, since it seems unlikely that there is only one underlying age-related process. This follows because most chronic diseases, including OA, a number of carcinomas, and the clinical manifestations of arteriosclerosis, show an increased incidence with age, which suggests the presence of aging processes. These aging processes may occur because older cells are more susceptible to disease, or because only a limited amount of "damage" can be tolerated and the relevant threshold is reached at the higher ages. Moreover, these aging processes for different chronic diseases may not be identical, although they may be synchronized. In addition to aging processes for different diseases there may also be more "basic" aging processes that occur in the absence of disease as the organism becomes more frail. These basic aging processes are of particular interest to gerontologists and may differ from the aging processes associated with at least some chronic diseases. Some aging processes may be interrelated and may involve similar mechanisms because the consequences of all aging processes are similar, in that these consequences (clinical manifestations of disease and general frailty) occur later in life and tend to occur together. Because of this interrelationship, a better understanding of the aging process relevant to OA (and to other chronic diseases) may also lead to a better understanding of more basic aging processes. There is also the related issue of identifying the risk factors for conditions of frailty (e.g., OA, sensory impairments, and Alzheimer disease), which are often nonfatal. These risk factors may not be the same as those for the fatal degenerative diseases, and it has been argued that an understanding of these nonfatal age-dependent conditions that are prevalent in the oldest age groups should be given priority (Olshansky et al., 1990).

Measurement Issues

From the above discussion, it follows that it would be of considerable interest to investigate, in a quantitative manner, the relationship between various postulated aging processes and different diseases. However, there are a number of difficulties. These difficulties become apparent when we examine the associations between chronological age and particular characteristics of groups of individuals. If this is done, one finds that many phenomena, such as loss of teeth and graying of hair, are strongly associated with chronological age. It would then seem reasonable to take these variables that are strongly associated with age, and combine them in some way to arrive at a measure of aging. Unfortunately, a strong association with age is neither a necessary nor a sufficient condition to justify the conclusion that a particular process represents an aging process (Brown and Forbes, 1976). It is possible that a particular variable maintains its level for a considerable length of time but that eventually there occurs a marked change that leads to disability or death. If this were the case the relation of this variable with age would not be strong, although the variable would represent an important aging process because of its strong association with the probability of death. Also, an association with age is not a sufficient condition. For example, the graying of hair becomes more common with age, and hence there is a strong association with age. However, the graying of hair on its own does not affect appreciably the probability of the occurrence of disease or death. Thus, any particular value of a variable, or change in a variable, must be associated with an increased probability of disease or death if it is to be considered an aging process. Such information is harder to obtain and may require a longitudinal study.

If one wants to measure aging processes, it is necessary to have data on individuals for whom no disease is present; otherwise one cannot be sure whether one is measuring aging processes or disease. However, particularly in older age groups, this would be extremely difficult because many chronic diseases, or their underlying pathological manifestations (such as arteriosclerosis), occur to some extent in most individuals, without necessarily giving rise to clinical symptoms. In fact, we generally do not know when many diseases, such as malignancies or even OA, start, and what determines the first stage of the progression of such diseases. Consequently, it is almost impossible to identify older individuals who are free from any preclinical signs of disease.

The Example of Osteoarthritis

Difficulties in measuring aging processes and investigating their relationship to diseases can be illustrated further for a specific condition, namely, OA. As for many other chronic diseases, the prevalence of the clinical manifestations of OA increases with age (fig. 1.1), and mathematical studies have shown that this increase tends to be exponential (Brown and Forbes, 1974). This increase is based on averages, but the average prevalence values at different ages are not entirely satisfactory, since they neglect the variability that occurs at different ages or even for individuals of the same age. Moreover, the variability of OA at different ages would be expected to increase with age. It follows that in any age group there will be one group of persons with a low prevalence of symptoms, for whom the manifestations of OA are relatively small or nonexistent, while for another group, with a high prevalence of symptoms, the manifestations of OA are pronounced.

Apart from the association with age, there are other risk factors for OA (see chapter 4). Even if some of these known risk factors can be adjusted for, or can be controlled in some way, and the variability in the prevalence of OA can be reduced, there remains the variability related to other genetic and environmental factors. The aim is to identify these other genetic and environmental factors and to determine why some persons develop OA more rapidly than others, even after adjustments have been made for known risk factors. These other risk factors may be related to aging processes. As mentioned previously, risk factors for OA (or other chronic diseases) may not be the same as risk factors for aging processes, but both sets of risk factors may affect the incidence of OA.

Since aging processes play a part in the development of OA and of other chronic diseases, it is likely that at least some of these processes contribute to a variety of chronic diseases. This brings us back to the concept of aging being related to underlying unknown processes that give rise to a number of diseases. It follows that, if these underlying processes could be identified, the control of those that are environmental in nature might well be beneficial, and such control might have a greater effect on more than one chronic disease than it would have if there were no basic underlying aging processes.

This, in turn, relates to the search for the aging processes that have been postulated by biological gerontologists. Theories of biological aging are extensive (Greenstock, 1993), and there is no agreement as to which theory best explains the various observations about biological aging. These observations include the fact that different species have different life spans, that there is considerable variation in life span within a species (such as *homo sapiens*), that there is a linear decline of most measurable functions with age, and that although there are numerous ways of shortening the life span there are few, if any, methods of extending the maximum human life span, although some are emerging (see chapter 2).

The Relationship of Aging and Disease to Theories of Aging

There are a number of unresolved questions with regard to theories of aging. One of these is whether the life expectancy of populations will tend to approach the hypothetical maximum life span, as suggested by Fries (1980, 1984, 1988). However, it has been pointed out that the mortality rates for the oldest age group have been decreasing more rapidly than those for any other age group (Grundy, 1984); this points against the hypothesis of a maximum life span, since, if we were to approach a maximum life span, mortality rates at the highest ages would be expected to increase rather than decrease (see also Schneider and Brody, 1983; Myers and Manton, 1984; Olshansky et al., 1990).

Another controversy concerns whether elderly people within a certain age group are now healthier than persons of similar ages in an earlier cohort. One might have expected, when comparing different cohorts, that as more people attain higher ages, say the age of 70, these later cohorts will contain a larger proportion of individuals with various disabilities and hence will be less healthy (Manton, 1986; Palmore, 1986; Finsen, 1988). However, this does not always appear to be the case, and at least one study (not unexpectedly) has shown that the 70-year-old population is now healthier than people of the same age in previous cohorts (Svanborg, 1988). It is not known whether reduced disease incidence or reduced aging processes are responsible for this change.

It is likely that the manifestations of aging are apparent throughout the body. Modifications related to basic aging processes may occur in connective tissues, cell components (Kohn, 1978, 1982; Hamerman, 1993), the immune system (with the expression of autoimmune diseases), and the hormonal system, as well as in gene expression, protein degradation, and enzyme functions. There has been considerable speculation as to how these and other aging processes (e.g., processes involving specific free radicals or cross-linking) lead to age-related changes, and it would be of interest to carry out the appropriate experiments, which would, for example, investigate whether the degree of cross-linking or the presence of certain free radicals is associated with a greater prevalence of specific chronic diseases (Schneider and Reed, 1985). If measurements on as many parameters as possible could be made on individuals who are appreciably affected by OA and on appropriate control groups (namely, those for whom the incidence of OA is minimal, preferably matched for the known risk factors), one could investigate which of these parameters are most strongly associated with this difference in the prevalence of OA. For example, if certain changes in collagen structure could be shown to be associated with the prevalence of OA, this would suggest that these changes are important in the development of OA. Such experiments may identify risk factors for basic aging processes as well as risk factors not previously identified for OA.

Identification of risk factors for aging processes could be important for a better understanding of OA and a number of other chronic diseases. This could have profound effects on the incidence of chronic diseases and thus affect future health care needs, particularly for the elderly population. For example, if the incidence of many chronic diseases could be delayed by some 7 years, the age-specific morbidity from these diseases would be about halved. This follows because morbidity and mortality from a number of chronic diseases double about every 7 years between the ages of about 30 and 70.

In practical terms, we suggest that a priority for medical research should be the identification of modifiable risk factors for OA and other chronic diseases, because the likelihood is that this will lead to a reduced incidence of these diseases (see also chapter 10). An additional advantage of this approach is that it could lead to the identification of risk factors for, and information on, more basic aging processes. Such information may also help to provide answers to a number of unresolved questions, such as the issue of the maximum life span and why changes have occurred in the prevalence of at least some chronic diseases.

Conclusions

Considering the relationship between aging and disease, various chronic diseases such as osteoarthritis can be regarded either as aging or as a disease, depending on how aging is defined. The risk factors for the various chronic diseases are not identical, and these risk factors may also differ from the risk factors for aging processes. Although these various risk factors may not be identical, it is expected that at least some of them would be similar; hence, modifying the risk factors for one particular disease might lead not only to a reduction of that disease but also to a reduction of the prevalence of a number of other chronic diseases, and thus have important implications for health care.

ACKNOWLEDGMENT

I am indebted to Dr. Leroy O. Stone for a number of helpful comments.

REFERENCES

Adams O. 1990. Life expectancy in Canada—an overview. *Health Reports* 2:361–367.
Berg L. 1985. Does Alzheimer's disease represent an exaggeration of normal aging? *Arch Neurol* 42:737–739.
Bierman EL. 1978. Atherosclerosis and aging. *Fed Proc* 37:2832–2836.
Branch LG, Jette AM. 1984. Personal health practices and mortality among the elderly. *Am J Public Health* 74:1126–1129.
Brody JA. 1985. Prospects for an ageing population. *Nature* 315:463–466.
Brown KS, Forbes WF. 1974. A mathematical model of aging processes. *J Gerontol* 29:46–51.
Brown KS, Forbes WF. 1976. Concerning the estimation of biological age. *Gerontology* 22:428–437.
Davies AM. 1985. Epidemiology and the challenge of ageing. *Int J Epidemiol* 14:9–21.
Evans JG. 1993. The aging-disease dichotomy is alive, but is it well? *J Am Geriatr Soc* 41:1272–1273.
Finsen V. 1988. Improvements in general health among the elderly: A factor in the rising incidence of hip fractures? *J Epidemiol Community Health* 42:200–203.
Forbes WF, Hirdes JP. 1993. The relationship between aging and disease: Geriatric ideology and myths of senility. *J Am Geriatr Soc* 41:1267–1271.
Forbes WF, Thompson ME. 1990. Age-related diseases and normal aging: The nature of the relationship. *J Clin Epidemiol* 43:191–193.
Forbes WF, Thompson ME, Agwani N, Hayward LM. 1993. A log-linear relationship between reported impairments and age: Implications for the multistage hypothesis. *J Gerontol: Biol Sci* 48:B33-B40.
Fried LP, Bush TL. 1988. Morbidity as a focus of preventive health care in the elderly. *Epidemiol Rev* 10:48–64.
Fries JF. 1980. Aging, natural death, and the compression of morbidity. *N Engl J Med* 303:130–135.
———. 1984. The compression of morbidity: Miscellaneous comments about a theme. *Gerontologist* 24:354–359.
———. 1988. Aging, illness, and health policy: Implications of the compression of morbidity. *Perspect Biol Med* 31:407–428.
Greenstock CL. 1993. Radiation and aging: Free radical damage, biological response, and possible antioxidant intervention. *Med Hypotheses* 41:473–482.
Grundy E. 1984. Mortality and morbidity among the old. *Br Med J* 288:663–664.
Hamerman D. 1993. Aging and osteoarthritis: Basic mechanisms. *J Am Geriatr Soc* 41:760–770.
———. 1995. Clinical implications of osteoarthritis and ageing. *Ann Rheum Dis* 54:1–4.
Kohn RR. 1978. *Principles of mammalian aging.* 2d ed. Prentice-Hall Foundations of Developmental Biology Series. Englewood Cliffs, N.J.: Prentice-Hall.
———. 1982. Cause of death in very old people. *JAMA* 247:2793–2797.

Manton KG. 1986. Cause specific mortality patterns among the oldest old: Multiple cause of death trends 1968 to 1980. *J Gerontol* 41:282–289.

Myers GC, Manton KG. 1984. Compression of mortality: Myth or reality? *Gerontologist* 24:346–353.

Olshansky SJ, Carnes BA, Cassel C. 1990. In search of Methuselah: Estimating the upper limits to human longevity. *Science* 250:634–640.

Palmore EB. 1986. Trends in the health of the aged. *Gerontologist* 26:298–302.

Perls TT. 1995. The oldest old. *Scientific American,* January, pp. 70–75.

Schneider EL, Brody JA. 1983. Aging, natural death, and the compression of morbidity: Another view. *N Engl J Med* 309:854–856.

Schneider EL, Reed JD. 1985. Life extension. *N Engl J Med* 312:1159–1168.

Svanborg A. 1988. *Health and aging: Perspectives and prospects,* edited by JF Schroots, JE Birren, A Svanborg. New York: Springer.

Thompson ME, Forbes WF. 1990. The various definitions of biological aging. *Can J Aging* 9:91–94.

2

Implications of the Accrual of Chronic Nonfatal Conditions in Very Elderly Persons

S. Jay Olshansky, Ph.D., and Christine K. Cassel, M.D.

Although very old people have always existed, their absolute numbers and proportions relative to the younger population have increased dramatically in the twentieth century. Accompanying this demographic trend of increased individual and population aging has been an unexpected rise in the prevalence of people who experience diseases and disorders that are largely unrelated to their ultimate cause of death. These chronic nonfatal conditions (hereinafter referred to as CNF conditions), which include, for example, osteoporosis, osteoarthritis, vision and hearing impairments, dementia, and Parkinson disease, have become so prevalent that their contribution to overall frailty and disability among older people has surpassed that of fatal diseases (Verbrugge and Jette, 1994). The accrual of CNF conditions in the twentieth century is unprecedented. Such conditions are now being experienced with a frequency not likely ever to have been known before by any subgroup of the human population. In this chapter we document the rise in CNF conditions that has occurred among older people in the United States, discuss why the rise occurred, and consider prospects for the future.

The Rise of Chronic Nonfatal Conditions

The majority of the increase in life expectancy in the latter part of the twentieth century in the United States and other developed nations has resulted from the development of methods of postponing deaths from fatal diseases—heart disease, cancer, and stroke. Considerably less progress has been made in preventing, postponing, and treating the CNF conditions associated with old age. These are predominantly chronic musculoskeletal diseases such as osteo-arthritis and osteoporosis, degenerative neurologic disorders such as Alzheimer and Parkinson diseases, and sensory impairments such as hearing loss and blindness. There is no empirical evidence indicating that the onset of nonfatal, disabling diseases occurs later in life today than it did just 20–30 years ago. In addition, declining death rates from fatal diseases do not seem to have any beneficial effect on many of the CNF conditions—implying that longer lives put the saved population at greater risk of experiencing CNF conditions and increase the duration of such conditions. Until more progress is made in understanding the causes of and potential methods of preventing the disabilities of old age, increasing longevity will bring more years of disability to both individuals and populations.

One way to measure the health of the older population is to identify the diseases and conditions that affect that population. Table 2.1 lists the conditions most commonly affecting older persons, as obtained in one nationally representative sample of community-dwelling persons—the National Health Interview Survey (NHIS) (Adams and Benson, 1990). This study, like most others currently available, is incomplete because it does not include people who reside in institutions—the frailest segment of the population. But even these data show that among older individuals, the potentially disabling diseases of aging have prevalence rates as high as 50 percent (for arthritis) and are known to increase rapidly with age. Many of these disorders are not usually considered fatal; persons often live with these conditions and die from other causes. Because the NHIS was not designed to capture all CNF conditions, dementia, confusion, and depression are not listed in table 2.1 even though these conditions are known to affect large numbers of older persons. Thus, these numbers underestimate overall chronic illness in the population over age 65. In addition, the aggregate burden of these conditions is often more than the data in table 2.1 imply. For many older persons, multiple disabling conditions are the rule, and their effects combine to increase disability (Guralnik et al., 1989).

The presence of CNF conditions has major social implications. For example, 250,000 hip fractures occur every year in the United States (Kellie and Brody, 1990; Schneider and Guralnik, 1990). Twenty percent of the people who fracture a hip do not survive another year, and another 20 percent are never able to walk again without assistance. Furthermore, 50 percent of hip fracture patients are discharged from the hospital to a nursing home. A conservative pro-

Table 2.1.   Leading Self-Reported Chronic Conditions for Noninstitutionalized Adults, 1990

Condition	Age 65–74		Age 75 and Older	
	Men	Women	Men	Women
Arthritis	337.1 (1)	517.6 (1)	496.7 (1)	588.5 (1)
Hypertension	317.6 (2)	437.0 (2)	294.7 (4)	423.1 (2)
Hearing impairment	308.6 (3)	183.8 (4)	402.1 (2)	335.8 (4)
Heart disease	259.7 (4)	209.0 (3)	371.0 (3)	342.5 (3)
Chronic sinusitis	150.9 (5)	152.4 (5)	99.1 (9)	189.1 (7)
Deformity[a]	139.9 (6)	142.5 (6)	130.5 (6)	204.4 (6)
Tinnitus	84.8 (7)	—	—	—
Cataracts	76.0 (8)	132.4 (7)	182.7 (5)	264.5 (5)
Visual impairment	74.9 (9)	—	124.8 (7)	—
Diabetes	74.0 (10)	102.5 (8)	—	92.6 (10)
Varicose veins	—	89.3 (9)	—	107.8 (9)
Hemorrhoids	—	78.1 (10)	—	—
Diseases of the prostate	—	—	99.3 (8)	—
Frequent constipation	—	—	—	114.6 (8)
Emphysema	—	—	80.6 (10)	—

SOURCE: Adams and Benson, 1990.
NOTE: Rates are per thousand members of the civilian noninstitutional population. Rankings for each age/sex category are in parentheses.
[a]Deformity or orthopedic impairment; permanent stiffness so that the affected joint does not move.

jection of the number of hip fractures expected to occur in the year 2010 is 350,000, with an estimated cost of more than $3 billion for acute care alone (Schneider and Guralnik, 1990).

Dementia, caused primarily by Alzheimer disease and by strokes, is another age-associated disorder that in itself is not fatal but is known to cause severe dependency and disability. The Established Population for Epidemiologic Studies of the Elderly (EPESE) for East Boston indicates that 47 percent of the population aged 85 and older have Alzheimer disease (Evans et al., 1989). Current costs for the care of patients with moderate to severe dementia are estimated to be $35.8 billion per year, including long-term care expenses. It has been conservatively estimated that there will be 5 million cases of dementia in the United States in the year 2010, resulting in an annual cost of at least $80 billion (in 1985 dollars) (Schneider and Guralnik, 1990).

Although data are available on diseases affecting older persons, from a health and social service perspective individuals' functional abilities are a better predictor of medical and service needs. Despite the fact that some people remain independent throughout life, observed rates of dependence increase rapidly with age. For example, while 22.6 percent of the population aged 65 to

74 experience difficulty with activities of daily living (ADL), this increases to 44.5 percent of the population aged 85 and older. Further, activities such as shopping, paying bills, and cleaning house are more difficult to perform than are basic self-care activities. When one applies observed rates of disability (for example, from the Longitudinal Study of Aging) to the projected size of the future older population, it becomes clear that millions more disabled individuals in the United States will need support in the coming decades. Assuming there are no changes in the age-specific risk of disability, the number of people aged 65 and older experiencing difficulty with ADL will therefore increase from 8.7 million in 1990 to 11.5 million in 2010—a 32.2 percent increase in just 20 years. According to a recent Institute of Medicine report, medical spending per capita for those limited in activity because of two or more chronic conditions is five times the corresponding figure for persons not limited in activity (Pope and Tarlov, 1991).

In the future, unless there are major scientific breakthroughs, CNF conditions will continue to occur at the same high age-specific rates (Rudberg et al., 1996). If the present prevalence rates of these common conditions are applied to the projected growth of the older population, the prevalence of these conditions will increase dramatically in the coming decades. The challenge for researchers and medical practitioners is to understand the etiology and to prevent or delay the onset of CNF conditions, while at the same time developing devices, medications, and environments that will allow an optimal quality of life for the millions of elderly people who are thus affected.

Why Have Chronic Nonfatal Conditions Increased?

Two primary reasons exist for the rising prevalence and prevalence rate of CNF conditions among recent cohorts surviving to older ages. The first is based purely on demographic trends observed globally during the past 200 years. Before the middle of the eighteenth century, birth rates and death rates hovered between 30 and 50 per thousand—demographic conditions that, although fluctuating, probably had remained within those bounds since the origin of humans. Under those relatively stable demographic conditions, only a small proportion of any given birth cohort was able to survive to old age because of extremely high attrition during youth and middle age as a result of infectious and parasitic diseases. As improved lifestyles and medical technology during the past 200 years succeeded in reducing death rates during youth and middle age, survival into older age ranges (65–85 and older) became common.

The transition from high to low birth rates and death rates led not only to much greater prospects for the extended survival of individuals but also to the dual demographic phenomenon of rapid population growth and accelerated population aging (Olshansky et al., 1993). For example, the fact that declines in death rates outpaced declines in birth rates in the nineteenth and twentieth centuries led to growth rates that approached (and in some cases even exceeded) 3 percent. Since the size of the human population doubles about every 25 years when growth rates are at 3 percent, the number of people now alive (about 5.5 billion) is five times as great as it was just 100 years ago. Perhaps equally important, in low-mortality populations the age structure (i.e., the proportion of the population alive at every age) has been transformed from its historically stable pyramidal form to a squarelike or rectilinear form. The result of this demographic trend, referred to as population aging, was a rapid rise in the number and proportion of the population that reaches and exceeds the age of 65.

How did these historical demographic events influence the prevalence of CNF conditions today? First, the size of successive birth cohorts increased in the United States throughout most of the twentieth century, with particularly large increases observed during the post–World War II era. Changes in the size of birth cohorts are known to have a "ripple effect" on many aspects of society (Martin and Preston, 1994), causing (for example) increased demands on educational resources at younger ages, more competition in job and marriage markets, and ultimately, at older ages, the increased prevalence of CNF conditions even if the rates of their occurrence remain constant. During the same time that the birth cohorts increased in size, death rates from childhood diseases declined rapidly. Thus, not only were more babies being born, but those that were born had a much higher probability of surviving past their first few years of life into middle and older age. Increased individual survival, which contributed to population aging and the transformation of the age structure, led to an even more rapid acceleration in the rise in CNF conditions than would have otherwise occurred in the absence of larger birth cohorts.

In addition to these demographic forces, recent successful efforts to reduce the risk of death at older ages from fatal senescent diseases are the second primary factor contributing to the rise in the prevalence of CNF conditions. For example, Greunberg (1977) and Kramer (1980) developed the argument that if advances in medical treatment and technology postpone death from fatal diseases by successfully treating infectious diseases associated with them, the additional survival time may be disproportionately spent in a state of poor health. A modern perspective has been given to this argument (Verbrugge, 1984; Olshansky et al., 1991), and a considerable amount of empirical evidence has been amassed in support of what now may be referred to as *the expansion-of-*

morbidity hypothesis (e.g., see Crimmins et al., 1989, 1994; Rogers et al., 1990; Mathers, 1991). The logic behind this hypothesis is as follows: If the predisposing risk factors for fatal and CNF conditions are different from each other, and if the primary effort of medicine is to reduce the risk of death from fatal senescent diseases (with comparatively less effort placed on the CNF conditions), then the extended survival of individuals with fatal conditions would expose the "saved" population to a longer duration of time during which the CNF conditions have the opportunity to be expressed or progress to a more advanced stage. For example, if individuals predisposed to Alzheimer disease lived longer because of medical advances that reduced their risk of vascular diseases, this would permit the complications associated with Alzheimer disease to progress to a more advanced stage than would otherwise have been the case. The logic behind the expansion-of-morbidity hypothesis is that although progress may have been made in postponing the onset and age progression of fatal diseases, comparable progress has not been made against the CNF conditions.

An alternative school of thought, referred to as the *compression-of-morbidity hypothesis,* maintains that lifestyle changes and advances in medicine will continue to reduce the risk of death from fatal diseases and will simultaneously postpone the onset and age progression of the nonfatal disabling diseases. The underlying premise of this theory is that the human lifespan has a fixed biological limit of approximately 85 years, toward which populations are headed (Fries, 1980, 1989). As improved lifestyles postpone the onset and expression of fatal diseases and of nonfatal but highly disabling diseases and disorders, more people will be pushed toward their biological limits, and morbidity and disability within populations will be compressed into a shorter duration of time before death.

Although evidence supporting this view has been scarce, a recent study suggests that in the United States between 1984 and 1989 healthy life expectancy was increasing more quickly than was disabled life expectancy (Manton et al., 1995). Data from England (Bone, 1997) indicate that although the proportion of total life expectancy spent in a general state of disability has risen between 1976 and 1992, the duration of life spent severely disabled declined during this same period. This indicates that for some populations recently observed over short periods of time, there is evidence for a limited compression of morbidity within the overall trend of a rising prevalence of CNF conditions. Whether these short-term trends can be sustained is unknown at this time.

Prospects for the Future

If CNF conditions have been rising because of survival into an age range in which the risk of experiencing such conditions is high, then it stands to reason that continued reductions in death rates at older ages will lead to an increase in the prevalence of CNF conditions in the future. According to the expansion-of-morbidity hypothesis (Olshansky et al., 1991), this would occur as progress is made against the forces of senescent mortality without comparable progress in postponing the onset and age progression of CNF conditions. The implication of this hypothesis is that current efforts by the medical community to extend the lives of people with fatal conditions could have the inadvertent effect of escalating the prevalence of CNF conditions.

In addition to inevitable demographic forces operating to raise the prevalence of CNF conditions, there is a biological force that could also accelerate this phenomenon—increased genetic heterogeneity. Recall from our earlier discussion that in the twentieth century there has been a rapid increase in the proportion of each birth cohort that survives into older age ranges. This means that previous generations of older people were highly selected subpopulations of their original birth cohorts, and that this selection process is now operating with much less efficiency. The implication is that individuals possessing genes that, under harsher environmental conditions, would have precluded their survival to old age are now surviving into age ranges that have rarely or never before been experienced by such individuals. Examples include individuals with PKU, leukemia, and early onset diabetes, and many other diseases and disorders that used to be lethal early in life. If senescence is in fact a multigenic phenomenon involving the dual expression of genes during different parts of the lifespan (i.e., pleiotropy), as suggested by evolutionary biologists (Williams, 1957; Rose, 1991; Charlesworth, 1994), then increased genetic heterogeneity at older ages may lead to the expression of new or infrequently observed senescent diseases and disorders. As an example, consider the extended survival now experienced by individuals who carry the normally lethal gene that leads to early onset diabetes. In the coming decades, for the first time in human history, individuals who carry this gene will survive into older ages with great frequency. At this time it is too early to know whether, or even how, this gene might express itself at later ages. It is this uncertainty that leads to speculation about the possible expression of new diseases among the less selected older cohorts of the future.

In spite of the known demographic forces that inevitably place an upward pressure on the prevalence of CNF conditions, it is possible both to influence the expression of CNF conditions and to ameliorate some health problems associated with their presence (Rudberg and Cassel, 1993). Why is it that senescence-related diseases and disorders are inherently modifiable? The answer may be found in the biological literature.

The origin of modern evolutionary theories of senescence dates back to the theory of aging set forth by the biologist August Weismann (see Weismann, 1891). (Kirkwood and Cremer [1982] present a thorough review of the research of August Weismann and other evolutionary biologists.) Weismann viewed the aging (and eventual death) of individuals as an adaptive phenomenon that would benefit the species by eliminating the old who were competing with the young for limited resources. Perhaps more interesting, Weismann speculated on why it is that somatic cells (i.e., all the cells of the body with the exception of the germ cells and their progenitors) lose their ability to be immortal. Weisman's view, much like the modern view of Dawkins (1976), was that reproduction is the most critical function of life. Once an individual has reproduced and the reproductive success of the offspring has been assured, the function of that individual's life is complete and death can then occur. The question raised by Weismann was why it is that death occurs after the reproductive period—that is, what mechanisms might be involved in the demise of the individual?

According to Weismann, the one aspect of life that could not be avoided was the inevitable exposure of the individual to external forces that produced a constant barrage of small injuries to the body. Because the perfect repair of these injuries is simply not realistically possible, it became self-evident why older individuals should be replaced by new ones. This was the rationale supporting both the need for reproduction and the importance of death. Thus, even if immortality was theoretically possible, it could not be realized in the real world, where the external force of injury was ubiquitous and unavoidable.

Weismann argued that when a given characteristic of an organism became useless, natural selection would no longer operate on it and the trait would disappear (this was the non-adaptive theory of aging). This assertion was referred to as the principle of panmixia. (The example of panmixia presented in Kirkwood and Cremer [1982] is that of a species that eventually becomes adapted to living in dark caves—the eventual result of which is a progressive loss of vision while the development of other, more useful organs occurs.) Applying this principle to the postreproductive period, Weismann viewed that time in the lifespan as useless. If extended longevity was not necessary (or practically achievable) in an environment where external forces of injury were unavoidable, excess longevity would disappear (a phenomenon referred to as retrogression). Weismann then extended his line of reasoning to the limited replicative potential of somatic cells as a way of explaining the cellular mechanisms involved in the process of senescence.

The modern evolutionary theory of aging was provided by the Nobel laureate Sir Peter Medawar (1952), who was able to make extensive use of Mendelian genetics in his arguments. Like Weismann, Medawar invoked the importance of the ever-present external force of mortality, which was acknowledged to be the primary reason why most members of a population were unable to live long enough to experience senescence. Medawar's unique contribution to the evolutionary theory of senescence was the argument that genes that arise from mutation and whose expression is related to time would affect a different number of people depending on when in the lifespan the genes were expressed. If they were expressed early in the lifespan, a large number of individuals would be affected, while only a few would be influenced if they were expressed later in the lifespan. By implication, natural selection would favor and bring early into the lifespan those genes that were advantageous, while pushing genes with damaging effects into later portions of the lifespan, in which fewer individuals would normally be affected. Senescence is therefore a result of the accumulation of genes with damaging effects that have been pushed by natural selection into the postreproductive period of life (the "genetic dustbin"), and the extended survival of individuals (through protection from external sources of mortality) into an age range where these diseases have the opportunity to be expressed. Williams (1957) then extended the Medawarian view by hypothesizing that some of the genes that have damaging effects later in the lifespan may have positive effects early in the lifespan. This made senescence not just a product of deleterious genes expressed later in life but also an inadvertent consequence of selection favoring genes with early adaptive functions and late-acting damaging effects (referred to as pleiotropic genes).

This modern evolutionary theory of senescence was therefore fundamentally based on the presence of what may be referred to as a *selection gradient*. If lethal genes are expressed before the reproductive period begins (i.e., before sexual maturity), natural selection will prevent those genes from entering subsequent generations. If some lethal genes are expressed after the end of the reproductive period, then the ability of natural selection to eliminate these genes from subsequent generations is dramatically reduced because (1) the genetic contribution to the next generation has already been accomplished, and (2) the force of selection must be weak during portions of the lifespan in which few members of a birth cohort would normally survive. The resulting selection gradient fundamentally links attributes of a species' reproductive period to the effectiveness of selection in modifying the timing of expression of lethal genes.

The latest extension of the evolutionary theory of senescence appears in a series of articles published by Kirkwood and colleagues (see Kirkwood, 1977, 1992; Kirkwood and Holliday, 1979; Kirkwood and Rose, 1991; Kirkwood and Franceschi, 1992). Like Weismann and Medawar, Kirkwood argues that the inevitable force of external mortality plays a crucial role in the timing of senescence. However, in this case the logic supporting the existence of senescence is based more on its proximate causes—differential energy investments in somatic and germ cells, with the time-dependent decline in somatic maintenance. Species facing fewer external forces of mortality would be able to profit from, and take advantage of, a delayed and longer reproductive period. Senescence is therefore viewed as a product of accumulated damage to somatic cells which is indirectly regulated by the level of external forces of mortality present in a species' ecologic niche.

Consider the fact that most animals, including humans, evolved under a particularly hostile set of environmental conditions that killed most members of a cohort even before they reached sexual maturity. Survival in hostile environments requires highly efficient mechanisms to maintain the biological integrity of the organism. According to evolutionary biologists (Weismann, 1891; Kirkwood, 1977; Kirkwood and Holliday, 1979), immortality did not evolve because perfect maintenance and repair mechanisms would divert biological resources from more fruitful investments, such as reproduction. If organisms are even to survive to reproductive ages, these mechanisms have to operate with great efficiency. However, perfect maintenance and repair mechanisms for DNA are not required in a world where the force of extrinsic mortality is normally high. The inevitable damage that does occur, when accumulated over a lifetime, in turn leads to many of the diseases, disorders, and physiologic changes that are commonly known as aging. In other words, the biological forces that lead to senescence are likely to be a by-product of evolution operating on other attributes of a species that influence its survival—such as reproduction. If senescence is an inadvertent by-product of selection operating on reproduction, then its expression should be inherently modifiable because it has not been directly programmed into the genome. By contrast, if senescence was programmed directly (i.e., if specific death genes evolved), then altering senescence would require modifications to the genome itself—a technology that is not currently available and would be particularly controversial if developed.

All animals alive today are carriers of a genetic code that evolved under the environmental conditions present when each species arose. Humans also carry programmed biological responses that evolved under conditions that prevailed 100,000 years ago, when anatomically modern humans first appeared.

This genetic legacy is a dual-edged sword—with both advantages and disadvantages. For example, an extremely efficient fat storage mechanism is a disadvantage in today's world of plentiful food supplies. We are constantly reminded of our inability to compensate for this highly efficient fat storage mechanism as our waists, hips, and thighs absorb the excess calories we consume.

However, our genetic legacy also offers unique opportunities for extending the length and improving the quality of life. Remember, senescence is not programmed directly as a biological clock designed to go off at a predetermined time—it is a by-product of an evolved reproductive pattern and of survival into an age range that permits its expression. Thus, one of the most important biological properties of senescence is that its expression can be modified without manipulating the genetic code (genome) itself. This has important implications for medical and gerontologic research focused on extending life—particularly the healthy years of life.

Methods of manipulating the expression of senescence-related diseases and disorders fall into three categories. One approach is to identify senescence accelerators and avoid them. Senescence accelerators are behaviors or substances that hasten one or more components of the aging process—with premature death as a result. Known and suspected senescence accelerators include cigarette smoking, radiation (such as exposure to the sun), excessive alcohol consumption, stress, and environmental toxins. Other senescence accelerators will undoubtedly be identified in the future.

A second approach is to identify and favorably influence senescence decelerators. However, slowing the aging process is much more difficult than accelerating it. This is because decelerating the aging process requires an understanding of all, or certainly the most important, of the mechanisms of senescence. In spite of the difficulty of simultaneously decelerating senescence for all of the major systems in the body, scientists are rapidly learning how to manipulate some of the most important throttles governing senescence. For example, the immune system operates with great efficiency, in part, because it is capable of learning from experience. Training the immune system to combat infectious diseases was one of the most important medical advances of the twentieth century. Training the immune system to combat senescence may be an important medical advance in the twenty-first century. Modifying diets to include more fruits and vegetables, which are natural sources of antioxidants, may help to decelerate senescence at its source—at the cellular and molecular levels. Consuming more calcium when one is younger increases accumulated bone mass, so that when bone loss begins in the third decade of life there will be more bone to lose—which will postpone the onset of osteoporosis.

One of the most promising approaches for decelerating senescence is the development of pharmaceuticals that, like fruits and vegetables, operate at the molecular level to reduce the inevitable damage to nuclear and mitochondrial DNA. DNA damage has been implicated as an important factor influencing the eventual expression of senescence-related diseases and disorders (Harmon, 1992). Substances that protect DNA, reduce accumulated damage, or possibly even reverse previous damage would be important new methods of decelerating senescence.

Finally, considerable progress has already been made in delaying the onset and age progression of some senescent diseases and ameliorating the effects of senescent diseases and disorders once they have already been expressed (Verbrugge and Balaban, 1989; Rudberg and Cassel, 1993). For example, hip fractures are known to increase exponentially with age (Brody, 1985). The two major risk factors for this disorder are osteoporosis and falls—both of which can be altered by dietary modification and changes in the physical environment. Visual and hearing disorders are widely prevalent in older age groups. The second leading cause of blindness in the elderly population, glaucoma, can be treated if diagnosed early, and cataracts are a common condition that can be treated with surgery. It is also possible to ameliorate some symptoms of arthritis with medication and surgery. Many of the infectious diseases that proliferate in older people with compromised immune systems can be forestalled by immunizations (this is true of pneumococcal pneumonia and influenza; see Lavizzo-Mourey and Diserens, 1989). Manipulating the environment or specific behaviors can also delay the onset of, or possibly even prevent, some forms of disability. One form of primary prevention believed to reduce disability is weight reduction, which is thought to alter the progression of knee osteoarthritis (Felson et al., 1992) (see also chapter 10). In short, methods of intervening in the progression of disability associated with CNF conditions, as well as fatal conditions, have already been developed, and there is reason to be optimistic that additional gains are forthcoming.

Conclusions

The rise in chronic nonfatal conditions in the twentieth century in the United States and other developed nations is a product of dramatically improved survival at younger and middle ages, the survival of larger birth cohorts to older ages, and lifestyle modifications and advances in medicine that postpone death from fatal conditions. There is a considerable body of scientific literature suggesting that the modern rise in life expectancy may accelerate the rise in CNF conditions by exposing the saved population to a longer duration of time in which CNF conditions have the opportunity for expression or progression. However, other data imply that in some countries the prevalence of the most severe forms of disability actually may have declined in recent years. No matter what trends may be occurring in the short term, the anticipated rapid aging of the population after the year 2011, when the first members of the post–World War II baby boom cohorts reach age 65, will inevitably lead to a rapid rise in the prevalence of CNF conditions.

An important biological attribute of the process of senescence is that it has not been programmed directly by natural selection—a fact that implies that the timing of expression of senescent diseases and disorders (including CNF conditions) is inherently modifiable. It has been suggested here that progress has already been made in delaying the onset and age progression of fatal diseases, and that it is possible to make comparable gains against the CNF conditions that have already been expressed among recent cohorts of older persons. There is reason to be optimistic that gains of this sort can continue, although it should be emphasized that changes in genetic heterogeneity at older ages could provide the opportunity for new or infrequently observed diseases and disorders to be expressed. Monitoring the health status of the older population, with an emphasis on the development and use of new measures of health and disabled life expectancy, will permit scientists to provide important public policy information on the general health status of the population.

REFERENCES

Adams PF, Benson V. 1990. *Current estimates from the National Health Interview Survey, 1989.* Vital and Health Statistics, ser. 10, no. 176. Washington, D.C.: National Center for Health Statistics.

Brody J. 1985. Prospects for an ageing population. *Nature* 315:463–466.

Bone M. 1997. Policy applications of health expectancy. *J Aging Health*, in press.

Charlesworth B. 1994. *Evolution in age-structured populations.* Cambridge: Cambridge University Press.

Crimmins EM, Hayward MD, Saito Y. 1989. Changes in life expectancy and disability-free life expectancy in the United States. *Population Dev Review* 15:235–267.

Crimmins EM, Hayward MD, Saito Y. 1994. Changing mortality and morbidity rates and the health status and life expectancy of the older population. *Demography* 31:159–175.

Dawkins R. 1976. *The selfish gene.* Oxford: Oxford University Press.

Evans DE, Funkenstein H, Albert MS, Scherr PA, Cook NA, Chain MJ, Hebert LE, Hennekens CH, Taylor JO. 1989. Prevalence of Alzheimer's disease in a community population of older persons: Higher than previously reported. *JAMA* 262:2551–2556.

Felson DT, Zhang Y, Anthony JM, Naimark A, Anderson JJ. 1992. Weight loss reduces the risk for symptomatic knee osteoarthritis in women: The Framingham study. *Ann Intern Med* 116:535–539.

Fries JF. 1980. Aging, natural death, and the compression of morbidity. *N Engl J Med* 303:130–135.

————. 1989. The compression of morbidity: Near or far? *Milbank Q* 67:208–322.

Greunberg EM. 1977. The failures of success. *Milbank Q* 55:3–24.

Guralnik JM, LaCroix AZ, Everett DF, Kovar MG. 1989. *Aging in the eighties: The prevalence of comorbidity and its association with disability.* Advance Data from Vital and Health Statistics, no. 170. Hyattsville, Md.: National Center for Health Statistics.

Harmon D. 1992. Free radical theory of aging. *Mutat Res* 275:257–266.

Kellie SE, Brody JA. 1990. Sex-specific and race-specific hip fracture rates. *Am J Public Health* 80:326–328.

Kirkwood TBL. 1977. Evolution of aging. *Nature* 270:301–304.

————. 1992. Comparative life spans of species: Why do species have the life spans they do? *Am J Clin Nutr* 55:1191S–1195S.

Kirkwood TBL, Cremer T. 1982. Cytogerontology since 1881: A reappraisal of August Weismann and a review of modern progress. *Hum Genet* 60:101–121.

Kirkwood TBL, Franceschi C. 1992. Is aging as complex as it would appear? *Ann NY Acad Sci* 663:412–417.

Kirkwood TBL, Holliday R. 1979. The evolution of ageing and longevity. *Proc R Soc Lond [Biol]* 205:531–546.

Kirkwood TBL, Rose MR. 1991. Evolution of senescence: Late survival sacrificed for reproduction. *Phil Trans R Soc Lond [Biol]* 332:15–24.

Kramer M. 1980. The rising pandemic of mental disorders and associated chronic diseases and disabilities. *Acta Psychiatr Scand* 285:382–397.

Lavizzo-Mourey D, Diserens D. 1989. Preventative care in the elderly. In: *Practicing prevention for the elderly,* edited by D Lavizzo-Mourey, S Days, D Disernes, G Grisso. Pp. 1–9. Philadelphia: Hanley and Belfus.

Manton KG, Stallard E, Corder L. 1995. Changes in mortality and chronic disability in the US elderly population: Evidence from the 1982, 1984, and 1989 National Long Term Care Surveys. *J Gerontol: Soc Sciences* 58:S194-S204.

Martin LG, Preston SH, eds. 1994. *Demography of aging.* Washington, D.C.: National Academy Press.

Mathers CD. 1991. *Health expectancies in Australia, 1981 and 1988.* Australian Institute of Health, Health Differentials Series, no. 1. Canberra: Australian Institute of Health.

Medawar PB. 1952. An unsolved problem in biology. London: HK Lewis.

Olshansky SJ, Rudberg MA, Carnes BA, Cassel C, Brody J. 1991. Trading off longer life for worsening health: The expansion of morbidity hypothesis. *J Aging Health* 3:194–216.

Olshansky SJ, Carnes BA, Cassel CK. 1993. The aging of the human species. *Scientific American,* April, 46–52.

Pope AM, Tarlov AR, eds. 1991. Magnitude and dimensions of disability in the United States. In: *Disability in America: Toward a national agenda for prevention of disabilities.* Pp. 41–75. Washington, D.C.: National Academy Press.

Rogers A, Rogers RG, Belanger A. 1990. Longer life but worse health? Measurement and dynamics. *Gerontologist* 30:640–649.

Rose MR. 1991. *Evolutionary biology of aging.* New York: Oxford University Press.

Rudberg M, Cassel C. 1993. Are death and disability in old age preventable? *Facts Res Gerontol* 7:191–202.

Rudberg M, Parzen MA, Leonard L, Cassel C. 1996. Functional limitation pathways and transitions in older persons. *Gerontologist* 36:430–440.

Schneider EL, Guralnik JM. 1990. The aging of America: Impact on health care costs. *JAMA* 263: 235–240.

Verbrugge LM. 1984. Longer life but worsening health? Trends in health and mortality of middle-aged and older persons. *Milbank Q* 62:475–519.

Verbrugge LM, Balaban DJ. 1989. Patterns of change in disability and well-being. *Med Care* 27:S128-S147.

Verbrugge LM, Jette AM. 1994. The disablement process. *Soc Sci Med* 38:1–14.

Weismann A. 1891. The duration of life. In: *Essays upon heredity and kindred biological problems,* edited by EB Poulton, S Schonland, AE Shipley. Pp. 5–66. Oxford: Clarendon Press.

Williams GC. 1957. Pleiotropy, natural selection, and the evolution of senescence. *Evolution* 11:398–411.

3

Long-Term Home Health Care for Frail, Homebound Elderly Persons

Philip W. Brickner, M.D.

Old age is honored only on condition that it defends itself, maintains its rights, is subservient to no one, and to the last breath rules over its own domain.—Cicero, quoting Cato, in *Old Age* 11

Men and women of advanced age are an increasingly prominent component of the U.S. population. We know that, for each individual, biological rather than chronological age determines the ability to live and thrive, yet our plans for care of the elderly population in general require that we understand the major demographic shifts that are taking place. For instance, a half-century ago persons 85 years old were rarities in this country, but by 1990 there were 3 million men and women that age and older. One million were 90 or more, and there were about 36,000 centenarians. In 2030, the number of persons aged 85 and older is projected to reach 8.1 million (NCOA, 1995). These individuals of great age will need help most if they are to survive with dignity and in basic comfort. This is the demographic imperative (Maddox, 1982).

By law, regulation, and stereotype, the age of 65 years marks the beginning of old age. According to this definition, for those who live into their 90s fully one-third of life will have been spent being old. The long silent period of aging (chapter 7) will include, for many persons, years of sustained good health; for many others, it will include chronic disability and a need for long-term care.

This discussion is concerned with the latter group. The options for those who are very old and frail, with significant chronic disabilities and difficulty in conducting important activities of daily living, are limited to institutional placement, long-term home health care, and abandonment. That abandonment of aged persons could truly be considered an option had never occurred to me until I participated in a discussion at the Health Care Financing Administration (HCFA, the federal agency responsible for Medicare) about 15 years ago. I was speaking to several midlevel HCFA staff members about why Medicare regulations should be amended to pay for long-term care of elderly persons at home. I argued that this change would be wise because such care would be cheaper than nursing home care. One of the staffers interrupted me and said: "Why yes, I understand what you're saying. But wouldn't it be even cheaper yet to let them die unattended at home?"

I know better now. While care at home, in most cases, is in fact cheaper than care in institutions, the prime reason for developing long-term home health care services for aged persons is that home is where they want to be. A 76-year old woman, a patient in such a program, said:

> Why should I go to a nursing home? You see my shrine over there? When I wake up at night I sit in my rocker and say my rosary. When I feel like it I can go to the kitchen and make myself a cup of tea. Do you see this furniture and this rug? They're *mine*. Why should I give them up? No, I will have no part of a nursing home. (Brickner, 1978, p. 24)

Pressure to place older persons in institutions arises because no genuine system of long-term care for elderly persons exists in this country. Instead, we live with anachronistic and uncoordinated programs, policies, and funding methods. A systematic approach would allow a range of options. Older persons would be free to move between programs of varying comprehensiveness and cost as their health and social needs required. We should seek the least restrictive form of care that is appropriate. This principle allows for maximal individual responsibility and decreases dependency and infantilization of older persons.

Long-Term Home Health Care

Overall History

How did we come to accept institutions as the best way to care for frail aged persons and, at the same time, find that we can neither build nor pay for enough nursing homes to satisfy future needs? Why have we pressed for long-term institutional placement when the very people targeted for such care resist and resent the idea?

In the eighteenth and early nineteenth centuries, perceptions of old age were ambiguous, but the tendency of our society to shun elderly people was present even then. The practice of dumping poor old persons and younger paupers together into almshouses grew. It then became easy to think of aged persons, in general, as helpless and dependent on the charity of others. The attitudes of nineteenth-century physicians about life force and vital energy encouraged this view. Each human being was believed to be born with a limited quantity of vital energy; as it was consumed, the body became an empty husk—devoid, finally, of life force. It was logical, then, for advanced age to signify inevitable physical and mental decline, and aged persons themselves were perceived as disabled and useless. Enforced retirement was seen by most as the only sane and kind social policy.

It followed that treating the diseases of aged individuals was pointless. The notion of dependent superannuation developed, a view that has led directly to our current model of old-age dependency, advocacy of institutional care for aged paupers, and state financing for the arrangements.

However, at the same time that these general concepts were being translated into policy, individual and local efforts in opposition to institutional placement were growing. In 1796 the Boston Dispensary created a service that gave the impoverished sick the option of care at home rather than in the hospital. Hospitals of that era were akin to pesthouses, where the old and homeless went to die; the rich were treated at home by their own physicians (Spiegel and Domanowski, 1983). Thus, home care for the poor was an enlightened concept.

Shame in the face of need was a concern that Lillian Wald and Mary Brewster faced in the 1890s. Their efforts to help care for immigrant mothers and their infants on the Lower East Side of New York were at first hampered by the reluctance of the poor themselves to consider help. "And these women did not try to uplift them or sentimentalize over them or offer them charity . . . Practically the only concrete help they could give was nursing care for the sick" (Metropolitan Life, n.d.). The Visiting Nurse Service of New York was born from this small beginning. During the early 1900s, the number of visiting nurse agencies in the northeastern United States grew significantly (Steward, 1979; Buhler-Wilkerson, 1985; Roberts and Heinrich, 1985). These home health programs expanded to include nutrition and social services and occupational, physical, and speech therapies, as well as homemaker and home health aide care.

In 1909 the Metropolitan Life Insurance Company offered home health services to its policy holders; the John Hancock Insurance Company provided similar coverage (Steward, 1979). This benefit became so popular that by 1928 Metropolitan employed more than 500 home care nurses and had contractual relationships with almost 1,000 visiting nurse agencies around the country. These programs were phased out at the beginning of World War II, when hospitals became more widely used and inpatient insurance coverage became widely available.

In 1942 Michael Reese Hospital (in Chicago) and in 1947 Montefiore Hospital (in New York) founded the country's first major hospital-based home care programs, efforts that have served as prototypes (Levenson, 1981; Salzman et al., 1987). The rationale behind this concept was that "it must be clearly understood that the hospital bed is not the 'natural habitat' of a sick human being and that the alternatives to hospitalization not only may be economical of beds and money but may be beneficial as well as comforting to the patient" (Cherkasky, 1947).

Since 1947, common sense has led to the creation of a network of home care programs emanating from hospitals across the country. However, as these programs gradually became subject to government control, they were permitted to function only after certification by state authorities, a practice that continues to date. Certification has the virtue of controlling costs by imposing strict admission rules for patients, limiting services through the so-called skilled nursing and intermittent care requirements, and insisting on a limited stay in the program. But these very requirements render hospital home care programs powerless to meet a significant need: *long-term* care at home for frail aged persons, with assistance from both paraprofessionals and professional health workers.

Legislative History

Formal attempts on the part of government to develop a basis for long-term care services can be traced to the Social Security Act of 1935, which

> established the cash welfare payments for the old age, dependent children and blind categories. It also prohibited payments to "inmates of public institutions," which provided an impetus for placing people in private profit-oriented board and care homes rather than county service systems. These homes formed part of the provider-base when nursing home benefits subsequently were explicitly adopted. (Fox, 1983)

In 1950, states were permitted for the first time to pay the costs of health service for individuals receiving welfare benefits. Before this, such care was a local responsibility and was dealt with haphazardly. The Hill-Burton Act, as amended in 1954, authorized funding, in the form of grants, for nursing home construction in the not-for-profit sector. This critical development set a precedent for public support of nursing homes and is recognized as the initial impetus for the major and explosive growth of these institutions, both public and proprietary, during the third quarter of the twentieth century (Stevens and Stevens, 1974; Vladeck, 1980).

In 1960 the Kerr-Mills amendments to the Social Security Act provided federal funds, with matched state money, for health services to aged poor persons. Thus the concept of medical indigency was recognized in federal legislation. In large part the funds made available through this bill were used to house elderly persons in nursing homes.

It was in 1964 that, through Medicare, for the first time a significant portion of the population, largely comprising persons aged 65 years and more, received entitlement to health insurance protection on a basis other than indigency. Medicare is paid for by each individual through deductions from Social Security benefits. At present no means test is required for eligibility, although there are fiscal pressures on the program that could ultimately alter this basic principle. Current federal budget considerations may lead to block grants to the states and change it further.

The long-term health care needs of elderly persons receive minimal support under Medicare (AARP, 1994; Lubitz et al., 1995). This insurance program provides benefits instead largely for *acute* hospital inpatient care and physicians' fees, a concept that was established in the original legislation and regulations and remains unaltered today. Yet the demographic changes we have noted strongly support the view that the *chronic* health care needs of elderly persons are substantial, increasing, and unmet.

Medicaid, developed in 1965 as amendments to the Social Security Act, is more a compilation and summary of prior health care financing legislation than a new concept. The Medicaid amendments incorporated funding to pay the health care costs of the poor through a relationship to the welfare system. Medicaid is therefore strictly limited to those who pass a means test, and is supported by tax levy funds of federal, state, and some local governments. The Medicaid legislation resulted in a broadened definition of medical indigency and in implementation of payment for health care costs of all persons receiving welfare support; it stressed nursing home placement for eligible individuals, thus enhancing our country's pro-institutional bias for care of frail elderly persons (Folkemer, 1994; Kassner, 1995).

Programs at Work

Over the last quarter-century, programs have been developed by urban hospitals and community agencies to try to fill the gap in long-term home health care (LTHHC) for elderly persons. A number of reports are available (Schreiber and Hughes, 1982; Blackman et al., 1985; Perkel, 1987; Balaban et al., 1988; Herron, 1988; Finucane et al., 1994; Woods, 1995; Kiely, 1996). While there are important differences between these various efforts, one quality they have in common is that care for aged persons in their homes is provided by teams of health professionals, usually including a nurse and a physician, and often including a social worker (Goldberg, 1991; Heinemann et al., 1994).

LTHHC program staff may help patients find paraprofessional help, but home health aides, nurses' aides, and housekeepers are not usually employees of the program. This distinction is important in avoiding confusion between LTHHC programs and the large number of service agencies across the country that are in the business, often proprietary but sometimes not-for-profit, of dispensing paraprofessional services for hourly fees plus overhead. Help from family and friends, if any, may be vital in the network of care (Marks, 1987; Andolsek et al., 1988; Johnson and Troll, 1992; Logan and Spitze, 1994).

The Chelsea-Village Program of St. Vincent's Hospital (in New York City), with which I have been associated since its start, will serve as the prototype for this discussion.

The Chelsea-Village Program

In January 1973 a physician, a nurse, and a social worker from St. Vincent's made their first team visit to a homebound aged individual living in our community. We entitled this effort the Chelsea-Village Program (CVP) because St. Vincent's serves primarily the population of the Chelsea and Greenwich Village neighborhoods of Manhattan. Our objective was simply to help our homebound aged patients stay out of institutions, remain in their own homes and community, retain the maximum possible level of independence, and continue in the best attainable state of health.

We tried from the start to acknowledge that we existed to serve our patients and to fulfill their desires, rather than to impose upon them our preconceived views as to what was best for them. The value of this viewpoint was emphasized by one of our first patients, a 92-year-old woman who greeted us at the front door of her apartment saying, "Thank God you're here. The only thing I'm worrying about is keeping out of a nursing home."

Our criteria for accepting patients in the CVP remain unchanged:

— geographic accessibility (can we get there?);
— the patient's inability to leave home without extraordinary means;
— a lack of adequate health care at home; and
— the patient's willingness to receive us.

We have no financial eligibility requirements, and we do not accept money from patients. Since our purpose is to bypass obstacles that deny our patients access to health services, it is antithetical to create at the same time a financial barrier to care. Indeed, an unusual aspect of the CVP is the financial structure that has allowed it to thrive. Because we have chosen to give care without cost to our patients, we have looked elsewhere for financial support. We have had consistent help from private philanthropies, but most of the financial backing for the CVP comes from St. Vincent's Hospital, which has understood that the success of the CVP is in the institution's best interests. This is in part because the program has created a steady resource of patients who look to our hospital for care; in part because this work is a service that is appreciated by the community in which the hospital resides; and in part because the CVP fulfills St. Vincent's founding mission of care for the sick poor. We believe that financial support for similar programs in other institutions can reasonably be created on a similar basis.

The Genesis of the Concept

Observation in our hospital's emergency room in the late 1960s taught us that members of certain groups (e.g., homeless persons and frail elderly persons) characteristically arrive by ambulance too late for care, moribund or dead on arrival. In trying to understand why, we learned that aged persons, particularly those who are homebound and alone, are often barred from the health care system by their disabilities.

We recognized that in order to have a practical impact on their multifaceted problems, it would often be necessary to apply the skills of medicine, nursing, and social work together. By teaming these three major disciplines, we believed that we could establish and sustain a network of services sufficient to make a life at home viable for many of our patients and avoid creating unrealizable expectations. If there is no coordinated method of bringing professional health services into the home, there is either pressure for institutional placement or an unattended death. We have learned that the desperate wish of most of our aged patients is to remain at home despite all risks. Institutional transfer is equated with death.

The Program's Beginnings

We spent 6 months analyzing how to obtain referrals, meeting with community agencies, and clarifying our purposes with our hospital administration and departmental hierarchies. On our first home visit, on January 17, 1973, the team walked to the patient's apartment. We had no paid staff, no money, no vehicle for transportation. We had the formal support of our hospital, a telephone in the Department of Community Medicine, widespread support and interest throughout the local community, and good weather.

Financial Support

After 4 months of work, we prepared a position paper summarizing the intent of the CVP and its results to date. With this, we succeeded in raising from private philanthropic sources funds sufficient to employ a full-time social worker and driver, and to rent a van for efficient staff transportation. This means of support has been essential to the program's growth. In 1994, of the CVP's budget of about $420,000, approximately $210,000 was raised from private donors. Of the remainder, $30,000 was turned back to the program from Medicare fees to physicians for their home visits, $40,000 was estimated as the value of time volunteered by physicians, and $140,000 was hospital support for office, administration, and a share of professional staff costs.

In 1994, over the entire span of 12 months, the CVP cared for a total of 246 individuals in their own homes, and on December 31, 1994, there were 201 persons active in the program. The cost of the CVP's services over the entire year averaged $1,842 per person.

The relationship of the CVP and long-term home health care to Medicare and Medicaid must be understood: Those CVP physicians who are eligible send bills to Medicare and turn all such income back to support the CVP. The nurses and social workers cannot generate Medicare income for their home visits. Medicaid support for the CVP is not available, although paraprofessional services such as those of home health aides can occasionally be arranged through Medicaid.

The full-time salaried staff today consists of three social workers and three nurses, as well as a driver, a coordinator, and a translator (Chinese-English). Twenty physicians participate on a regular unsalaried basis. The CVP does not employ paraprofessional staff. It is the task of the social worker, in consultation with colleagues, the patient, and family members, if any, to plan this aspect of support for care at home; then the means of obtaining paraprofessional assistance are identified. The social worker's skill in obtaining entitlements is critical. Without such help at home, the plan for most frail homebound elderly persons will fail. It is also important to note, however, that in most instances an aide or a homemaker alone will not be adequate to sustain long-term home care. Paraprofessional assistance must be integrated with other services.

Through the 23 years ending in December 30, 1995 we have cared for 2,002 persons in the Chelsea-Village Program.

Services to Chinese-Speaking Patients

The Living at Home Program, a national foundation-supported grant effort (Bogdonoff et al., 1991), in 1987 gave the CVP the opportunity to start providing care at home for monolingual Chinese-speaking patients by funding Chinese-speaking staff. As a result of amendments (in 1965 and later) to the 1952 United States immigration law (*Immigration and Nationality Act of 1952; Act of October 3, 1965*), and subsequent legislation (*Immigration Reform and Control Act of 1986; Immigration Act of 1990*), substantial numbers of persons from mainland China, Taiwan, and Hong Kong arrived in New York City. Many frail elderly men and women are included, now living on the lower east side of Manhattan in the very same walk-up tenements that were the homes of nineteenth-century immigrants from Europe, and in the area called Little Italy. This component of our work has thrived. In 1994, 95 of the 246 aged persons who were active in our program during the year were monolingual Chinese men and women.

We have had much to learn about the notable cultural distinctions that influence the response of aged Chinese patients to our offer of services. In addition to the impact of the enormous geographical range of their origin, a general truth holds for almost all: they lack previous experience with any substantial medical care system. Fifteen of our patients were rural agricultural laborers. They may have been cared for during illness or trauma by a health worker with less training than a nurse in the United States, or they may have received obstetrical care from a person with less experience than a midwife, or from a female family member.

Significant characteristics of our Chinese-speaking patients stem from their immigrant status, their attitudes toward accepting help from outside the family unit, and language barriers. These factors tend to isolate them from the larger world around them in New York City. And unless help is given, these men and women, who are almost uniformly poor, often lack the knowledge and ex-

Table 3.1. Primary Causes of Homeboundness in Patients in Chelsea-Village
Program, 1994

Type of Disability	Number of Patients ($n = 246$)	Percentage of Patients
Medical	90	36.59
Generalized debility and weakness	21	
Cardiac disease	24	
Chronic pulmonary disease	12	
Peripheral vascular disease	8	
Obesity	7	
Cirrhosis	1	
Malignancies		
Breast	4	
Gastrointestinal tract	2	
Other	3	
Other medical	8	
Orthopedic	61	24.79
Arthritis	34	
Previous fractures	14	
Amputation(s)	2	
Intervertebral disc	2	
Other orthopedic	9	
Neurological	54	21.95
Cerebrovascular accident (stroke)	35	
Parkinson disease	8	
Multiple sclerosis	2	
Blindness	5	
Poliomyelitis, old	1	
Other	3	
Psychiatric-psychosocial	41	16.67
Dementia	35	
Anxiety	2	
Other psychiatric	4	
Total	246	100.00

perience to access benefits to which they are entitled, including Medicare, Medicaid, food stamps, and paraprofessional assistance.

Who Are Our Homebound Aged Patients?

The average age of our patients is 83 years. Two-thirds are women. Two-thirds live alone. All are homebound. Most are poor. This combination of circumstances, threatening and challenging for many, is dealt with by most of our

Table 3.2.   Status of Patients in Chelsea-Village Program, Year Ending 1994

	Number of Patients	Percentage of Total
Active in care at home	178	72.36
Discharged from program	68	27.64
Total	246	100.00
Reasons for discharge		
Died in hospital	21	
Discharged to nursing home	17	
No longer needs CVP service	13	
Transferred to LTHHCP	7	
Refuses further contact	0	
Died at home	10	
Relocated	0	
In hospital over 3 months	0	
Total	68	

patients through grit and humor, and a determination to remain independent.

The clinical disorders that cause home-boundness in CVP patients are summarized in table 3.1. While there are no surprises, it is notable that osteoarthritis is the prime cause in 14 percent. Osteoarthritis, stroke, and dementia constitute the three most common reasons for being homebound. The cumulative length of stay in the program, patient status for the year 1994, and the age of patients in 1994 are shown in table 3.2 and in figures 3.1 and 3.2.

While the CVP knows a thousand stories, the following case history illustrates well the value of teamwork, and the determination of older persons to retain independence and control.

Doris

The CVP team first met Doris in 1975. When the nurse and social worker approached her in the hallway of her SRO hotel, she was guarded but did accept them. What Doris wanted was "someone to care about me now and when I die." Over the years the team came to know her well and became her surrogate family.

Born in eastern Europe, she immigrated here at the age of 19. While living with her aunt and sister, she worked in factories and sweat shops. She married at the age of 40, but soon left her abusive husband to move back with her sister. At age 49, her family had her committed to a state mental institution because she was a "trouble maker." Twenty years later, at age 70, she was released to live in an SRO hotel room. Widowed, without children, and rejected by her family, she was alone. Although not literally homeless, she was certainly living in isolation on the margins.

Doris was an eccentric woman with her own garish style, always well dressed, donning bright red lipstick and costume jewelry. Her tiny room was crammed with furniture, but she kept it clean and colorfully decorated with curtains and plastic flowers. Although she was often anxious, she derived strength from her religious practices and her newfound independence. Over the years the team promoted these strengths and intervened when she needed support.

Our program cared for Doris for 15 years. This long-term relationship was sustained despite changes of CVP staff. She always felt comfortable with at least one team member, and so able to accept new personnel as they were acquired. With each change, the senior team member bridged the gap and eased the transition for Doris. She was cared for continuously by the team entity and felt secure about this long-term arrangement.

She needed persistent medical attention for chronic congestive heart failure and hearing loss. For Doris our care also entailed ongoing emotional support as she dealt with her loneliness and inexorable aging. She longed to be reunited with her sister but was rejected when the team attempted a reconciliation. Day-to-day interventions entailed monitoring her health status, checking her mail, attending to her bills and shopping for her groceries. In addition, team members would celebrate with her on holidays. Eventually, as her health declined, the team coordinated a comprehensive array of services for her. Continuity was maintained as the team served as liaison between Doris and the other agencies providing hot meals, and visiting companions. Eventually, she could not manage alone. She often left food burning on her hot plate. Her safety was in jeopardy. The landlord initiated a process to have her deemed incompetent and removed to a nursing home. The outreach team was in conflict. They were torn, realizing her fear of being institutionalized again, yet appreciating the unsafe nature of her present state. Team members supported her through an ordeal that lasted six months. Advocating on her behalf, they secured a lawyer as she wished, and made plans for a second

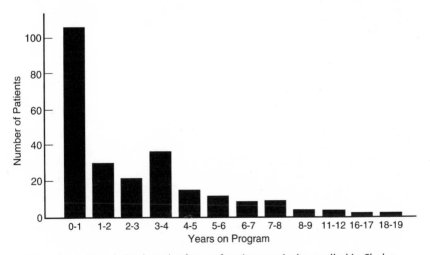

Figure 3.1.   Cumulative length of stay of patients actively enrolled in Chelsea-Village Program, 1994 (*n* = 246).

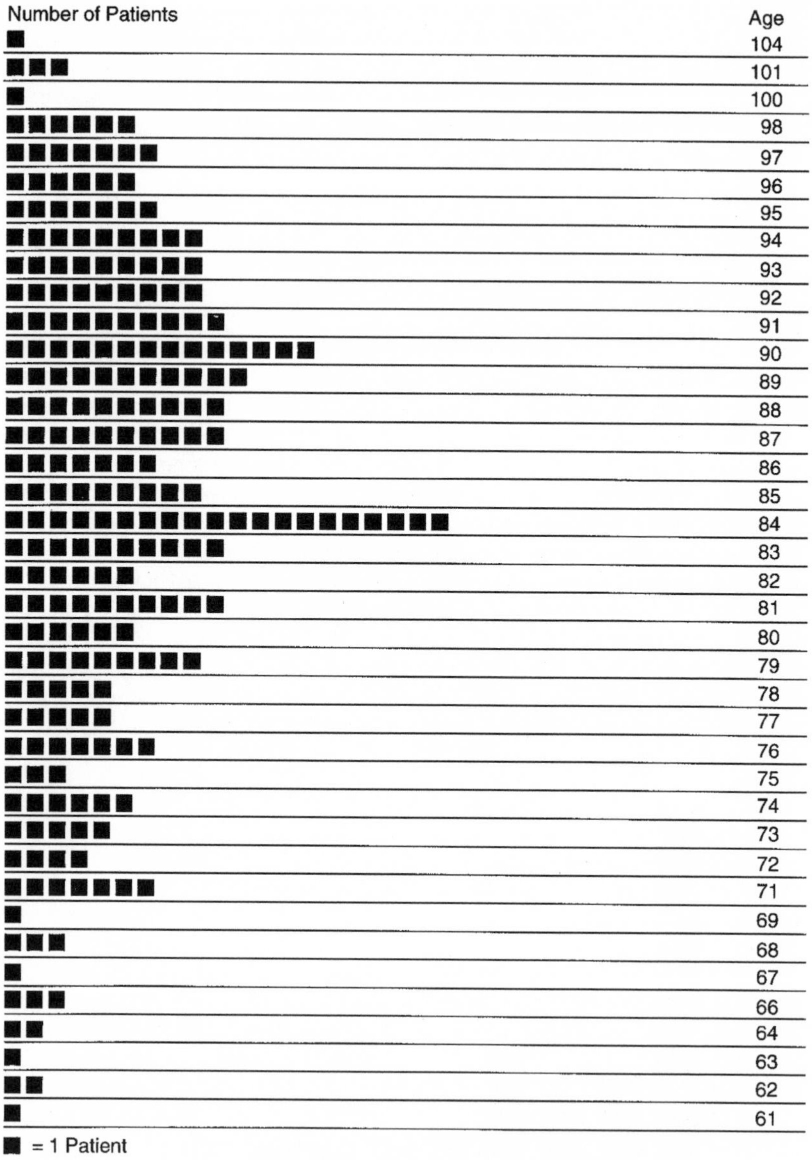

Number of Patients   **Age**

Number of Patients	Age
■	104
■■■	101
■	100
■■■■■■	98
■■■■■■■	97
■■■■■	96
■■■■■■	95
■■■■■■■■	94
■■■■■■■■	93
■■■■■■■■	92
■■■■■■■■■	91
■■■■■■■■■■■■	90
■■■■■■■■■■	89
■■■■■■■■■	88
■■■■■■■■■	87
■■■■■■	86
■■■■■■■■	85
■■■■■■■■■■■■■■■■■■■■	84
■■■■■■■■■	83
■■■■■■	82
■■■■■■■■■■	81
■■■■■	80
■■■■■■■■	79
■■■■■	78
■■■■■	77
■■■■■■	76
■■■	75
■■■■■■	74
■■■■■	73
■■■■	72
■■■■■■■	71
■	69
■■■	68
■	67
■■■	66
■■	64
■	63
■■	62
■	61

■ = 1 Patient

Figure 3.2.   Ages of patients actively enrolled in Chelsea-Village Program, 1994 (*n* = 246).

psychiatric opinion. But she was assessed, examined, and interrogated too many times. Exhausted and frantic she confided in the social worker whom she had met that first day in 1975, "I won't move . . . I'll die first." On the day of the scheduled court hearing, Doris was found dead in her room. She was 90 years old. The team notified her niece who assured them that Doris would be buried, as she had wished, in sacred ground. (Savarese and Weber, 1993, pp. 6–7)

Projections for Long-Term Home Health Care after the Year 2000

Physicians think in terms of prognosis and prescription, and we hope to cure or salve. When there is no salvation, we at least try to find a supportive way to admit the truth. We do not understand what will happen to our country's ability to care for persons of advanced age. There is no political or financial cure in sight, no salvation. What remains is the last resort: to tell the truth.

In truth, the supply of money to support care of frail aged persons is shrinking (Gold, 1995), while the numbers of those who need help grow (Manton and Vaupel, 1995). The prognosis for adequate tax-based support through the year 2000 is bad. Is there a realistic hope of assistance being provided to homebound elderly persons from other sources?

Volunteer efforts have always been vibrant in our country. Today, such programs as friendly visitors programs, services for shopping and delivery of food, foster grandparents' programs, immunization programs, and legal counsel are available to frail aged persons who have the knowledge and energy to search them out.

The religious community has already started to increase its efforts. Schrock (1996) notes that "on the practical side, there are many kinds of hands-on care . . . provided by congregations and ecumenical agencies. Churches are increasingly becoming community centers. Kitchens built for church suppers . . . are producing meals on wheels for the elderly. Many congregations provide elder health care programs [of] education, counseling support and clinics . . . [to] . . . address health care needs, . . . training for better nutrition, detect early signs of illness, address loneliness, depression, and often the failure of the elderly to care for themselves" (p. 58).

Philanthropic organizations will continue to put dollars into care of frail aged persons, but the resources of foundations and wealthy individuals are extremely modest compared to the financial need.

What about managed Medicare? Driven first by considerations of finances, proprietors of the new Medicare HMOs will focus on reducing hospital costs. Managed Medicare programs, in fact, will identify long-term home health care as a bad use of resources. "If denying home care leads to . . . a nursing home, that does not involve a medical expense, and Medicare does not pay for it. Once the patient is impoverished, the bills fall to Medicaid, to charity, or to no one" (Campion, 1995, p. 1214).

Thus, the truth is that the prognosis for health care for frail elderly people at home is bad. Many of these older men and women in the United States are likely to be thought of as ballast, to be tossed overboard to keep the ship of state afloat.

What shall we do? We must seek amelioration, since cure is not feasible. The adage Don't just stand there, do something! applies. To care for as many frail older persons as possible at home calls for

— combining the forces of all available community groups, particularly religious organizations, to provide services;

— emphasizing to philanthropic resources that frail aged people are at risk, and encouraging increased support of programs that serve them in their own homes;

— expecting hospitals and medical schools to develop long-term home health care programs to serve their local areas, both for the teaching value this work offers to students and house officers and in the spirit of community service. If the Chelsea-Village Program can thrive based at an academic medical center such as St. Vincent's, in New York, many other institutions can do the same.

Conclusion

It has been argued that after a person has lived out a natural life span, medical care should no longer be oriented to resisting death (Callahan, 1987, 1990). But this does not allow us to bar the frail aged from holding on to what, for most, is their last desperate wish: to be near friends and family, to remain independent and in their own homes, to be in control of their own lives. This requires long-term home health care.

Human beings have intrinsic worth. As a fundamental ethical principle, we cannot accept that some living persons are more valuable than others, or that advanced age is a marker for abandonment. What will we have achieved as a society if those among the least able to defend themselves, frail homebound aged persons, are abandoned?

Perhaps each of us must sacrifice some benefits to sustain essential and equitable care for all. That is rationing. If, however, some lose everything so that others may gain, that is triage; and triage of the frail elderly population should not be accepted.

REFERENCES

Act of October 3, 1965. PL 89-236, 79 Stat 911.

American Association of Retired Persons (AARP). 1994. *The cost of long-term care.* Washington, D.C.: AARP, Public Policy Institute.

Andolsek KM, Clapp-Channing NE, Gehlbach SH, Moore I, Proffitt VS, Sigmon A, Warshaw GA. 1988. Caregivers and elderly relatives: The prevalence of caregiving in a family practice. *Arch Intern Med* 148:2177–2180.

Balaban DJ, Goldfarb N, Perkel RL, Carlson BL. 1988. Follow-up study of an urban family medicine home visit program. *J Fam Pract* 26:307–312.

Blackman DK, Brown TE, Learner RM. 1985. Four years of a community long term care project: The South Carolina experience. *PRIDE Inst J* 4:3–12.

Bogdonoff MD, Hughes SL, Weissert WG, Paulsen E. 1991. *The Living at Home Program.* New York: Springer.

Brickner PW. 1978. *Home health care for the aged.* P. 24. New York: Appleton-Century-Crofts.

Buhler-Wilkerson K. 1985. Public health nursing: In sickness or in health? *Am J Public Health* 75: 1155–1161.

Callahan D. 1987. *Setting limits.* New York: Simon and Schuster.

———. 1990. *What kind of life.* New York: Simon and Schuster.

Campion EW. 1995. New hope for home care [editorial]. *N Engl J Med* 333:1213–1214.

Cherkasky M. 1947. Hospital service goes home. *Modern Hospital,* May.

Finucane TE, Fox-Whalen S, Burton R. 1994. The elder housecall program at Johns Hopkins. *J Long Term Home Health Care* 13:29–36.

Folkemer D. 1994. *State use of home and community-based services for the aged under Medicaid.* Washington, D.C.: AARP, Public Policy Institute.

Fox PD. 1983. Long term care: A bird's eye view. *PRIDE Inst J* 2:23–30.

Gold SD. 1995. Cuts that grow and grow. *New York Times,* November 14.

Goldberg AI. 1991. What is a home care physician? *Am Acad Home Care Physicians Newsletter* 3:1–7.

Heinemann GD, Schmitt MH, Farrell MP. 1994. Characteristics of geriatric health care teams [abstract]. *Gerontologist* 34:270.

Herron CM. 1988. Bringing health care home. *Health Prog* 69:48–51.

Immigration act of 1990. PL 101-649.

Immigration and nationality act of 1952. (McCarran-Walter act). Act of June 27, 1952. 66 Stat 163, Title 8, USCS.

Immigration reform and control act of 1986. PL 100-568.

Johnson CL, Troll L. 1992. Family functioning in late late life. *J Gerontol* 47:S66–S72.

Kassner E. 1995. *Long-term care: Measuring the impact of a Medicaid cap.* Washington, D.C.: AARP, Public Policy Institute.

Kiely SC. West Penn Hospital home visit program. 1996. In: *Geriatric home health care,* edited by PW Brickner, FR Kellogg, AJ Lechich, R Lipsman, LK Scharer. New York: Springer.

Levenson D. 1981. Martin Cherkasky at Montefiore. *Montefiore Medicine* 2:47.

Logan JR, Spitze G. 1994. Informal support and the use of formal services by older Americans. *Social Sciences* 49:S25-S34.

Lubitz J, Beebe J, Baker C. 1995. Longevity and medicine expenditures. *N Engl J Med* 332:999–1003.

Maddox GL. 1982. Challenges for health policy and planning. In: *International perspectives on aging: Population and policy challenges,* edited by RH Binstock, WS Chow, JH Schulz. Pp. 127–158. New York: United Nations Fund for Population Activities.

Manton KG, Vaupel JW. 1995. Survival after the age of 80 in the United States, Sweden, France, England, and Japan. *N Eng J Med* 333:1232–1235.

Marks R. 1987. The family dimension in long term care: An assessment of stress and intervention. *PRIDE Inst J* 6:18–26.

Metropolitan Life Insurance Company, Health and Welfare Division. N.d. *Lillian D. Wald: Pioneer in public health nursing.* Pp. 1–2. New York: Metropolitan Life Insurance.

National Council on Aging (NCOA). 1995. *Perspectives on aging—January-March 1995.* Washington, D.C.: NCOA.

Perkel R. 1987. Home visits. In: *Urban family medicine,* edited by RB Birrer. New York: Springer-Verlag.

Roberts DE, Heinrich J. 1985. Public health nursing comes of age. *Am J Public Health* 75:1162–1172.

Salzman H, Langendorf R, Ravenna P. 1987. Home health care (Michael Reese Hospital, Chicago) [letter to the editor]. *N Engl J Med* 106:168.

Savarese M, Weber CM. 1993. Case management for persons who are homeless. *J Case Management* 2:3–8.

Schreiber MS, Hughes S. 1982. The Chicago five hospital homebound elderly program: A long term home care model. *PRIDE Inst J* 1(1):12–20.

Schrock J. 1996. The role of the religious community in shaping community. *J Long Term Home Health Care* 15:57–59.

Spiegel AD, Domanowski GF. 1983. Beginnings of home health care: A brief history. *PRIDE Inst J* 2:28.

Stevens R, Stevens R. 1974. *Welfare medicine in America: A case study of Medicaid.* New York: Free Press.

Steward JE. 1979. *Home health care.* St. Louis, Mo.: CV Mosby.

Vladeck BC. 1980. *Unloving care.* New York: Basic Books.

Woods J. 1995. House calls. *Catholic New York,* September 7:16–17.

PART II

Osteoarthritis in an Aging Population

4

Evidence for the Increasing Prevalence of Osteoarthritis with Aging
Does This Pertain to the Oldest Old?

Flavia M. Cicuttini, M.B., Ph.D., and Tim D. Spector, M.D.

Osteoarthritis (OA) is one of the most common chronic diseases and the most frequent cause of rheumatic complaints in the older population. Once thought to be a result of normal aging, OA is now recognized to be a manifestation of complex and dynamic events. Although epidemiologic studies have identified a strong association of OA with age during the late adult years, it is still unclear whether this association continues into very old age. In this chapter we review the issues relating to the definition of OA in epidemiologic studies, and the evidence for an age effect, particularly as it relates to the oldest old, and consider some of the factors associated with OA.

Defining Osteoarthritis for Epidemiologic Studies: Clinical versus Radiologic Criteria

Epidemiologic studies of OA require explicit diagnostic criteria to classify the disease in the general population. Classification of OA remains a problem. There is no absolute clinical, radiologic, or pathologic standard against which the epidemiology of OA can be tested (Spector and Cooper, 1993). The available evidence suggests that radiography is less subject to bias than is clinical examination in defining OA in population-based epidemiologic studies (Dieppe and Cushnaghan, 1992; Hart et al., 1994).

Most studies to date have used a system of grading radiographic severity that was developed by Kellgren and Lawrence (1963). This system assigns one of five grades (0–4) to OA at various joint sites: knee, hip, hand, and spine. Grading is performed by comparing the index radiograph with reproductions in a radiographic atlas. The criteria for increasing severity of OA relate to the sequential appearance of osteophytes, joint space loss, subchondral sclerosis, and cyst formation.

There are a number of problems with this system. The main ones include inconsistencies in the interpretation of the grading system and the prominence given to the osteophyte at all joint sites. Although the original intention of the system was that grades be defined by standard radiographs, the films finally chosen as the standards did not easily conform to the written descriptions. There has also been variation in the descriptions provided by the authors at various times, which has resulted in poor reproducibility between observers and centers (Kellgren and Lawrence 1963; Lawrence, 1977).

Another potential problem with the system lies in its emphasis on the osteophyte. While the precise chronological sequence of events in OA remains uncertain, the majority of current data point to a primary loss of articular cartilage, which is then followed by a variable subchondral bony reaction. Two of the four grades in the revised Kellgren/Lawrence scheme refer only to osteophytes. An individual with joint space narrowing but no visible osteophytes cannot be classified as having OA using the Kellgren/Lawrence system. The system therefore assumes that joint space loss occurs after osteophytosis. Some joints do not easily fit into this grading system. Hand joints, for example, may be narrowed and sclerotic without the presence of osteophytes.

The widespread realization of these deficiencies in the current procedure for the radiographic assessment of OA has lead to a reappraisal. One approach has been to break up the radiographic definition system into its component features, quantify each feature more precisely, and assess the reproducibility and clinical correlates of each. The available studies suggest that no single grading system (e.g., measurement of joint space alone) is suitable for the assessment of OA at all sites and that any radiographic grading system for OA should be joint specific. Different measures might be appropriate in different circumstances. At the hip, therefore, measurement of minimal joint space is simple and reproducible and might suffice for the assignment of OA in epidemiologic studies (Croft et al., 1990). However, at the knee, where the precise location for any joint space measurement and the tricompartmental structure of the joint make assessment of joint space more difficult, assessment of osteophytes performs better (Hart et al., 1991).

Aging and Osteoarthritis

Age is regarded as one of the most important risk factors for OA. Epidemiologic studies have shown an increased prevalence of OA with increasing age (Lawrence, 1969; Mikkelson et al., 1970). The rate of OA in three different age groups—individuals less than 45 years old, those 45–64 years old, and those older than 65—has been shown to be 2 percent, 30 percent, and 68 percent, respectively, for women, and 3 percent, 24.5 percent, and 58 percent for men (Lawrence et al., 1966). This increase tends to be arithmetic until 50–55 years of age and geometric thereafter. This is particularly so in women and in those with multiple joint involvement, especially involvement of the interphalangeal joints (Allander, 1974; Lawrence, 1977). The greatest incidence of OA occurs at 45 years, when OA develops in the interphalangeal joints and the carpometacarpal (CMC) joint. This is then followed by tibiofemoral joint involvement and finally hip disease. The mechanism for this age-related development of OA is unknown.

Although the prevalence of OA increases through middle age, there is controversy as to whether it continues to increase in those aged 70 years and beyond, especially among the oldest old, beyond the age of 85 years. One reason for the view that the prevalence of OA increases with age is based on the literature that compares the young with the old, without analyzing the elderly population by more narrowly defined age groups. For example, the Health and Nutrition Examination Survey (HANES), the largest of the population-based surveys and one that used non-weight-bearing radiography, included subjects aged 25–74 years of age (DHEW National Center for Disease Statistics, 1979). An increase in knee OA with each 10-year increment in age was found, but more detailed information on what happens in those more than 70 years of age was not available.

Two early studies that divided elderly persons into narrower age bands suggested an increase in OA with age. One study of chronic illness in nursing homes reported the percentage of residents with "impairments (arthritis)" among those aged 65–74, 75–84, and 85+ to be 23.2 percent, 36.3 percent, and 43.1 percent, respectively (DHEW National Center for Health Statistics, 1978). However, "arthritis" was not further defined. In another study, in which OA of the hands and feet was evaluated, the prevalence did approach 100 percent (DHEW National Center for Health Statistics, 1966b). In this study, the percentage of women with OA of the hand was 65.4 percent, 76.4 percent, and 85.5 percent among those aged 55–64, 65–74, and 85.55, respectively. These findings were based on a clinical definition of the disease.

In contrast, a study that evaluated the signs and symptoms suggestive of

OA of the knee in 682 elderly people demonstrated that both the frequency of signs and symptoms and the degree of severity of disease remained constant in the seventh, eighth, and ninth decades (Forman et al., 1983). This study has been criticized as not being representative of the general population, as subjects were drawn from senior citizen centers and from hospital inpatients who were acutely ill, and not from the population at large. In addition, radiologic assessment of disease was not used. However, within these limitations, this study showed that the percentage of those with significant, objective knee abnormalities remained approximately constant in the seventh, eighth, and ninth decades at 48 percent, 54 percent, and 48 percent, respectively. Furthermore, among those with knee abnormalities, the severity did not increase with age. Among whites, women had significantly more abnormalities than did men, and more severe disease. In black men and women, the disease prevalence was more comparable. These findings were consistent with those of another study based on clinical definition of disease which also found little difference in knee disease when groups of individuals aged 55–64 and 65–74 were compared (DHEW National Center for Health Statistics, 1979). In a study examining radiologic disease, Lawrence et al. (1966) showed that 28 percent of "nonrheumatoid" men aged 55–64 had grade 2–4 OA radiologic changes at the knee, compared to 26 percent of men aged 65 and over. The figures for "nonrheumatoid" women were 40 percent and 49 percent, respectively. Furthermore, among those with significant radiologic changes, the percentage of those with the most marked abnormalities did not increase with age. In a Japanese population, the severity of disease, as assessed by radiologic criteria, was shown to be similar in those aged 66–70 and in those 71 and older (Suzuki et al., 1967).

A major problem in interpreting the early studies is that, in the main, they were not population based, so bias in the selection of subjects may have affected the results. Recently, within the framework of a population-based study of 70-year-old people in Goteborg, a cross-sectional study examined OA in subsamples of three cohorts: those aged 70, those aged 75, and those aged 79 (Bergstrom et al., 1986). In this study, the prevalence of clinical OA of the knee joint was shown to decrease with age in females but to remain similar in males aged 70 and 79 years. The prevalence of radiologic OA of the knee joints was higher (but not to a statistically significant extent) in those aged 70 than in those aged 75 and 79. In contrast, the severity of radiographic OA in the wrists and hands increased with age in all groups. It is important to note that this study was based on relatively small numbers in each subgroup. When joint complaints and clinical and radiologic findings of OA in wrist, hand, and knee joints were studied in a subsample of 79 and 85 year olds in the same population, once again, age-related differences in the prevalence of OA were not found (Bagge et al., 1991a). On the contrary, a lower prevalence of radiographic OA in the wrists and hand joints was noted in 85-year-old men and women, and a lower prevalence of radiographic OA in the knees was noted in 85-year-old men. An increased mortality has previously been described in women with radiographic knee OA (Hochberg et al., 1989), which might in part explain these results. Against this explanation, however, is the failure to demonstrate any association between mortality and OA in this population (Bergstrom et al., 1986).

In contrast, the results of the Framingham Osteoarthritis Study, a population-based study of independently living elderly people, which examined the prevalence of radiographic and symptomatic knee OA, suggested that knee OA increases in prevalence throughout the elderly years, more so in women than in men (Felson et al., 1987). Radiographs were obtained on 1,424 subjects whose ages ranged from 63 to 94 years (the mean age was 73). Among this cohort, 206 were more than 85 years of age. Osteoarthritis was defined as grade 2 changes (definite osteophytes), or higher, in either knee. Radiographic evidence of OA increased with age, from 27 percent in subjects younger than age 70, to 44 percent in subjects aged 80 or older (Felson et al., 1987). The age-associated increase in OA was almost entirely the result of a marked age-associated increase in the incidence of OA in the women studied (Felson et al., 1987). One possible criticism of this study is that the population selected for the study may not be representative of the population of this age, as only people who were living independently were included in the study.

Most studies to date are consistent in showing an age-associated increase in the prevalence of both radiologic and clinical OA at least up to the age of 70 (Lawrence, 1969; Mikkelson et al., 1970; Felson et al., 1987; Verbrugge, 1992). Recently it was shown that incident OA of the knees continued to occur during the elderly years (Felson et al., 1995). The evidence for what happens to the prevalence of OA after the age of 70 is less clear. Hand OA appears to increase with age (DHEW National Center for Health Statistics, 1966b; Bergstrom et al., 1986), but the findings for knee OA are less consistent (table 4.1) (Bergstrom et al., 1986; Felson, 1990; Felson et al., 1987; Bagge et al., 1991b). In studies on very elderly subjects, the prevalence of radiologic OA may increase but disability and clinical symptoms may not, perhaps due to a selection of survivors with less comorbidity and decreased pain perception in aging joints (Acheson, 1983).

Table 4.1.   The Prevalence of Knee Osteoarthritis in the Older Age Groups

Source	Group(s) Studied	Disease Definition	Age Range (years)	Prevalence (%)
Forman et al., 1983	clients of senior citizen centers, and acutely ill hospital inpatients	clinical	60–69 70–79 80–89	48 54 48
Bergstrom et al., 1986	subgroups from population-based study	radiologic	70 75 79	20 14 13
Felson et al., 1987	general population, independently living	radiologic	< 70 70–79 > 80	27 34 44

Generalized Osteoarthritis

The question of whether polyarticular involvement exists in OA more frequently than would be expected on the basis of increasing age or chance alone remains uncertain. Although several hospital studies have documented the female preponderance and symmetrical pattern of involvement in polyarticular OA, there have been only two population-based studies addressing the issue of whether generalized OA comprises a specific disease subset (Acheson and Collart, 1975; Cooper et al., 1996). The first study, which was confined to the hand, assessed 1,334 men and women age 21 years and over in New Haven, Connecticut (Acheson et al., 1970). Following examination of the frequency distribution of affected joints, no evidence was found for the existence of generalized OA. However, radiographs of other joint groups were obtained in a small number of subjects, and the authors found that multiple joint involvement was positively associated with serum C-reactive protein, the weight-height ratio, and serum urate and antistreptolysin O (ASO) titers. On this basis, they proposed that systemic factors must underlie the development of OA (Acheson and Collart, 1975).

In contrast, evidence that generalized OA is a distinct entity was found in a recent study (Cooper et al., 1996). Attempts to define polyarticular disease are complicated by the steep age-related increase in joint involvement at each particular site. The problem was addressed in this study by examining the age-adjusted ratio of observed to expected joint groups and using a ratio of 2:1 or more as the cut-off for allocating an individual with multiple joint group involvement to the polyarticular subset. Using this method, evidence for generalized OA was found, with a predilection for symmetrical hand, knee, and spine involvement, independent of an age effect (Cooper et al., 1996).

Risk Factors for Osteoarthritis

Genetic Factors

For more than 50 years a strong genetic component has been thought to be present in certain forms of OA. Early studies by Stecher (1941) demonstrated that Heberden nodes (i.e., OA of the distal interphalangeal [DIP] joints) were three times as common in the sisters of 64 affected subjects as in the general population. Family studies in the early 1960s of individuals with generalized OA suggested that first-degree relatives of such persons were twice as likely as controls to also have radiographic generalized disease (Kellgren et al., 1963).

Recently, a clear genetic influence on OA was demonstrated in a study of 500 unselected female twins aged 45–70 years who were screened radiologically for OA of the hands and knees (Spector et al., 1996). The correlations of OA disease status were consistently twice as high in 130 pairs of identical twins as in a corresponding group of nonidentical twins. The influence of genetic factors was estimated to be between 50 and 65 percent, independent of known environmental or demographic confounders. The nature of the genetic influence in OA is speculative and may involve either a structural defect (i.e., collagen) or alterations in cartilage or bone metabolism. Exciting work has identified mutations in type 2 collagen as important in some rare, familial forms of OA (Palotie et al., 1989; Alla-Kokko et al., 1990), but the genetic basis of the common forms of OA is currently unknown (Ritvaniemi et al., 1995).

Obesity

In 1958 Kellgren and Lawrence found that knee OA was more common in obese people than in nonobese people and twice as common in females as in males. Heberden nodes have also been associated with obesity in some studies, although principally in men (Kellgren and Lawrence, 1958). No consistent association has been noted for hip OA. In 1960, the New Haven Survey found similar relationships between obesity and finger OA, and this association was stronger in females (Acheson and Collart, 1975). Other studies have found an association between OA of the knee and obesity (Leach et al., 1973; Hartz et al., 1986; Masse et al., 1988; also see chapter 10). A study in Zoetermeer, in the Netherlands, also found no association with hip OA but found a significant association with the commonly affected joints such as the DIP joints or the knee (van Saase et al., 1988). Data from the large National Health and Nutrition Examination Survey (NHANES I) found that the risk of OA increases with degree of obesity, and long-term obesity was significantly associated with knee

OA (Anderson and Felson, 1988; Davis et al., 1988). Davis et al. (1988) found that the body mass index (BMI) correlated with the presence of OA better than did other anthropomorphic measurements. They also found that waist circumference was inversely associated with combined hand and foot OA. Prospective data from the Framingham study confirmed that obesity precedes by 30 years the appearance of radiologic knee OA (Felson et al., 1988). Analysis of the NHANES I data has also shown that obesity is a strong predictor of bilateral knee disease (Davis et al., 1989).

Overall, the results to date suggest that the link between obesity and OA is more consistent in women, and is strongest in OA of the knees and less conclusive in other joints. Data from two subsamples of 79 year olds within the prospective study of 70-year-old people in Goteborg further confirmed obesity as a risk factor for OA in an aged population (Bagge et al., 1991b). In this study, a significant correlation between BMI and knee OA was found in both men ($P < 0.01$) and women ($P < 0.001$). A significant correlation between BMI and OA in hand joints was also found in men ($P < 0.01$) but not in women.

A recent population-based twin study showed that twins with osteoarthritis were generally 3–5 kilograms heavier than their co-twins with no disease. Significant increases in the risk of developing radiologic features of OA were observed for every kilogram increase in body weight (a 14% increase for tibiofemoral osteophytes, a 32% increase for patellofemoral osteophytes, and a 10% increase for CMC osteophytes). This result persisted even when only twins with asymptomatic radiologic OA were examined. This study emphasizes the potential importance of even minor weight gain as a risk factor for OA (Cicuttini et al., 1996).

Obesity has been shown to be the most important factor in the development of contralateral knee OA in middle-aged women in the general population with existing unilateral OA in the other knee (Spector et al., 1994). Over the course of a 2-year study, one-third of the women developed incident disease in the contralateral knee (based on a Kellgren and Lawrence score of 2+ or osteophyte change), and about one-fifth progressed radiologically in the index knee. Obesity at baseline was the most important factor related to incident disease, since about one-half of the women in the top BMI tertile developed OA, compared with one-tenth in the lowest tertile (relative risk 4.69, with confidence intervals 0.63–34.75). Interestingly, the associations of obesity with hip OA are much weaker and are inconsistent (Heliovaara et al., 1993; Tepper and Hochberg, 1993). Since both the hip and the knee are weight-bearing joints, more than mechanical factors may contribute to the development of OA in the knee (see chapter 10).

Studies show that obesity is likely to be the cause, rather than a result, of OA. One mechanism by which obesity may predispose an individual to OA is excess mechanical stress on joints. This mechanism is easy to understand in relation to weight-bearing joints. However, it is more difficult to understand how this mechanism may explain the association of obesity with OA in non-weight-bearing joints such as the DIP and the CMC. It is possible that the association is due in part to a metabolic effect.

Few studies have looked at the effect of weight loss in subjects who have established OA. Felson et al. (1991, 1995), studying the Framingham cohort, observed that weight loss in middle and later adult life substantially reduced the risk of symptomatic OA of the knee. Also, a recent study of middle-aged women has suggested that risk of knee OA increases by 35 percent for every 5 kilograms of weight gain (Spector et al., 1994). It appears, therefore, that reduction or maintenance of weight should be an important part of prevention of knee OA, and more work is needed on weight reduction studies and OA.

Physical Activity

The influence of prolonged loading of joints on the development of OA is unclear. There is considerable indirect evidence to support a relationship between long-duration, high-intensity weight-bearing exercise and OA of the hip and knee (Lane, 1993). Excessive bending of the hips in farmers (Croft et al., 1992a) and occupational knee bending in men have been shown to increase the risk of OA (Croft et al., 1992b).

The evidence in athletes, however, is conflicting. Most of the early studies on athletes were uncontrolled surveys on small numbers of current athletes which produced discrepant results (Panush et al., 1986; Marti et al., 1989). Other studies of soccer players have only included players who were symptomatic and in whom radiographs were requested. A recent large-scale record linkage study from Finland identified 2,049 male athletes and found an approximately two-fold increase in hospital admissions with an International Classification of Disease (ICD) code of OA (Kujala et al., 1994). While this was a powerful study in terms of sample size it had disadvantages, as it could not exclude referral bias or diagnostic bias as an explanation of the results.

Little information is available on the effect of physical activity on OA in elderly persons. In the cross-sectional study of 79 year olds in Goteberg, the individual's history of physical activity and occupational activity was assessed (Bagge et al., 1991b). There was no evidence that a history of heavy occupational and/or spare-time physical activity preceded the development of OA. However, the numbers of individuals with a history of heavy occupational and/or spare-time physical activity was small, thus limiting the extent to which this question could be examined in the study.

Hormonal Factors

Gender has been clearly associated with OA, with an effect particularly related to OA at specific sites. For example, below the age of 45 years OA is more common in men, and in these men it usually involves one or two joints (DHEW National Center for Health Statistics, 1966a; Lawrence, 1977). However, over the age of 55 years it is more common in women, usually involving several joints, mostly the interphalangeals, the first metacarpal, and the knees (DHEW National Center for Health Statistics, 1966a; Lawrence, 1977). Furthermore, the prevalence of OA of the knee among adults aged 55 to 74 years is greater in women than in men (Felson, 1988). Gender differences in the prevalence of OA of the hip, however, remain unclear. Some studies have demonstrated comparable rates between the two sexes in the same age group (Danielsson et al., 1984), while others have suggested a male predominance (Kellgren, 1961; Lawrence et al., 1966).

There is good epidemiologic and clinical evidence to link generalized OA (GOA) with hormonal factors. In the population surveys of Lawrence, x-ray evidence of nodal GOA was three times higher in women in the age range 45–64 (Kellgren and Moore, 1952). Other hospital-based studies have shown a female-to-male ratio as high as 10:1, with a marked peak of age of onset at 50 years in women for nodal GOA (Wood, 1982). Joint symptoms are also one of the principal components of the climacteric (Neugarten and Kraines, 1965) and may be associated with higher estradiol levels (Nordin and Polley, 1987). Other studies have found higher rates of hysterectomy in women developing OA, suggesting hormonal differences (Spector et al., 1988). In females, obesity has been found to correlate with generalized and knee OA and also with OA of a number of non-weight-bearing sites (Spector, 1990). It appears to be related to excess body weight rather than muscle bulk (Davis et al., 1988). Obesity in women is a known cause of hyperestrogenism via the peripheral formation of estrogen from androstenedione in the fat tissues. After the menopause, this route becomes the principal source of estrogens. Thus the association between OA and obesity also suggests a role of endocrine influences in the development of OA.

Smoking

Smokers appear to have a lower prevalence of OA than do nonsmokers, even after adjusting for weight. This has been observed in a number of studies including the NHANES I (Anderson and Felson, 1988) and the Framingham study (Felson et al., 1989), both of which suggested that smoking is protective. This was further confirmed in a subsample analysis of elderly persons for the knee but not the hand (Bagge et al., 1991b). In middle-aged community-dwelling women, no clear protective effect of smoking was observed for OA of the hands and knees, although there was a possible modest protective effect on the generalized form of OA (Hart and Spector, 1993).

Conclusions

Most studies to date are consistent in showing an increase in the prevalence of both radiologic and clinical OA with increasing age, at least up to the age of 70. The evidence for what happens to the prevalence of OA after this age is less clear. Hand OA appears to increase with age, but the findings for knee OA are less consistent. Obesity is likely to be the most important preventable risk factor for OA, and weight loss has been shown to be helpful even in elderly persons. The concern of this book with the oldest old should be reflected in future population studies seeking to determine the prevalence of OA in those 85 years of age and older, an issue that to date has not been sufficiently explored.

REFERENCES

Acheson, RM. 1983. Osteoarthritis: The mystery crippler [editorial]. *J Rheumatol* 10:180–183.
Acheson RM, Collart AB. 1975. New Haven Survey of joint diseases: Relationship between some systemic characteristics and osteoarthritis in a general population. *Ann Rheum Dis* 34:379–385.
Acheson RN, Chan Y, Clemett. 1970. New Haven survey of joint diseases: XII. Distribution of symptoms of osteoarthritis in the hand with reference to handedness. *Ann Rheum Dis* 29:275–285.
Alla-Kokko L, Baldwin CT, Moskowitz RW, Prockop DJ. 1990. A single base mutation in the type II procollagen gene (COL2A1) as cause of primary osteoarthritis associated with a mild chondrodysplasia. *Proc Natl Acad Sci USA* 87:6565–6568.
Allander E. 1974. Prevalence, incidence, and remission rates of some common rheumatic diseases or syndromes. *Scand J Rheumatol* 3:145–148.
Anderson JJ, Felson DT. 1988. Factors associated with osteoarthritis of the knee in the first national health and nutrition examination survey (NHANES I). *Am J Epidemiol* 128:179–189.
Bagge E, Bjelle A, Eden S, Svanborg A. 1991a. Osteoarthritis in the elderly: Clinical and radiological findings in 79 and 85 year olds. *Ann Rheum Dis* 50:535–539.
Bagge E, Bjelle A, Eden S, Svanborg A. 1991b. Factors associated with radiographic osteoarthritis: Results from the population study 70-year-old people in Goteborg. *J Rheumatol* 18:1218–1222.
Bergstrom G, Bjelle A, Sundh V, Svanborg A. 1986. Joint disorders at ages 70, 75, and 79 years—a cross-sectional comparison. *Br J Rheumatol* 25:333–341.

Cicuttini FM, Baker JR, Spector TD. 1996. Association of obesity with osteoarthritis of the hand and knee in women: A twin study. *J Rheumatol* 23:1221–1226.

Cooper C, Egger P, Coggon D, Hart DJ, Masud T, Cicuttini FM, Doyle DV, Spector TD. 1996. Generalised osteoarthritis in women: Definition for epidemiological studies and pattern of joint involvement. *J Rheumatol* 23:1938–1942.

Croft P, Cooper C, Wickham C. 1990. Defining osteoarthritis of the hip for epidemiological studies. *Am J Epidemiol* 132:514–522.

Croft P, Coggon D, Cruddas M, Cooper C. 1992a. Osteoarthritis of the hip: An occupational disease in farmers. *Br Med J* 304:1269–1272.

Croft P, Coggon D, Cruddas M, Cooper C. 1992b. Osteoarthritis of the hip and occupational activity. *Scand J Work Environ Health* 18:59–63.

Danielsson L, Lindberg H, Nilsson B. 1984. Prevalence of coxarthrosis. *Clin Orthop* 191:110–115.

Davis MA, Ettinger WH, Neuhaus JM, Hauck WW. 1988. Sex differences in osteoarthritis of the knee: The role of obesity. *Am J Epidemiol* 127:1019–1030.

Davis MA, Ettinger WH, Neuhaus JM, Sangsook AC, Hauck WW. 1989. The association of knee injury and obesity with unilateral and bilateral osteoarthritis of the knee. *Am J Epidemiol* 128:278–288.

Department of Health, Education, and Welfare (DHEW), National Center for Health Statistics. 1966a. *Osteoarthritis in adults by selective demographic characteristics, United States 1960–1962.* Rockville, Md.: DHEW.

———. 1966b. *Prevalence of osteoarthritis in adults by age, sex, race, and geographical area: United States, 1960–1962.* Ser. 11, no. 15. Rockville, Md.: DHEW.

———. 1978. *Profile of chronic illness in nursing homes.* P. 25, table 1. DHEW Publication no. (PHS) 78-1780. Rockville, Md.: DHEW.

Department of Health, Education, and Welfare (DHEW), National Center for Disease Statistics. 1979. *Basic data on arthritis of the knee, hip, and sacroiliac joints in adults ages 25–74 years: United States, 1971–1975.* DHEW Publication no. (PHS) 79-1661. Ser. 11, no. 213.

Dieppe P, Cushnaghan J. 1992. The natural course and prognosis of osteoarthritis. In: *Osteoarthritis: Diagnosis and medical/surgical management,* edited by RW Moskowitz, DJ Howell, VM Goldberg, HJ Mankin. 2d ed. Pp. 399–412. London: Saunders.

Felson DT. 1988. Epidemiology of hip and knee osteoarthritis. *Epidemiol Rev* 10:1–28.

———. 1990. The epidemiology of knee osteoarthritis: Results from the Framingham Osteoarthritis Study. *Semin Arthritis Rheum* 20(3, suppl. 1):42–50.

Felson DT, Naimark A, Anderson J, Kazis L, Castelli W, Meenan RF. 1987. The prevalence of knee osteoarthritis in the elderly: The Framingham Osteoarthritis Study. *Arthritis Rheum* 30:914–918.

Felson DT, Anderson JJ, Naimark A, Walker AM, Meenan RF. 1988. Obesity and knee osteoarthritis: The Framingham study. *Ann Intern Med* 109:18–24.

Felson DT, Anderson JJ, Naimark A, Hannan MT, Kannel WB, Meenan RF. 1989. Does smoking protect against osteoarthritis? *Arthritis Rheum* 32:166–171.

Felson DT, Zhang YO, Anthony JM, Naimark A, Anderson JJ. 1991. Weight loss reduces the risk of symptomatic knee OA in women: The Framingham study [abstract]. *Arthritis Rheum* 34:9.

Felson DT, Zhang Y, Hannan MT, Naimark A, Weissman BN, Aliabadi P, Levy D. 1995. The incidence and natural history of knee osteoarthritis in the elderly: The Framingham Osteoarthritis Study. *Arthritis Rheum* 38:1500–1505.

Forman MD, Malamet R, Kaplan D. 1983. A survey of osteoarthritis of the knee in the elderly. *J Rheumatol* 10:282–287.

Hart DJ, Spector TD. 1993. Cigarette smoking and risk of osteoarthritis in women in the general population: The Chingford Study. *Ann Rheum Dis* 52:93–96.

Hart DJ, Spector TD, Brown P, Wilson P, Doyle DV, Silman AJ. 1991. Clinical signs of early osteoarthritis: Reproducibility and relation to x-ray changes in 541 women in the general population. *Ann Rheum Dis* 50:467–470.

Hart DJ, Spector TD, Egger P, Coggon D, Cooper C. 1994. Defining osteoarthritis of the hand for epidemiologic studies: The Chingford Study. *Ann Rheum Dis* 53:220–223.

Hartz AJ, Fischer ME, Bril G. 1986. The association of obesity with joint pain and osteoarthritis in the HANES data. *J Chronic Dis* 39:311–319.

Heliovaara M, Makela M, Impivaara O, Knekt B, Oromaa A, Sievers K. 1993. Association of overweight, trauma, and workload with coxarthrosis: A health survey of 7,217 persons. *Acta Orthop Scand* 64:513–518.

Hochberg M, Lawrence RC, Everett DF, Comoni-Huntley J. 1989. Epidemiological association of pain in osteoarthritis of the knee: Data from the national health and nutrition examination survey and the national health and nutrition–1 epidemiologic follow-up survey. *Semin Arthritis Rheum* 18(suppl. 2):4–9.

Kellgren JH. 1961. Osteoarthritis in patients and populations. *Br Med J* 1:1–16.

Kellgren JH, Lawrence JS. 1958. Osteoarthritis and disk degeneration in an urban population. *Ann Rheum Dis* 17:388–396.

Kellgren JH, Lawrence JS. 1963. *The epidemiology of chronic rheumatism: Atlas of standard radiographs.* Vol 2. Oxford: Blackwell Scientific.

Kellgren JH, Moore R. 1952. Generalised osteoarthritis and Heberden's nodes. *Br Med J* 1:181–187.

Kellgren JH, Lawrence JS, Bier F. 1963. Genetic factors in generalized osteoarthritis. *Ann Rheum Dis* 22:237–255.

Kujala UM, Kaprio J, Sama S. 1994. Osteoarthritis of weight bearing joints of lower limbs in former elite male athletes. *Br Med J* 308:231–234.

Lane N. 1993. Exercise: A cause of osteoarthritis. *Rheum Dis Clin North Am* 19:617.

Lawrence JS. 1969. Generalised osteoarthritis in a population-based sample. *Am J Epidemiol* 90:381–389.

———. 1977. *Rheumatism in populations.* Pp. 98–155. London: W Heinemann Medical Books.

Lawrence JS, Bremner JM, Biers F. 1966. Osteoarthritis: Prevalence in the population and relationship between symptoms and x-ray changes. *Ann Rheum Dis* 25:1–24.

Leach RE, Baumgard S, Broom J. 1973. Obesity: Its relationship to osteoarthritis of the knee. *Clin Orthop* 93:271–273.

Marti B, Knobloch M, Tschoop A, Jucker A, Howald H. 1989. Is excessive running predictive of degenerative hip disease? Controlled study of former elite athletes. *Br Med J* 299:91–93.

Masse JP, Glimet T, Kuntz D. 1988. Gonarthrose et obésité. *Rev Rhum Mal Osteoartic* 55:973–978.

Mikkelson WM, Duff IF, Dodge HD. 1970. Age-specific prevalence of radiological abnormalities of the joints of the hands, wrists, and cervical spine of adult residents of the Tecumseh, Michigan, community health area, 1962–1965. *J Chronic Dis* 123:151–159.

Neugarten BL, Kraines RJ. 1965. "Menopausal symptoms" in women of various ages. *Psychosom Med* 27:266–273.

Nordin EC, Polley KJ. 1987. Metabolic consequences of the menopause. *Calcif Tissue Int* 41:s1-s59.

Palotie A, Väisänen P, Ott J, Ryhänen L, Elima K, Vikkula M, Cheah K, Vuorio E, Peltonen L. 1989. Predisposition to familial osteoarthritis linked to type II collagen gene. *Lancet* 1:924–927.

Panush RS, Schmidt C, Caldwell JR, Edwards NL, Longley S, Yonker R, Webster E, Nauman J, Stork J, Pettersson H. 1986. Is running associated with degenerative joint disease? *JAMA* 255:1152–1154.

Ritvaniemi P, Korkko J, Bonaventure J, Vikkula M, Hyland J, Paassilta P, Kaitila I, Kaariainen H, Sokolov BP, Hakala M, et al. 1995. Identification of COL2A1 gene mutations in patients with chondrodysplasias and familial osteoarthritis. *Arthritis Rheum* 38:999–1004.

Spector TD. 1990. The fat on the joint: Obesity and osteoarthritis. *J Rheumatol* 17:283–284.

Spector TD, Cooper C. 1993. Radiological assessment of osteoarthritis in population studies: Whither Kellgren and Lawrence? *Osteoarthritis and Cartilage* 1:203–206.

Spector TD, Brown GC, Silman AJ. 1988. Increased rates of prior hysterectomy and gynaecological operations in women with osteoarthritis. *Br Med J* 297:899–900.

Spector TD, Hart DJ, Doyle DV. 1994. Incidence and progression of osteoarthritis in women with unilateral knee disease in the general population: The effect of obesity. *Ann Rheum Dis* 53:565–568.

Spector TD, Cicuttini F, Baker J, Hart DJ. 1996. Genetic influences on osteoarthritis: A twin study. *Br Med J* 312:940–944.

Stecher RM. 1941. Heberden's nodes: Heredity in hypertrophic arthritis of the finger joints. *Am J Med Sci* 201:801.

Suzuki R, Kimura F, Kiman T. 1967. Etiology of osteoarthritis of the knee joint. *Fukushima J Med Sci* 14:55–87.

Tepper S, Hochberg MC. 1993. Factors associated with hip osteoarthritis: Data from the first National Health and Nutrition Examination Survey (NHANES-I). *Am J Epidemiol* 137:1081–1088.

van Saase JLC, Vandenbrouke JP, van Romunde LK, Valkenberg HA. 1988. Osteoarthritis and obesity in the general population: A relationship calling for an explanation. *J Rheumatol* 15:1152–1158.

Verbrugge L. 1992. Disability transitions for older persons with arthritis. *J Aging Health* 4:212–243.

Wood PH. 1982. Age and the rheumatic diseases. In: *Population studies of the rheumatic diseases*, edited by PH Bennett and PH Wood. Amsterdam: Excerpta Medica, 4:26–37.

5

General Concepts of Disablement

*Jean-Marie Robine, Jean-François Ravaud, M.D., and
Emmanuelle Cambois*

In memoriam: Pierre Minaire

Disability, as defined by the World Health Organization (WHO), is any restriction of an individual's "ability to perform an activity in the manner or within the range considered normal for a human being" (WHO, 1980, p. 143). The existence of such disability is perhaps as old as the human race itself, but the fossils remaining from prehistoric sites, and showing deformities, signs of bone disease, injuries, fractures, and the like, are not formal proof of this. They simply indicate the presence of numerous physical impairments but do not provide information on what was considered, at the time, to be the normal manner of carrying out different human activities or the normal way of behaving—in other words, how one lived.

On a historical scale, varieties of disablement quickly acquired names, as witnessed by the profusion of terms used (in various languages) in ancient texts—*impotent, invalid, incapable, inept, crippled, infirm, deficient, limited, feeble, simple, idiot, backward, retarded, degenerate,* and so on. In contrast, the use of the term *handicap* in the field of disablement is very recent (Stiker, 1982). Thus, in the nineteenth century, the first studies devoted to the state of health of the population (Committee of the Highland Society of Scotland, 1824; Chadwick, 1842) focused essentially on the number of work-loss days due to illness, a measure that still remains one of the main indicators of short-term disability in a population (Riley, 1991).

Only very recently has the disablement process been of interest theoretically. This contemporary approach was marked principally by the works of Saad Nagi (1965, 1976) and of Philip Wood (1975) in relation to the development of the WHO *International Classification of Impairments, Disabilities, and Handicaps* (ICIDH) (WHO, 1980), and, among francophone publications, by the works of Pierre Minaire (1983, 1993). All these works attempt to clarify the concepts used in this field of research in order to develop classifications or models that establish links between them and describe the disablement process. Numerous models were proposed during the 1960s and 1970s, in the United States and the United Kingdom; the works of Susser (1973, 1990) and Duckworth (1983, 1984) provide an interesting and detailed review of those models that contributed, more or less, to the current models.

One of the major difficulties, as will be demonstrated below, is the matter of terminology—for example, differences of meaning between French and English vocabularies. For an understanding of the precision of the current terminology, a bilingual dictionary (Harrap's or Larousse's, for example) can be used as a simple, effective, and excellent method of researching the correspondence of different terms, their translations, and their synonyms. This exercise, applied to the terms concerning the disablement process, shows both a great abundance of words and the absence of clear boundaries between them. One can go from one term to another by means of definitions, examples, or synonyms. As a whole, the terminology seems to comprise not a spectrum of precise states but rather, a dense, multidimensional universe. Note, however, that in the dictionaries used, both French and English, and in a larger context than strictly health, the term *handicap* is commonly synonymous with a *disadvantage* that makes success more difficult to achieve.

For a long time, the measurement of the number of work-loss days due to illness was enough to estimate disability. Before the epidemiologic transition, infectious diseases were the dominant health problem (Omran, 1971). It had essentially been a question of acute diseases, whose relatively short course led spontaneously either to death or to survival with serious sequelae, or more rarely to a cure. Rest (manifested as work-loss days) was the principal response during the wait for one of these three outcomes. With the epidemiologic transition and the massive decline in mortality, infectious diseases have been replaced by degenerative diseases, which now dominate the health scene. These newly dominant diseases are primarily chronic diseases, whose progress is much slower and more complex, with periods of acuity, remission, stability, and exacerbation and complications. Work-loss days due to illness no longer suffice to assess disability within an increasingly long-lived population, a growing proportion of whose members have retired from economic activity.

This chapter continues the theme developed thus far in the book—the consideration of chronic conditions, including osteoarthritis (OA), that affect elderly persons. Our review will be a general consideration of disablement, leading to chapter 6, which focuses on disability arising from OA and the interactions of other co-morbid conditions. In the first part of this chapter we will attempt to define the scope of disablement by presenting the main conceptual works dealing with definitions, measurements, classifications, or models. In light of the evolution of a number of these concepts over time, this requires an extensive discussion to present the broad aspects of the disablement process, so that in the second part of the chapter we can achieve a convergence of the gathered information. We conclude with a general model of the disablement process which seeks to integrate these different concepts.

Reflections on the Disablement Process

In this first part we follow, overall, a chronological order that distinguishes between works that appeared prior to the *International Classification of Impairments, Disabilities, and Handicaps;* the ICIDH itself and works that appeared after its publication; and works that are part of the current ICIDH revision process. Note that the vocabulary originally used by each author has been retained deliberately in this part.

Works Published prior to the ICIDH

When Katz and collaborators proposed their Index of Independence in Activities of Daily Living (Index of ADL) in 1963 as a measurement of biological and psychosocial functions to allow assessment of the results of treatments for elderly and chronically ill persons, they referred to the theoretical plan of child development and the work of pediatricians who distinguished between vegetative and culturally learned behaviors. The activities of daily living (bathing, dressing, going to the toilet, transferring [e.g., getting in and out of bed, or to a chair], continence, and feeding oneself) are simply defined as activities that people perform habitually and universally. Katz and his co-workers saw great parallels between the way in which an adult recovers from disabling illness and the development of functional independence in the child. They believed that independence in activities of daily living is important in terms of physical, emotional, and social well-being, and must, in fact, be a basic component in any definition of health applicable to aged persons.

Thus, it is paradoxical that one of the main current indicators in the field of disablement, if not the main one, was put together without reference to a theoretical framework of disablement. It must be noted that the reversible nature of disability is evident for Katz and his collaborators, since their indicator was precisely intended to measure the recovery of lost functions.

The complementary scale—the Instrumental Activities of Daily Living Scale (IADL)—was developed within the theoretical framework of a schema of competence (Lawton and Brody, 1969). This schema distinguishes human behaviors according to the degree of functional complexity required by the different tasks. The lowest level is called life maintenance; it is followed by successively more complex levels of functional health, perception-cognition, physical self-maintenance (i.e., ADL), instrumental self-maintenance, and effective activity emanating from the motivation to explore social behavior.

Because of the great diversity of the tasks a normal adult can perform, measuring the instrumental competence is extremely complicated. The IADL are a selection of instrumental activities accepted as indicating general competencies in elderly people. They concern the minimum instrumental competencies to be conserved during aging: the ability to use the telephone, to shop, to prepare food, to keep house, to do the laundry, to take transportation, to assume responsibility for self-medication, and to handle finances.

The first conceptual works directly devoted to the disablement process were published by Nagi in 1965 and in 1976. Nagi's objectives are very clear. He noted in 1965 that "a brief review of the literature reveals a great deal of inconsistency in the use of terms such as illness, sickness, impairment, disability, and handicap" (Nagi, 1965, p. 100). His objectives are to clarify the terms and concepts surrounding the phenomenon of disability.

He proposed to distinguish five "phenomena which are closely related and often overlapping but analytically separable" (Nagi, 1965, p. 101): (1) active pathology or disease, with (a) the onset of disease involving the interruption of normal processes, and (b) the simultaneous efforts of the organism to restore itself to a normal state of existence; (2) impairments (every disease involves an impairment, but not every impairment involves a disease); (3) functional limitations imposed by impairments on the individual's ability to perform the tasks and obligations of his usual roles and normal daily activities (e.g., roles within the family, peer groups, community, work, and other interactional settings, as well as activities involved in self-care); (4) forms of behavior associated with sickness and illness; and (5) disability, a pattern of behavior that evolves in situations in which there are long-term or continued impairments associated with functional limitations (Nagi, 1965, pp. 101–3).

In 1976, Nagi proposed a first important revision of this conceptual framework. He henceforth distinguished between (1) pathology, (2) impairment, (3) limitations in the functioning of performance of the human organism, and (4) disability. An impairment is defined as an anatomical, physiological, intellectual, or emotional abnormality or loss. At the level of organismic performances, Nagi distinguished three dimensions—physical, emotional, and mental; the first refers to sensory-motor functioning of the organism, the second to the effectiveness of psychological coping with life stress, and the last to the intellectual and reasoning capabilities. For him, disability henceforth concerned inability or limitations in performing social roles and activities in relation to work, family life, or independent living (Nagi, 1976, p. 441). Nagi clearly found that the same limitation in organismic performance does not always lead to the same disability, as disability depends on the requirements of the social roles in question. Finally, he specified that work and independent living are two of the most significant spheres of social roles and activities. (Versions of the Nagi model appear in chapters 6 and 8.)

Nagi's contribution, which does not include a classification system, was revised again at the beginning of the 1990s, with the publication of *Disability in America* (Pope and Tarlov, 1991), as presented below. Meanwhile, the World Health Organization published major works on the concepts relating to the disablement process, with a new classification.

The ICIDH and Contemporaneous Works

The WHO *International Classification of Impairments, Disabilities, and Handicaps* (1980), essentially developed by Wood (1975), distinguishes between (1) diseases and disorders, (2) impairments, (3) disabilities, and (4) handicaps. These distinctions correspond to the succession of events that can follow from a disease: (1) Something abnormal (i.e., a disease or disorder) occurs within the individual. (2) Someone becomes aware of this occurrence. The pathologic state is exteriorized by an impairment. (3) The performance or behavior of the individual may be altered, and the resulting disabilities reflect the consequences of impairments in terms of functional performance and activity; the pathologic state is objectivized. (4) Either the awareness itself, or the altered behavior or performance to which this gives rise, can lead to a handicap as the affected individual is disadvantaged relative to others; the pathologic state is socialized.

It is interesting to point out that before this reference work was published, Susser (1973) seems to have first proposed these distinctions. He wrote, "Thus, disease, illness, and sickness are not synonymous. *Disease* is best thought of as a process that creates a state of physiological and psychological dysfunction confined to the individual. *Illness* is best thought of as a subjective state, a psychological awareness of dysfunction, also confined to the individual. *Sickness* is best thought of as a state of social dysfunction, a social role assumed by the individual that is defined by the expectations of society and that, thereby, affects the state of his relation with others. Impairment, disability, and handicap are analogous terms, but they are not synonymous either. They refer to established, stable, and persisting states rather than to unstable evolving processes. *Impairment* refers to a persisting physical and psychological defect in the individual. *Disability* refers to persisting physical and psychological dysfunction, also confined to the individual. *Handicap,* like sickness, refers to persisting social dysfunction, a social role assumed by the impaired and disabled that is defined by the expectations of the society" (pp. 4–5). Unfortunately, neither this prescient statement nor Susser's subsequent work has been sufficiently quoted in the relevant literature in the field.

According to WHO: (1) *impairment* corresponds to any loss or abnormality of psychological, physiologic, or anatomical structure or function; (2) *disability* corresponds to any restriction or lack (resulting from an impairment) or ability to perform an activity in the manner or within the range considered normal for a human being; (3) the *social handicap* for a given individual results from an impairment or a disability that limits or prevents the fulfillment of a *normal role* (depending on age, sex and social and cultural factors).

The definition of these concepts has received considerable attention. According to WHO, *handicap* is characterized by a discordance between the individual's performance or status and the expectations of the particular group to which he belongs. The evaluation of handicap rests on the fact that one judges whether there is such a discrepancy or not. However, in the opinion of WHO, there are six fundamental dimensions for which "an individual with reduced competence in any of these dimensions of existence is, ipso facto, disadvantaged in relation to his peers" (WHO, 1980, p. 38). These dimensions, known as survival roles, comprise the ability of the individual to (1) "orient himself in regard to his surroundings, and to respond to these inputs; (2) maintain an effective independent existence in regard to the more immediate physical needs of his body, including feeding and personal hygiene; (3) move around effectively in his environment; (4) occupy time in a fashion customary to his sex, age, and culture, including following an occupation (such as tilling the soil, running a household, or bringing up children), or carrying our physical activities such as play and recreation; (5) participate in and maintain social relationships with others; and (6) sustain socioeconomic activity and independence by virtue of labor and the exploitation of material possessions" (WHO, 1980, pp. 38–39). It is clear, for WHO, that higher-level needs, such as self-fulfillment, are more difficult to measure and may have to remain secondary to the more fundamental needs corresponding to survival roles.

The problems of drawing boundaries between impairment and disability are evident. Thus, without otherwise defining the notion of functional limitation, WHO notes that "in reaching agreement on terminology with other international agencies, it has been necessary to make certain modifications to the definitions included in a preliminary draft of this manual (Wood, 1975). In the draft, *functional limitations* were regarded as being elements of disability, whereas they have now been assimilated with impairments" (WHO, 1980, p. 27). For WHO, "disability is concerned with compound or integrated activities expected of a person or of a body as a whole, such as are represented by tasks, skills, and behaviors" (WHO, 1980, p. 28). Thus, difficulty in using stairs would be classed by Nagi as a limitation in physical performance (a difficulty in going up and down stairs) and by WHO as a disability (a stair-climbing disability). This discrepancy, as we shall see later on, will only be resolved by the introduction of new concepts that allow distinctions to be made between purposeful activities and simple actions (climbing stairs, for example, is only an action and does not constitute an activity in itself), and by clarification of disabilities with respect to precise actions or restrictions of activity.

The World Health Organization stresses that the descriptive adjectives *mental* and *physical* can be applied only to impairments and that it is incorrect to use them for disabilities and handicaps. This point is valid for the organismic performances as defined by Nagi. In effect, climbing stairs, for example, summons up physical, mental, and sensory abilities at the same time: a disability in climbing stairs may be a consequence of a physical impairment, a mental impairment, or a sensory impairment. Beyond this detailed comparison, Granger (1984) stressed the similarity between the models of Nagi and of WHO, and the latter's emphasis on the possible reversibility of disability.

With respect to handicaps, WHO pointed out that disadvantage (handicap) has often been identified, incorrectly, with dependence. While it is important to have fundamental self-sufficiency in regard to the physical functions of daily living, the confusion of *handicap* with the term *dependence* obscured social needs. In integrated societies, individuals are extremely interdependent, be it for social relationships or for employment opportunities and economic self-sufficiency. Insufficient independence is only one of the dimensions of handicap, according to WHO; the absence of social relationships is another.

Grimley Evans (1983), for his part, stressed that one must not confuse independence with autonomy. Autonomy is the ability to set and follow one's own rules—in other words, to decide what one wants to do—while the notion of independence refers back to the independent realization of a whole series of activities. Thus, for example, a person who is dependent on others to get around may remain autonomous if he makes the decisions regarding his itineraries.

After the publication of the WHO classification, Pierre Minaire developed the *situational handicap* concept (1983). A situation is "all the concrete relations which, at a given moment, bring a subject or a group into unity with the circumstances in which they must live and react" (Minaire et al., 1991, p. 287). In Minaire's opinion, handicap is the result of confrontation between the disability of the person (by which he meant the functional deficiency, disfigurement, or psychological impairment) and the environmental situation. The process of handicap therefore includes environmental aspects analyzed in terms of situations. Minaire specified that, without exception, one is handicapped not *in the absolute,* but *with reference to something.* In his opinion, the situational handicap model completes the three dimensions of the WHO model, by integrating the person within the environment (Minaire, 1993). Thus, the handicap is a characteristic not of the person but of the interaction between him and his environment. In that way Minaire refutes the linearity of the WHO classification. Notice, finally, that for him, the quality of life corresponds to an assessment by the person himself of all the handicaps that he encounters in daily life due to his dysfunctions within his surroundings (Minaire, 1993).

In 1990, while drawing up a review of the use of the *International Classification of Impairments, Disabilities, and Handicaps,* the Council of Europe noticed that the notion of disability contains two elements, namely, *functional limitation* (which is close to "impairment") and *activity restriction* (which is close to "handicap"). No definitions were given, but some examples were proposed. Thus, difficulties in performing actions such as "bending" or "reaching for an object" are functional limitations, while difficulties in performing activities of daily living (e.g., dressing or domestic chores) are activity restrictions. The term *action,* introduced here for clarity, does not occur in the document of the Council of Europe. From now on, it seems more logical to measure functional limitations in terms of ability (ability or inability to carry out an action) and to measure activity restrictions in terms of performance (performance or nonperformance of specific activities)—(see Colvez and Robine, 1986). These terminological clarifications, indeed, allow one to see that in the ICIDH, functional limitations in locomotion are classified as disabilities, and functional limitations in cognition are classified as impairments.

It must be noted that the distinction, within disability, between functional limitations and activity restrictions figures very clearly in the first proposals of Wood. (See, in particular, "Wood's terminological scheme" due to Taylor [1977] and reproduced in Duckworth [1983].) "Wood's terminological scheme" clearly explains the sequence: disease (disorder or injury) → impairment → functional limitation → activity restriction → handicap. In 1990, the Réseau Espérance de Vie en Santé (REVES) committee on conceptual harmonization clearly recommended that, within the term *disability,* the distinction should be made between functional limitation and activity restriction (Chamie, 1990).

In 1991, the text *Disability in America* (Pope and Tarlov, 1991) presented a revised version of Nagi's scheme as a conceptual model. The terminology was changed slightly, and it showed the disablement process as consisting of the four following stages: (1) pathology, (2) impairment, (3) functional limitation, and (4) disability. For this text, the definitions of the ICIDH appeared to be confusing, and the term *handicap* was not acceptable. The model proposed by this text introduced risk factors that are biological, environmental (social and physical), lifestyle-related, and behavioral. The model also introduced the notion of quality of life. According to the model, environmental modification (e.g., elimination of physical obstacles and barriers) is an important form of disability prevention.

In the same year, LaPlante (1991) adopted a working definition of *disability* as a limitation in the performance of actions and/or activities resulting from impairments. He noted that the question of whether the term *disability* concerns actions or activities is at the heart of the debate about the meaning of the term. He cited the statement by Homans (1974) that actions are the basic units of human performance. For LaPlante, there are an indefinite number of physical and mental actions in which an individual interacts with the physical and social world. In fact, LaPlante defined actions and activities using the following examples: Talking, thinking, remembering, walking, and seeing are *actions;* playing, working, and reading a newspaper are *activities.* LaPlante pointed out that activities are very often components of the roles an individual occupies. The point of these conceptual distinctions is that one specific activity can be accomplished by means of different groups of actions; this explains why impairments do not inevitably have an impact on activity. Furthermore, LaPlante comes back to differences between Nagi's model and that of WHO.

Nagi refers to problems in performing actions as functional limitations, and to problems in performing activities as disability. In the WHO framework, the term *disability* refers to problems in performing actions (i.e., functional limitations) and to problems in activity, but problems in performing highly valued roles are defined separately as handicaps. In the *Americans with Disabilities Act of 1990*, reference is made to the major life activities.

Finally, one should note the appearance during the last few years of movements such as the Independent Living Movement, which analyzes disability as a consequence of an unsuitable environment and not as a consequence of disease (see, e.g., Reiser and Mason, 1992).

It is clear that the concepts used with reference to social roles and activities relating to work, family, or independent living (Nagi, 1976), and to major life activities such as caring for oneself, performing manual tasks, walking, seeing, hearing, speaking, breathing, learning, working, and participating in community activities *(ADA, 1990)* are very ill-defined. An attempt at clarification by way of a revision process will be discussed next.

Works Belonging to the Current ICIDH Revision Process

Although the ICIDH revision process, which will end in a revised classification in 1998–99 (de Kleijn–de Vrankrijker, 1995), officially began in 1993, the Quebec Committee and Canadian Society for ICIDH prepared their proposals for the revision much earlier. It was they who took the further step of attempting to establish the importance of the environment in the handicap creation process; they propose to introduce this as a new dimension of the ICIDH. The environment has social, cultural, and physical aspects, which may either be obstacles to or supports for the functioning of the individual (Bolduc, 1993; Fougeyrollas, 1995). Their proposal for nomenclature is composed of (1) social factors, subdivided into (a) socioeconomic organizations and (b) social roles; and (2) environmental factors, subdivided into (a) nature and (b) development. In their opinion, a "handicap situation is a disruption in the accomplishment of a person's life habits taking into account age, sex and socio-cultural identity, resulting, on the one hand from impairments or disabilities and, on the other hand from obstacles caused by environmental factors." The life habits "ensure the survival and development of a person in society throughout the person's life. There are daily and domestic activities as well as social roles recognized in a socio-cultural context for a person according to age, sex, and social and personal identity" (Fougeyrollas and Majeau, 1991, p. 17). Thirteen life habits, the perturbation of which leads to situations of handicap, were listed: (1) nutrition,

(2) fitness, (3) personal care, (4) communication, (5) residence, (6) mobility, (7) responsibility, (8) family relations, (9) interpersonal relations, (10) community, (11) education, (12) employment, and (13) recreational and other habits. This rather long list is a good description of all the situations in which a handicap might arise.

Within the framework of the ICIDH revision process, some researchers are concentrating on the applicability of disablement concepts to the field of mental health (Ustün et al., 1995). One of the major concerns of the ICIDH is to avoid the false, but still commonly accepted, dichotomy between the mind and the body. The WHO/MNH Disability Working Group, which treats aspects of mental health in the revision process of the ICIDH, notes that the current definitions of disablement concepts must be clarified as to their content and extent. Impairments currently are defined as involving structures and functions, which leads to confusion. This particular point is explained in detail by Brandsma et al. (1995). Disability concerns activity and ability simultaneously; abilities are abstract aptitudes, while activities are observable performances. Finally, handicaps refer both to societal circumstances that hinder people from performing their activities and to individual limitations. In the current definition of handicap, the term *role* encompasses both survival roles and social roles (e.g., self-care, family, partner, parental, citizenship, and occupational roles), thus creating some confusion; there is also the problem of boundaries between handicaps and disabilities. The WHO Group on Mental Health, Behavioral, and Developmental aspects of the ICIDH proposes new definitions as a working basis for the revision of the classification. In the context of health experience, an *impairment* is any abnormality of psychological or physical functions or of appearance; a *disability* is an interference with an individual's performance of an activity in relation to the environment; and a *handicap* is a societal disadvantage for a given individual which limits or prevents the fulfillment of a social role that is normal for that individual (Ustün et al., 1995).

Classification of the Disablement Process

Three points become evident when one analyzes the component elements of the universe of disablement: the first is the strong convergence, despite appearances, of the different models; the second is that the dynamic aspect of the disablement process is an essential element; and the third is that all the difficulties surrounding definitions seem to come from the fact that, in all the studied works, at least five well-identified concepts have been rearranged in three levels, in differing ways.

Throughout the various documents reviewed, the disablement process appears to be extremely dynamic. Thus, in Nagi's opinion (1976) a given functional limitation does not always lead to the same disability; the extent of disability depends in part on the level of demands required by different roles. In the opinion of WHO (1980), not all impairments lead to disability, and not all disabilities lead to handicap. However, an impairment can lead directly to a handicap, although there is no disability. A handicap can even exist as a result of the simple recollection of a mental impairment—for example, hospitalization in a psychiatric clinic. In the opinion of LaPlante (1991), impairments do not inevitably affect an activity if the activity can be performed using different groups of actions. In Minaire's opinion (1993) there is no such thing as an absolute handicap; rather, handicaps exist with regard to a role to fulfill in a specific situation or in a particular environment. One may refer with interest to the work of Ville et al. (1992) on the relationships between different concepts of the disablement process, social identity, and perceived handicap.

In addition to this stochastic character (not totally determined) of disablement models, numerous authors also emphasize the inseparability of the concepts of disability. There is a continuum of states (Martin et al., 1988) ranging from simple discomfort or limitation to total incapacity in performing the activities of daily living (Verbrugge, 1990). The dynamic and convergent aspects of disablement then lead to a third concept that seems to have been rediscovered—namely, reversibility, a characteristic that was the basis of the work of Katz and colleagues in 1963 and was quoted in the ICIDH in 1980.

The dynamic aspect of disablement was studied particularly by Verbrugge, through analysis of the models of Nagi and WHO (Verbrugge, 1990). Verbrugge clearly distinguished disability from the disablement process itself (Verbrugge and Jette, 1994; Verbrugge, 1995). This notion of disablement has no equivalent in French. It was proposed by Philip Wood himself that a unitary conception be presented, whereas hitherto, impairment, disability, and handicap were separate entities (Wood and Badley, 1978; Wood, 1980), but this proposal has not been retained by WHO. In fact, the reintroduction of the notion of disablement by Verbrugge corresponds to the evident need to have a generic term at our disposal encompassing the different concepts of the field: impairments, functional limitations, and disability in the scheme of Nagi; impairments, disabilities, and handicaps in the WHO classification. One of the current difficulties in the definition of *disability* is that the term refers to a group of concepts and, at the same time, to one of the precise concepts contained within the group. That is why we, too, now prefer the title "General Concepts of Disablement" to the title initially planned for this chapter, "General Concepts of

Disability." For the same reason, the French have translated *International Classification of Impairments, Disabilities, and Handicaps* (WHO, 1980) as *"Classification Internationale des Handicaps: Déficiences, Incapacités et Désavantages"* (Organisation Mondiale de la Santé, 1988), *impairment* being translated by *déficience, disability* by *incapacité,* and *handicap* by *désavantage.* The term *handicap* is then reintroduced as a global term referring to all three concepts, ranging from impairment (corresponding to the initial biological handicap that will or will not be overcome) to disadvantage (the social handicap). It is probable that WHO moved away from the concept of disablement to avoid difficulties of translation in languages other than English, but, as emphasized by Duckworth (1983), the usefulness of such a concept is evident if one does not wish to be either specific or pedantic. Today, the United Nations Statistical Division uses the initials IDH in its working documents when it wants to deal with all three concepts (impairment, disability, and handicap)—which is perhaps a bit too technocratic.

Attempts to Organize the Concepts of the Disablement Process

According to WHO, disability concerns actions and/or activities (WHO, 1980), while for Nagi disability concerns activities and social roles (Nagi, 1976). It seems evident that resolving this divergence requires definitions of different concepts of human activity. Most authors never define the concepts of human activity but instead give two or three examples intended to help the reader to understand, for example, what distinguishes a role from an activity. Thus, differentiating an activity from an action, Homans (1974) distinguished between "gross units of action, which we shall call *activities* ('fishing' is an example), and . . . the finer units of which the gross are composed, which we shall simply call *acts* or *actions* ('baiting a hook' is an example)" (p. 20). The need for clarification of terminology, which is the starting point of Nagi's work in 1965, is at the heart of the current debate, as Hutchinson mischievously pointed out, citing Lewis Carroll: "When I use a word . . . it means just what I choose it to mean, neither more nor less" (Hutchinson, 1995, p. 91).

Below, we successively reintroduce the different concepts of disablement, independently presented in the first part of this chapter, by defining them in relation to each other in order to extract a common or unifying language that would allow us to propose a general model of the disablement process. We will reintroduce first the concepts of human activity and then those of the disablement process.

The Concepts of Human Activity

In the everyday environment, the real world with its social, economic, and physical dimensions, each person has one or more roles to fulfill (with regard to the people around him or her—family, social group, colleagues, etc.— or with regard to society in general), leading to different situations and implying various obligations. The everyday environment can be more or less favorable, or more or less hostile (in which case one talks of *obstacles* or *barriers*), to the fulfillment of these different roles. This actual environment is in contrast to the laboratory setting, in which a subject is observed in a controlled environment.

The individual's roles are decisive because they provide him with a place and status within the different groups that make up society. Two types of role can be distinguished:

(1) *Survival roles.* These refer to what the subject must do for daily survival: the performance of a combination of basic activities that permit one to achieve independence in daily life. The most frequent measurements are made by using (a) minimal independence, which is the ability to perform, without help, the activities that are strictly necessary for an individual's survival and that nobody else can do in that individual's place; and (b) the ability to live alone in a normal household.

(2) *Social roles.* These refer to what the subject must do to live in society: the performance of a combination of activities that allow him to ensure his social integration. Individuals integrate themselves into society by performing activities consistent with their age (e.g., going to school, or carrying out professional and domestic tasks). One role that is certainly ancient but that has a new importance today is that of caregiver. Thus, children more and more often have to take charge of elderly parents who have become dependent and/or have lost their autonomy.

Among occupations, professional activity deserves particular mention, as it contributes to the performance of both types of role: the remuneration derived from the occupation permits assurance of the economic part of *survival* roles, and the place and the social status that professional activity provides allows much *social* integration.

Human activities are innumerable. They allow different objectives to be attained. They are distinguished from simple actions (or acts) by the fact that they are useful in themselves. The notion of "a task" is close enough to that of "an activity." We have already discussed (1) the elementary activities of daily living, which are a set of activities considered necessary to permit minimal independence; and (2) the instrumental activities of daily life, which are all the instrumental activities considered necessary to live alone in a normal household. It is generally considered that an individual who needs help from another person to carry out the elementary or instrumental activities of daily living is dependent, particularly if that individual is elderly. This "dependence" is most often evaluated by means of scales of ADL and IADL. In theory, dependence must be distinguished from loss of autonomy (Grimley Evans, 1983), but in practice the two notions are often confused.

Actions (or acts) constitute the basic units of human activity. An action can be considered an intermediary or fragmentary part of an activity, not useful in itself, but contributing to the performance of a useful activity. Actions can be broken down in turn to finer units. Thus, one may consider gestures as body movements without purpose, which, once combined, allow the performance of precise actions. It must also be noted that the same gesture can be used for the performance of several actions and that certain actions can be performed by combinations of various gestures.

The Concepts of the Disablement Process

In the field of locomotor functions, the introduction of the concepts of human activity allows the establishment of correspondences between the four types of disablement identified in Part One: impairments, functional limitations, activity restrictions, and handicaps. (1) Difficulty in performing or inability to perform a gesture is an impairment; (2) difficulty in performing or inability to perform an action is a functional limitation; (3) difficulty in performing or inability to perform an activity is an activity restriction; and (4) difficulty in performing or inability to perform a role is a handicap. Disablement, or the disablement process, describes the processes that lead from the disease (or disorder) to the handicap via impairments, functional limitations, and activity restrictions. If the environment, with its social, economic, and physical dimensions, does not constitute an actual link in the process, it is still an essential explanatory element: obligations and expectations that are part of the environment relate to activity restrictions and the formation of judgments concerning the presence of a handicap.

1. *Impairments* concern both structures and functions. According to Brandsma et al. (1995), an impairment is any loss or deviation of an anatomical structure, a physiologic function, or a psychological function. It must be stressed that impairments, like functional limitations or activity restrictions, are often inappropriately restricted to losses or reductions, which is incorrect, as they cor-

respond also to deviations, including all inappropriate forms of structure, function, or performance—in particular excessive forms, such as delirium, epilepsy, or obesity. However, the words used—*impairment, limitations, restrictions*—themselves add to this confusion.

2. *Functional limitations* are difficulties in performing actions. Functional limitations are generally measured by a questionnaire that seeks to learn about abilities to perform some specific actions. While often confronted with identical daily activities, individuals do not inevitably perform them by means of the same actions. Thus, in the field of health, a functional limitation corresponds to any loss or deviation (resulting from an impairment) in the ability to perform an action.

3. *Activity restriction* is difficulty in performing an activity. It is generally measured by asking about performance of the major activities of daily life. Thus, in the field of health, the term *activity restriction* refers to any loss or deviation (resulting from an impairment and/or a functional limitation) in the capacity to perform an activity in the manner, or within the range, that is normal for a human being in light of his environment.

The environment has a different role in the concept of functional limitations than it has in the concept of activity restrictions. Functional limitations are normally measured for a fixed environment (climbing stairs of 10 steps, walking 200 meters, carrying 5 kilograms), while activity restrictions depend on the actual environment of the individual. Indeed, functional limitations being equal, activity restrictions depend on the environment.

4. *Handicaps* are difficulties in performing various roles. The World Health Organization defined this in the ICIDH as follows: "In the context of health experience, a handicap is a disadvantage for a given individual, resulting from an impairment or a disability, that limits or prevents the fulfillment of a role that is normal (depending on age, sex, and social and cultural factors) for that individual" (WHO, 1980, p. 183). Such a handicap is assessed on the basis of a judgment concerning the extent to which an individual's performance in daily living is consistent with the activities required by his obligations (i.e., the expected performance taking account of the role examined). The existence of a handicap resulting from an impairment, from a functional limitation, and/or from an activity restriction depends, then, on the environment.

Finally, for each of the four concepts—impairment, functional limitation, activity restriction, and handicap—one can define degrees of severity on the basis of the importance of the difficulties encountered in performing various gestures, actions, or activities, or in fulfilling different roles, on a continuum ranging from mere discomfort to complete inability.

Conclusion: A General Model of Disablement

All the difficulties with the definitions discussed above seem to come from the tendency of authors to regroup in three levels at least five well-identified concepts. In a very recent work, Hutchinson (1995) proposed a model permitting the combination of different approaches. First of all, he identified six concepts: (A) disease or disorder, (B) impairment, (C) disability, (D) disadvantage due to impairment or disability, (E) disadvantage due to social environment, and (F) social environment. Next, he distinguished between the medical model—that of the ICIDH—which concentrates on (A), (B), (C), and (D) and leaves out (E); and the social model, which concerns (A), (B), (E), and (F) and ignores (C) and (D). (Hutchinson used "→" to describe the action of every element in the disablement process.) The schemes are (A) → (B) → (C) → (D) for the medical model, and (A) → (B) → the person ← (E) ← (F) for the social model. He then proposed a combined model: (A) → (B) → (C) → (D) ← (E) ← (F), where (A) is condition, (B) impairment, (C) disability, (D) disadvantage, (E) discrimination, and (F) environment; and, thinking positively, (A) is condition, (B) strength, (C) ability, (D) advantage, (E) privilege, and (F) environment.

With the same concern for integrating the different concepts and approaches, we propose, in conclusion, a general model of disablement (fig. 5.1). It is organized in four levels, which are (1) "the person," (2) "the environment," (3) "the situation," and (4) "the judgment." At the individual level, we will distinguish the person taken alone, his or her environment, the situation of the person in the environment, and the assessment made of this situation; at the collective level (populations, groups), we will distinguish persons, the environment, the situations of persons, and the assessment made of these situations.

With respect to figure 5.1 as a general model of disablement:

1. The characteristics of "the person" that may intervene in the process of disablement, apart from diseases or disorders at the origin of the process, are his global health state (comorbidity, etc.); his physical, intellectual, or emotional abilities; the presence or absence of impairments and functional limitations; and his various abilities and potentialities; to which are added his habits (playing sports, consuming alcohol, etc.), his socioeconomic characteristics, such as level of education, and his psychosocial identity.

2. The "environmental" characteristics that influence the process of disablement are physical (e.g., physical obstacles such as steps), economic (e.g., cost of care), and social (e.g., law, expectations, discrimination).

3. The "situation" refers to the meeting of a person and an environment,

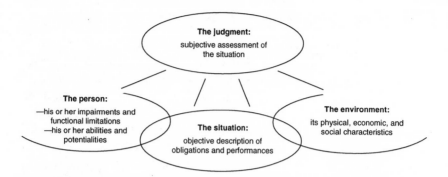

Figure 5.1.   The four levels of a general model of disablement. The *judgment* is the subjective assessment of the situation. It is based on the perception of the gaps between obligations and performances. The judgment can be made by an individual on the basis of his or her own expectations, or by the society according to the expectations it has for the individual. The judgment states whether the individual has a handicap or not, and whether the environment is handicapping or not.

as defined in (1) and (2). It is within the framework of this situation that the roles of the individual are determined (by expectations, obligations, and objectives), and (b) the person's activity is carried out. It is also within this framework that performances in daily life, as well as possible activity restrictions, are observed. One sees, in this way, that an action directed toward the person can change the characteristics of the person and the situation; in the same way, an action directed toward the environment can change the characteristics of the environment and of the situation.

4. The "judgment" consists of assessing whether the person, as defined in (1), has a social handicap or not, as a result of a disease (or disorder). The judgment depends on the situation as defined in (3) and therefore also depends on the environment as defined in (2). It is based on the gaps observed and/or perceived between obligations and performances. It is, in fact, an implicit judgment on the quality of life related to observed, perceived, or experienced health. A recent study showed that limitations of activity are some of the key determinants of the health-related quality of life (Hennessy et al., 1994).

The judgment can be formulated either by the person, on the basis of his expectations, or by the environment (i.e., other people) in relation to the expectations of society, and with the possibility of discord between the different judgments. The handicap can then be perceived by the person, and/or perceived and recognized by society. The model also allows an evaluation of whether the environment imposes a handicap or not, particularly at a collective level.

Clearly, this is a general model of disablement which aims to describe the dynamic way in which the process leads from disease (congenital malformation, chronic diseases and disorders, sequelae of accidents or of disease) to handicap. Figure 5.1 represents the situation at any time. An action between time t and $t + 1$ toward the person or the environment, for example, can modify the situation at $t + 1$ and consequently the judgment made about it.

The model simply arranges—in an operational way—the different concepts linked to the disablement process in four levels: (1) the characteristics of the person at any moment; (2) the characteristics of the environment at the same moment; (3) the situation that arises from the meeting between the person and the environment; and finally, (4) the judgment made about this situation. It considers all the different models examined in the first part of this chapter. Thus, for example, the diagram of Nagi (1976) (see chapter 6) is based on two of these levels (the person and the situation), and the diagram of WHO (1980) is based on three of these levels. Finally, Minaire's model (1993)—centered on the situation—is based on four levels. (A first version of the general model of the disablement process was discussed at length with Pierre Minaire at St. Etienne in 1993.)

We believe that our general model of the disablement process—which may appear simple—is in fact very powerful in organizing the different concepts in relation to each other. The model clearly distinguishes (on the one hand), between the characteristics of the person, the environment, and the situation arising at this interface; and (on the other hand) between objective descriptions and subjective judgments.

ACKNOWLEDGMENT

Michel Thuriaux and Yvon Brunelle made helpful comments that contributed to the preparation of this chapter in its final form.

REFERENCES

Americans with Disabilities Act (ADA) of 1990. PL 101-336, 104 Stat. 42 USC, 12101 ff. 101st Congress.

Bolduc M. 1993. For a conceptual model that better reflects the environment. In: *Calculation of health expectancies,* edited by JM Robine, CD Mathers, MR Bone, I Romieu. Pp. 81–98. Montrouge: John Libbey Eurotext.

Brandsma JW, Lakerveld-Heyl K, van Ravensberg, et al. 1995. Reflection on the definition of impairment and disability as defined by the World Health Organization. *Disability and Rehabilitation* 17:119–127.

Chadwick E. 1842. *Report on the sanitary condition of the labouring population of Great Britain.* Edinburgh: Edinburgh University Press.

Chamie M. 1990. *Report of the committee on the conceptual harmonization of statistics for the study of disability-free life expectancy.* Montpellier, INSERM, REVES paper no. 41. New York and Strasbourg.

Colvez A, Robine JM. 1986. Problems encountered in using the concepts of impairment, disability, and handicap in a health assessment survey of the elderly in Upper Normandy. *Int Rehabil Med* 8:18–22.

Committee of the Highland Society of Scotland. 1824. Report on friendly or benefit societies, exhibiting the law of sickness, as deduced from returns by friendly societies in different parts of Scotland. Edinburgh.

Council of Europe. 1990. *Evaluation of the use of the International Classification of Impairments, Disabilities, and Handicaps (ICIDH) in surveys and health-related statistics.* Strasbourg: Council of Europe.

de Kleijn–de Vrankrijker MW, ed. 1995. The International Classification of Impairments, Disabilities, and Handicaps (ICIDH): Perspectives and developments (Part I). *Disability and Rehabilitation.* Special issue.

Duckworth D. 1983. *The classification and measurement of disablement.* Department of Health and Social Security, Research report no. 10. London: Her Majesty's Stationery Office.

———. 1984. The need for a standard terminology and classification of disablement. In: *Functional assessment in rehabilitation medicine,* edited by CV Granger and GE Gresham. Pp. 1–13. Baltimore: Williams and Wilkins.

Fougeyrollas P. 1995. Documenting environmental factors for preventing the handicap creation process: Quebec contributions relating to ICIDH and social participation of people with functional differences. *Disability Rehabilitation* 17:145–153.

Fougeyrollas P, Majeau P. 1991. The handicap creation process: How to use the conceptual model examples. *ICIDH International Network* 4(3):1–62.

Granger CV. 1984. A conceptual model for functional assessment. In: *Functional assessment in rehabilitation medicine,* edited by CV Granger, GE Gresham. Pp. 14–25. Baltimore: Williams and Wilkins.

Grimley Evans J. 1983. Prevention of age-associated loss of autonomy: Epidemiological approaches. *J Chronic Dis* 37:353–363.

Hennessy CH, Moriarty DG, Scherr PA, Brackbill R. 1994. Measuring health-related quality of life for public health surveillance. *Public Health Rep* 109:665–672.

Homans GC. 1974. *Social behavior: Its elementary forms.* Rev. ed. New York: Harcourt Brace Jovanovich.

Hutchinson T. 1995. The classification of disability. *Arch Dis Child* 73:91–99.

Katz S, Ford AB, Moskowitz RW, Jackson BA, Jaffe MW. 1963. Studies of illness in the aged: The Index of ADL. A standardized measure of biological and psychosocial function. *JAMA* 185:914–919.

LaPlante MP. 1991. The demographics of disability. *Milbank Q* 69(suppl. 2):55–77.

Lawton MP, Brody EM. 1969. Assessment of older people: Self-maintenance and instrumental activities of daily living. *Gerontologist* 9:179–186.

Martin J, Meltzer H, Eliot D. 1988. *The prevalence of disability among adults.* Office of Population Censuses and Surveys. London: Her Majesty's Stationery Office.

Minaire P. 1983. Le handicap en porte-à-faux. *Prospective et Santé* 26:39–46.

———. 1993. Models of disability. In: *Proceedings of the 1991 International Symposium on Data on Aging,* edited by M Feinleib. National Center for Health Statistics. Vital and Health Statistics, ser. 5, no. 7, 9–17.

Minaire P, Cherpin J, Flores JL, Weber D. 1991. Le handicap de situation. *Perspectives Psychiatriques* 30:286–290.

Nagi SZ. 1965. Some conceptual issues in disability and rehabilitation. In: *Sociology and rehabilitation,* edited by MB Sussman. Pp. 100–113. Washington, D.C.: American Sociological Association.

————. 1976. An epidemiology of disability among adults in the United States. *Milbank Q* 54: 439–467.

Omran AR. 1971. The epidemiologic transition: A theory of epidemiology of population change. *Milbank Q* 49:509–538.

Organisation Mondiale de la Santé, CTNERHI-INSERM. 1988. *Classification internationale des handicaps: Déficiences, incapacités, et désavantages.* CTNERHI—INSERM. Reprint, 1993.

Pope AM, Tarlov AR, eds. 1991. *Disability in America: Toward a national agenda for prevention.* Washington, D.C.: Institute of Medicine, National Academy Press.

Reiser R, Mason M. 1992. *Disability equality in the classroom: A human rights issue.* London: Disability Equality in Education.

Riley JC. 1991. Working health time: A comparison of preindustrial, industrial, and postindustrial experience in life and health. *Explorations in Economic History* 28:169–191.

Stiker H-J. 1982. *Corps infirme et sociétés.* Paris: Aubier/Montaigne.

Susser M. 1973. *Causal thinking in the health sciences: Concepts and strategies of epidemiology.* New York: Oxford University Press.

————. 1990. Disease, illness, sickness, impairment, disability, and handicap [editorial]. *Psychol Med* 20:471–473.

Taylor D. 1977. *Physical impairment: Social handicap.* London: Office of Health Economics.

Ustün TB, Cooper JE, van Duuren-Kristen, Kennedy C, Hendershot G, Sartorius N. 1995. Revision of the ICIDH: Mental health aspects. *Disability Rehabilitation* 17:202–209.

Verbrugge LM. 1990. The iceberg of disability. In: *The legacy of longevity,* edited by SM Stahl. Pp. 55–75. Newbury Park, Calif.: Sage.

————. 1995. New thinking and science on disability in mid- and late life. *Eur J Public Health* 5:20–28.

Verbrugge LM, Jette AM. 1994. The disablement process. *Soc Sci Med* 38:1–14.

Ville I, Ravaud JF, Marchal F, Paicheler H, Fardeau M. 1992. International Classification of Impairments, Disabilities, and Handicaps: An evaluation of the consequences of facioscapulohumeral muscular dystrophy. *Disability Rehabilitation* 14:168–175.

Wood PHN. 1975. Classification of impairments and handicaps. WHO/ICD 9/REV.CONF/75.15. World Health Organization.

————. 1980. The language of disablement: A glossary relating to disease and its consequences. *Int Rehab Med* 2:86–92.

Wood PHN, Badley EM. 1978. An epidemiological appraisal of disablement. In: *Recent advances in community medicine,* edited by AE Bennett. Edinburgh: Churchill Livingstone.

World Health Organization (WHO). 1980. *International classification of impairments, disabilities, and handicaps.* Geneva: World Health Organization.

6

Osteoarthritis, Comorbidity, and Physical Disability

Andrew A. Guccione, Ph.D., P.T.

To some, the role of osteoarthritis in precipitating functional decline in an elderly population is obvious and simple to grasp. However, several considerations belie the simplicity of this notion and in fact complicate the study of osteoarthritis (OA) and physical disability among elders. The first consideration is whether the presence of arthritis is regarded as problematic by either the patient or the clinician. Even though radiographic evidence of OA is extremely common in persons over 40 years of age, OA is not always symptomatic when present (Moskowitz, 1992). If the condition is sufficiently symptomatic to provoke a clinical visit, however, the individual with OA typically exhibits a cluster of complaints including pain, muscle and joint impairments, and functional limitations in activities of daily living (ADL) that need to be addressed (Cunningham and Kelsey, 1984; Lee et al., 1985; Felson, 1988).

A second consideration that has hindered the study of OA and disability is that, in the past, the prevalence of the condition may have made OA seem too "common" in the view of many clinicians and investigators to be viewed as a "serious" ailment relative to other medical problems of the geriatric patient. But recent studies have shown that OA and its functional burden are a major public health problem of elders (Verbrugge and Patrick, 1995). It is likely that more than 60 million adults in the United States have OA (Felson, 1990). Osteoarthritis is widespread in adults over the age of 65 and is found in women more often than in men, a sex difference that widens with each decade. Although aging is indeed strongly statistically associated with OA, aging in itself does not cause OA, nor should OA be considered a "normal" aging process (Brandt and

Fife, 1986; Mankin and Brandt, 1989; and chapter 1). The risk of disability attributable to knee OA alone is as large as the risk due to any other common medical condition of elderly persons (Guccione et al., 1994). The magnitude of the burden of arthritis is even greater when all sites of OA are considered. Furthermore, the impacts of arthritis on women are especially troublesome. Davis et al. (1991) provided evidence that the impact of knee OA on the physical functioning is greater in older women than in all other age and sex subgroups. In light of the magnitude of its functional impact and its prevalence, chronic arthritis represents a major impact on the health of female elders and their quality of life.

The third consideration, which has major implications for the measurement of disability, is the interrelationship of OA and comorbidity. Few elders have a single medical problem, and an increase in the number of coexistent conditions among elders is directly associated with an increase in limitations of ADL (Guralnik et al., 1989; Verbrugge et al., 1989). Associations between disease and physical disability in elderly persons have been found for arthritis (Guccione et al., 1990; Yelin and Spitz, 1990; Verbrugge et al., 1991a, 1991b; Guccione et al., 1994), hip fracture (Magaziner et al., 1990), low back pain (Lavsky-Shulan et al., 1985; Guralnik and Kaplan, 1989), diabetes (Pinsky et al., 1985; Mor et al., 1989; Barrett-Connor and Wingard, 1991), hypertension (Pinsky et al., 1985; Guralnik and Kaplan, 1989), coronary heart disease (Nickel and Chirikos, 1990; Pinsky et al., 1990), cardiovascular disease (Harris et al., 1989), depression (Berkman et al., 1986), stroke (Jette et al., 1988; Kelly-Hayes et al., 1988), visual impairment (Mor et al., 1989), breast cancer (Satariano et al., 1990), and cognitive deficits (Scherr et al., 1988).

Because OA is one of the most prevalent diseases of elderly persons, the measurement of its functional consequences must always contend with the various impacts of other conditions on an elder's functional level. There is, however, no reason to assume that each disease has a similar impact on function. Building upon a previous study of the task-specific relationship between arthritis and physical functional limitations in elderly persons, Guccione et al. (1994) showed that other diseases also have task-specific impacts on function. Thus, in a disabled elder with multiple chronic conditions, the inability to perform certain tasks may be related either to the broad effects of a single disease (e.g., a stroke) on most or all basic ADL and instrumental ADL (IADL) (these terms are described in chapter 5), or to the independent, and sometimes interactive, effects of several diseases, each of which affects only a few activities (Guccione et al., 1994; Furner et al., 1995). The effects of OA on function are specific to the affected joint and the functional task to be accomplished. Knee OA, for example, clearly affects functional activities related to transfers and ambulation (Ettinger et al., 1994). Furthermore, the interactive effects of OA and other medical conditions may be synergistic and may propel the trajectory of disability even further (Verbrugge et al., 1989).

This chapter will summarize what is known about the relationship between OA and physical disability in elderly persons and describe the various methods currently available to assess physical disability in individuals with OA and other age-associated comorbidities.

A Model for the Process of Disablement

Unraveling the interrelated processes that lead to physical disability in the individual with OA and other potentially disabling conditions first requires both the clinician and the investigator to sort through the various factors that contribute to disablement. An expanded model of the process of disablement (fig. 6.1), originally articulated by Nagi (1976, 1991), discussed in chapters 5 and 8, can be used to illuminate the process of disablement in OA by sorting patient data into four categories: disease, impairment, functional limitation, and disability (Guccione, 1994). Furthermore, regarding disease, impairment, functional limitations, and disability the model suggests three interconnected hypotheses that are useful in the study of the functional impacts of OA and comorbidity.

1. *The first hypothesis* is that disablement begins with a specific disease and its active pathology. Osteoarthritis can be described as a localized process marked by joint space narrowing due to progressive destruction of articular cartilage and the formation of osteophytes at the joint margin (Mankin, 1989). Disease produces primary impairments of the body system that is the particular locus of the pathologic state. Therefore, the primary impairments that are associated with OA are found chiefly in the alterations of the normal structures and functions of bones, muscles, and joints of the musculoskeletal system, which are expressed clinically as losses of range of motion (ROM) and strength. Although the period of active disease may be relatively brief in an individual's life, the impairments that a person experiences may not be similarly confined. Impairments of one system may also contribute to secondary impairments of other systems as part of the total picture of the process of disablement. For example, Philbin et al. (1995) demonstrated impairments of the cardiopulmonary system in severely deconditioned individuals with advanced OA.

2. *The second hypothesis* about the process of disablement in arthritis is that the magnitude of some primary and secondary impairments is sufficient to alter the performance of routine functional tasks or activities. Functional limi-

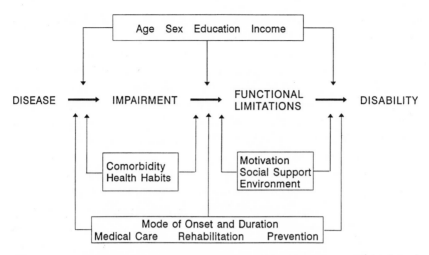

Figure 6.1. An expanded model of the process of disablement in arthritis based upon the Nagi model. *Source:* Reprinted from *Physical Therapy.* A. A. Guccione, "Arthritis and the process of disablement," *Phys Ther* 1994;74:408–414, with permission of the American Physical Therapy Association.

tations indicate deviation from what is normally expected, whereas an individual's impairments indicate aberrant conditions of tissues, organs, and systems. In an individual with OA, the functional limitations in ADL and the loss of the ability to work result from anatomical changes within cartilage and subchondral bone, impaired joint mobility, and muscle weakness and atrophy.

Although the relationship between OA and physical disability is mediated precisely by the exact nature of the disease-related impairments (Guccione et al., 1990; Davis et al., 1991), only a very small number of studies have attempted to discern the degree to which musculoskeletal impairments, including those related to OA, are associated with limitations in physical functional activities. Some of our understanding of the impact of OA on function must be inferred from the general literature on musculoskeletal impairment in elders. In a series of studies, Bergstrom et al. (1985a, 1985b) reported on the connection between joint impairment and function in a group of 79-year-old men and women. They found that lower-extremity joint complaints were more common than upper-extremity complaints. Among those elders who had upper-extremity complaints, ROM was most restricted in the wrists and shoulders. Hip motion was limited in 84 percent of the individuals who had lower-extremity complaints. When elders with symptoms and joint complaints were compared to elders without such problems, significant differences were found in the ability to use public transportation and climb stairs. Elders with musculoskeletal impairments were also more likely to use ambulation aids.

The impact of musculoskeletal impairments is not limited only to current level of functional status. In a group of elderly persons in Massachusetts, Jette and colleagues (1985, 1990) identified strong predictive relationships between musculoskeletal impairment, its progression, and future functional decline in elderly persons. They also noted that the impact of musculoskeletal impairment of the hand was chiefly on basic ADL, while lower-extremity impairment affected IADL to a greater extent.

In a descriptive study of 95 patients with arthritis, Badley and coworkers (1984) investigated the association of limited ROM with difficulty in performing basic ADL. Subjects had difficulty walking to a toilet, transferring to a toilet, getting in and out of a bath, and walking up and down stairs if they could not flex their knees at least 70 degrees, and even greater ROM was required for some activities. The degree of functional limitation among individuals with arthritis has been directly linked to the severity of the disease, but this relationship may be dependent on both the particular joint studied and the measure of function used. The connection between radiographic grade of OA and function is strong for knee OA (Guccione et al., 1990; Davis et al., 1991; Mattson and Brostrom, 1993) but much weaker for hand OA (Baron et al., 1987). Functional loss in hand OA has been shown to be more closely associated with strength loss than the OA itself (Baron et al., 1987). Muscle weakness has also been related to disability in persons with knee OA (McAlindon et al., 1993).

On first glance, the assumption that pain, secondary to pathologic changes in normal joint structures, would be the primary factor limiting function appears almost self-evident (Moskowitz, 1992; Mattson and Brostrom, 1993). Pain is strongly linked to the radiographic severity of the disease (Lethbridge-Cejku et al., 1995). However, pain alone is not sufficient to explain functional limitations in individuals with OA. Guccione and coworkers (1990) showed that functional deficits in elders are more likely in individuals with severe radiographic OA but with fewer painful symptoms than in individuals with milder radiographic changes but more symptomatic disease. In terms of clinical complaints, it is likely that some individuals with OA remain asymptomatic precisely by avoiding those activities that elicit pain on motion. However, it is also known that moderate to severe radiographic disease accompanied by symptoms is likely to limit functional activities broadly (Davis et al., 1991). Therefore, any complete investigation of OA and function in elders must adequately account both for radiographic severity of the disease and for the presence of pain.

The first awareness of the impact of OA as a disabling disease is often noted when the older person reports limitations in performing some or all activities in his or her daily routine. Several studies have established both a cross-sectional and a longitudinal relationship between arthritis and functional limitations. Yelin et al. (1987) found that, by comparison with a non-OA control group, individuals with OA were restricted in their ability to do household chores, shopping, and errands, and to engage in leisure activities. Knee OA (the knee is the site of OA most frequently studied in the epidemiologic literature) has been shown to have specific impacts on a person's performance of an array of basic ADL and IADL involving the lower extremity (Guccione et al., 1990, 1994; Davis et al., 1991; Mattson and Brostrom, 1993; Ettinger et al., 1994). In a study of nursing home residents with arthritis, Guccione et al. (1989) found, even when controlling for age, that residents with arthritis had more pain and were more likely to require assistance with dressing, bringing a glass to the mouth, turning a faucet, getting in and out of bed, bending down, and walking. They were also more likely to use a wheelchair daily than were other residents without arthritis.

Individuals with arthritis experience most of their functional limitations in physical activities, but the concept of function has psychological and social dimensions as well. Although each of these dimensions is distinct, the physical function of the individual with arthritis may very well influence psychological and social functioning, and physical performance in turn will be influenced by psychological and social functions (Mattson and Brostrom, 1991). For example, difficulty in getting out into the community may curtail an elder's social activity and interactions, thereby contributing to a sense of isolation and loneliness. As depression has already been linked to physical disability in elderly persons (Berkman et al., 1986; Bruce et al., 1994; Guccione et al., 1994), it is clear that individuals with OA can benefit from social activities that promote a sense of well-being (Zimmer et al., 1995).

3. *The third hypothesis* about disablement proposes that functional limitations generally underlie disability. Persistent limitations across the spectrum of functional tasks and activities generally expected of independent adults in specific social roles qualify an individual as disabled. Osteoarthritis places a substantial burden of disability on affected individuals who attempt to confront their inability to fulfill social roles and interpersonal relationships successfully as members of a family and/or of the work force.

Although the process of disablement is depicted heuristically as a linear progression, there are several reasons why one cannot assume that an individual will be disabled merely by virtue of having an impairment or functional limitation. For example, minor losses of shoulder ROM might barely affect the ability to comb one's hair. When more substantial losses of ROM affect the performance of this activity, there are still alternative methods for accomplishing the activity and thus avoiding disability. An individual may learn to compensate for lost shoulder ROM by using the available ROM in other joints to best advantage. In other instances, the performance of the task itself may be adapted using special equipment. When Hughes et al. (1993) rated joint impairment on the basis of the presence of tenderness, swelling, pain on motion, decreased ROM, crepitus, and deformity in 541 elders, they found that musculoskeletal impairment explained only 15 percent of the variance in scores on an index of functional limitations.

Furthermore, each of the steps in the process of disablement can be modified by a host of factors in addition to comorbidity, such as age, sex, education, income, personal and health habits, motivation, social support, and physical environment. Anxiety, depression, and coping style have been related to functional limitations in individuals with hip or knee OA (Summers et al., 1988).

Finally, the evidence suggests that functional limitations among people with arthritis are not static. Although chronic arthritis would appear to have a progressive impact on function (Furner et al., 1995), Verbrugge (1992) provided evidence that over a period of 2 years, at least some individuals with arthritis improve functionally, even if their musculoskeletal impairments endure.

Functional Consequences of Arthritis

Studies on the functional consequences of arthritis proceed in several methodological directions. Some studies demonstrate an independent effect of OA while controlling for other coexistent conditions. Guccione et al. (1994), in the Framingham study cohort, investigated the cross-sectional association of 10 medical conditions with functional limitations in stair climbing, walking a mile, doing heavy home chores, keeping house, cooking, grocery shopping, and carrying bundles. Specifically, data were analyzed on prevalent knee OA, hip fracture, diabetes, stroke, heart disease, congestive heart failure, intermittent claudication, chronic obstructive pulmonary disease, depressive symptomatology, and cognitive impairment. Even when the study controlled for all the other comorbid conditions, individuals with knee OA had a substantial likelihood of needing assistance for stair climbing, walking a mile, keeping house, and carrying bundles. Limitations in these particular activities are also consistent with the specific musculoskeletal impairments of OA. Furthermore, Guccione et al. (1994) found that the sheer prevalence of knee OA, coupled with its moderate impact on function, accounted for a substantial proportion of the burden of disability in the community.

Other studies have examined the likelihood of disability longitudinally. Using data on 5,210 participants in the Longitudinal Study of Aging (LSOA), Boult et al. (1994) demonstrated that arthritis was as likely to lead to limited capacity for seven ADL and IADL over a 4-year period of study as were any of eight other chronic conditions, with the exception of cerebrovascular disease. Interestingly, age, education, and social interaction also predicted functional limitations, supporting research models that account for a broad range of factors that influence the trajectory of disability in elderly persons.

Besides examining the direct effects of arthritis on impairment and function, studies have also confirmed that the functional impacts of chronic arthritis are enhanced when the individual with arthritis has another comorbid condition. Although their analyses combined subjects with OA with subjects with other forms of arthritis, Verbrugge et al. (1991a) presented compelling evidence from the National Health Interview Survey Supplement on Aging (SOA) that those subjects with arthritis coupled with comorbidity had substantially greater odds of physical disability in walking, shopping, grasp, and light housework than did individuals with arthritis alone. Using data on 2,946 participants aged 55 or older from the National Health and Nutrition Examination Survey (NHANES I) Epidemiologic Follow-up Study, Ettinger et al. (1994) explored the associations of knee OA and four comorbid conditions (heart disease, pulmonary disease, obesity, and hypertension) with physical disability 10 years after the start of the study. The odds of reporting difficulty with ambulation and transfers among individuals with knee OA and heart disease, knee OA and pulmonary disease, or knee OA and obesity were substantially greater than were the odds of functional difficulty among individuals without knee OA or a comorbid condition.

Methodological Considerations

In considering the study of OA, comorbidity, and physical disability, the first task is to specify the criteria for identifying cases of OA for epidemiologic and clinical studies. The specific pathologic processes of OA may be manifest in radiographs that can be used to grade severity (Felson, 1990). Ideally, to evaluate knee OA one should use standing, anterior-posterior films of the tibiofemoral compartment which are graded according to the criteria of the Kellgren-Lawrence scale (Kellgren and Lawrence, 1963), although limitations on this grading system are discussed in chapter 4. It has been suggested that films of the patellofemoral joint be included, as OA of this joint is associated with knee pain in the absence of tibiofemoral disease (McAlindon et al., 1992). The requirement that a weight-bearing radiograph be used complicates the logistics of a community-based study as well as increasing its cost. Therefore, some studies (e.g., the NHANES I study) have had to be done using non-weight-bearing films (Davis et al., 1991; Ettinger et al., 1994); others (e.g., the SOA study) merely used self-reported "arthritis" (Verbrugge et al., 1991a, 1991b). Prospects for technological advances in imaging are discussed in chapter 12.

The second methodological task required for studies on OA is to create an appropriate question with which to ascertain the presence of pain. For example, a common question asked in the study of pain and knee OA is, "Have you had pain in or around the knee for most days of a month within the last year?" This phrasing was used in the Framingham study (Felson et al., 1987; Guccione et al., 1990) and the NHANES I study (Davis et al., 1991; Ettinger et al., 1994).

Ascertaining comorbidity raises similar issues with respect to defining various medical conditions and establishing a feasible method of data collection. What criteria should be used to define the condition, what is the nature of the research question, and what inferences are to be made from the data analysis? Criteria sets that require extensive laboratory tests and imaging are likely to increase the precision of a study. However, in a large study of community-dwelling elders, this increase in precision is likely to come at the expense of feasibility. Self-reported disease may be the only feasible alternative method of case ascertainment in these instances.

Investigation of physical disability poses at least as many research challenges as does the epidemiologic study of disease itself. Functional activities for the person with OA encompass all those tasks, activities, and roles that identify a person as an independent adult, and require the integration of both cognitive and affective abilities with motor skills. These include eating, sleeping, elimination, hygiene, bipedal locomotion, and complex hand activities, all of which permit independence in a personal environment; as well as home chores, community ambulation, work, and recreation, which permit independence in the social world. Another approach records the self-reported ability to perform 10 particular physical tasks that were first described by Nagi (1976) as associated with work disability: (1) walking up 10 steps without resting; (2) walking a quarter of a mile; (3) sitting for 2 hours; (4) standing for 2 hours; (5) stooping, crouching, or kneeling; (6) reaching up over one's head; (7) reaching out to shake hands; (8) grasping with the fingers; (9) lifting or carrying 10 pounds; and (10) lifting or carrying 25 pounds. Appropriate functional assessment of the individual with OA for the purposes of research or clinical care must adequately sample activities and tasks representing this broad range of human physical function.

There are two distinct modes of functional assessment: self-report and performance-based assessment. Large population-based studies of function have routinely used self-report data to gather information on ADL and IADL by questioning individuals directly or through a trained interviewer. There appears to be little difference in quality between data obtained by self-report and data obtained by a face-to-face interviewer (Morris and Boutelle, 1985). Self-report is considered by many to be the more feasible and cost-effective means of gathering standardized functional status data on large numbers of individuals. A number of instruments have been developed for this purpose, and there has been substantial examination of their psychometric properties with respect to reliability, validity, and clinical utility in their application to arthritis research (Guccione and Jette, 1988, 1990). The reliability of self-assessment depends upon whether the instrument is able to capture function in clearly worded questions without language bias, whether there are concise directions on completing the questions, and whether the format encourages accurate reporting of answers to all questions.

Some self-report instruments use the phrase "Could you . . . ?" in its questions, while others query about the same activity by asking "Do you . . . ?" These are not equivalent forms of a single question and do not yield the same information. It is extremely important to distinguish between questions that identify a person's perceived capacity to perform a task (e.g., "If you had to, *could* you cook your own meals?") and those that indicate a person's habitual performance (e.g., "*Do* you cook your own meals?"). The first way of phrasing a question taps into an elder's beliefs about his or her personal abilities, which may be based only partially on actual current experience. The second approach establishes whether the individual does the activity habitually. Thus, an elder might truthfully respond to a question about stair climbing in the following way: "I could climb the stairs to the second floor of my home (if I had to), but I do not climb the stairs (because it hurts my knee and I don't want to)."

The time frame reference of self-assessment is also a relevant consideration. Commonly used self-report instruments differ from each other in the "window" employed to gauge a person's functional level (i.e., the past 24 hours, the previous week, the previous month, or the previous year). Typically, a respondent's functional level is measured by the degree of difficulty experienced in performing an activity or the degree of dependence upon human assistance in performing the activity.

In contrast to self-report, a performance-based functional assessment consists of direct observations of an elder's ability to perform motor routines or discrete tasks under specific test conditions. Commonly, this approach to assessment of physical function requires observation of a subject's performance of predetermined upper- or lower-extremity activities related to various combinations of reaching, turning, twisting, lifting, carrying, bending, stooping, kneeling, sitting, standing, transferring, and walking. Some performance measures also include observations of simulated ADL or IADL. Performance-based assessments apply specific, objective criteria for grading performance according to time, distance, accuracy, or completion. Although few specific uses of these performance batteries on elders with OA have been reported (Marks, 1994), their value in geriatric research is emerging (Guralnik et al., 1994, 1995; Daltroy et al., 1995). The major advantage of this approach is that the professional judgment of functional status is based on clear-cut objective evidence of the ability to perform the task rather than on subjective interpretations and criteria for success that may vary from individual to individual (Guralnik et al., 1989). Directly relevant to the study of OA in the lower extremity, this task-oriented approach particularly examines the complex integration of systems that permits an individual to maintain a posture, to make transitions to other postures, or to sustain safe and efficient movement. As summative indexes of the combined effects of impairments on a person's ability to function, these measures may very well become standard examinations for planning rehabilitation programs (Guccione, 1991).

Direct, structured observations of function also have some drawbacks (Meyers et al., 1993). When the performance battery includes items that directly mimic ADL or IADL, an assumption is made that the controlled environment of a structured situation is reasonably similar to the environment in which a person functions. Some individuals, however, may not be able to transfer out of a chair as part of a research study but may be totally independent in transferring from any chair in their own homes. Individuals with OA usually have a substantial period of time in which to adapt to decrements in function. Thus, these individuals can be quite resourceful in adapting the manner in which they perform functional activities. Furthermore, performance-based assessments quantify capacity but not habit. Observation can indicate what an elder has the capacity to do but may not reveal what that person *will* do any more accurately than would asking the person directly. Thus, there may be some disparity between what elders regard as their capabilities and what they habitually do at home under specific conditions. Finally, there is no guarantee that a performance-based assessment of function will adequately capture the impact of disease on function. It is clear that the impact of OA on physical disability is specific to the particular joint involved and the particular task or activity to be performed. A timed test of manual dexterity might be quite informative with respect to hand OA but provide no insight as to the impact of OA in other upper-extremity joints. Similarly, while current lower-extremity batteries of function might describe the effects of knee OA on activities such as transferring or walking, their ability to discern the impacts of OA of the hip, ankle, and foot are far less certain. For these reasons, self-report and performance-based assessments of function should be considered complementary approaches in arthritis research, rather than mutually exclusive techniques.

Conclusion

Osteoarthritis is a highly prevalent medical condition of elderly persons and has substantial impacts on functional activities which are specific to the affected joints. Our understanding of the disease-specific effects of OA has been confounded by the disease-specific impacts of other common medical conditions in elderly persons with OA. The evidence strongly suggests that while the impact of arthritis on function may not be as great as that of some other conditions, the combined effects of arthritis and comorbidity is generally greater than the impact on function of either alone. The technology of functional assessment continues to grow in response to both clinical and research needs, first with the development of psychometrically tested self-report methods, and more recently, with the emergence of performance-based functional batteries. Combining both self-report and performance-based approaches in the future is likely to enhance our understanding of the personal impact of OA.

REFERENCES

Badley EM, Wagstaff S, Wood PHN. 1984. Measures of functional ability (disability) in arthritis in relation to impairment of range of joint movement. *Ann Rheum Dis* 43:563–569.
Baron M, Dutil E, Berkson L, Lander P, Becker R. 1987. Hand function in the elderly: Relation to osteoarthritis. *J Rheumatol* 14:815–819.
Barrett-Connor E, Wingard DL. 1991. Heart disease risk factors as determinants of dependency and death in an older cohort. *J Aging Health* 3:247–261.
Bergstrom G, Anaiansson A, Bjelle A, Grimby G, Lundgren-Lindquist B, Svanborg A. 1985a. Functional consequences of joint impairment at age 79. *Scand J Rehabil Med* 17:183–190.
Bergstrom G, Bjelle A, Sorensen LB, Sundh V, Svanborg A. 1985b. Prevalence of symptoms and signs of joint impairment at age 79. *Scand J Rehab Med* 17:173–182.
Berkman LF, Berkman CS, Kasl S, Freeman DH, Leo L, Ostfeld AM, Cornoni-Huntley J, Brody JA. 1986. Depressive symptoms in relation to physical health and functioning in the elderly. *Am J Epidemiol* 124:372–388.
Boult C, Kane RL, Louis TA, Boult L, McCaffrey D. 1994. Chronic conditions that lead to functional limitation in the elderly. *J Gerontol* 49:M28–M36.

Brandt KD, Fife RS. 1986. Ageing in relation to the pathogenesis of osteoarthritis. *Clin Rheum Dis* 12:117–130.

Bruce ML, Seeman TE, Merrill SS, Blazer DG. 1994. The impact of depressive symptomatology on physical disability: MacArthur Studies of Successful Aging. *Am J Public Health* 84:1796–1799.

Cunningham LS, Kelsey JL. 1984. Epidemiology of musculoskeletal impairments and associated disability. *Am J Public Health* 74:574–579.

Daltroy LH, Phillips CB, Eaton HM, Larson MG, Partridge AJ, Logigian M, Liang MH. 1995. Objectively measuring physical ability in elderly persons: The Physical Capacity Evaluation. *Am J Public Health* 85:558–560.

Davis MA, Ettinger WH, Neuhaus JM, Mallon KP. 1991. Knee osteoarthritis and physical functioning: Evidence from the NHANES I epidemiologic follow-up study. *J Rheumatol* 18:591–598.

Ettinger WH, Davis MA, Neuhaus JM, Mallon KP. 1994. Long-term physical functioning in persons with knee osteoarthritis from NHANES I: Effects of comorbid medical conditions. *J Clin Epidemiol* 47:809–815.

Felson DT. 1988. Epidemiology of hip and knee osteoarthritis. *Epidemiol Rev* 10:1–28.

———. 1990. Osteoarthritis. *Rheum Dis Clin North Am* 16:499–512.

Felson DT, Naimark A, Anderson J, Kazis L, Castelli W, Meenan RF. 1987. The prevalence of knee osteoarthritis in the elderly: The Framingham Osteoarthritis Study. *Arthritis Rheum* 30:914–918.

Furner SE, Rudberg MA, Cassel CK. 1995. Medical conditions differentially affect the development of IADL disability: Implications for medical care and research. *Gerontologist* 35:444–450.

Guccione AA. 1991. Physical therapy diagnosis and the relationship between impairments and function. *Phys Ther* 71:499–703.

———. 1994. Arthritis and the process of disablement. *Phys Ther* 74:408–414.

Guccione AA, Jette AM. 1988. Assessing limitations in physical function in patients with arthritis. *Arthritis Care Res* 1:170–176.

Guccione AA, Jette AM. 1990. Multidimensional assessment of functional limitations in patients with arthritis. *Arthritis Care Res* 3:44–52.

Guccione AA, Meenan RF, Anderson JJ. 1989. Arthritis in nursing home residents: A validation of its prevalence and examination of its impact on institutionalization and functional status. *Arthritis Rheum* 31:1546–1553.

Guccione AA, Felson DT, Anderson JJ. 1990. Defining arthritis and measuring functional status in elders: Methodological issues in the study of disease and disability. *Am J Public Health* 80:945–949.

Guccione AA, Felson DT, Anderson JJ, Anthony JA, Zhang Y, Wilson PWF, Kelly-Hayes M, Wold PA, Kreger BE, Kannel WB. 1994. Specific diseases and their effects on the functional limitations of elders in the Framingham study. *Am J Public Health* 84:351–358.

Guralnik JM, Kaplan GA. 1989. Predictors of healthy aging: Prospective evidence from the Alameda County Study. *Am J Public Health* 79:703–708.

Guralnik JM, LaCroix AZ, Everett DF, Kovar MG. 1989. *Aging in the eighties: The prevalence of co-morbidity and its association with disability*. Advance Data from Vital and Health Statistics, no. 170. Hyattsville, Md.: National Center for Health Statistics.

Guralnik JM, Branch LG, Cummings SR, Curb JD. 1989. Physical performance measures in aging research. *J Gerontol* 44:M141–M146.

Guralnik JM, Simonsick EM, Ferrucci L, Glynn RJ, Berkman LF, Blazer DG, Scherr PA, Wallace RB. 1994. A short physical performance battery assessing lower extremity function: Association with self-reported disability and prediction of mortality and nursing home admission. *J Gerontol* 49:M85–M94.

Guralnik JM, Ferrucci L, Simonsick EM, Salive ME, Wallace RB. 1995. Lower-extremity function in persons over the age of 70 years as a predictor of subsequent disability. *N Engl J Med* 332:556–561.

Harris T, Kovar MG, Suzman R, Kleinman JC, Feldman JJ. 1989. Longitudinal study of physical ability in the oldest-old. *Am J Public Health* 79:698–702.

Hughes SL, Edelman PL, Singer RH, Chang RW. 1993. Joint impairment and self-reported disability in elderly persons. *J Gerontol* 48:S84–S92.

Jette AM, Branch LG. 1985. Impairment and disability in the aged. *J Chronic Dis* 38:59–65.

Jette AM, Pinsky JL, Branch LG, Wolf PA, Feinleib M. 1988. The Framingham Disability Study: Physical disability among community-dwelling survivors of stroke. *J Clin Epidemiol* 41:719–726.

Jette AM, Branch LG, Berlin J. 1990. Musculoskeletal impairments and physical disablement among the aged. *J Gerontol* 45:M203–M208.

Kellgren JH, Lawrence JS. 1963. *Atlas of standard radiographs: The epidemiology of chronic rheumatism.* Vol 2. Oxford: Blackwell Scientific Publications.

Kelly-Hayes M, Wolf PA, Kannel WB, Sytkowski P, D'Agostino RB, Gresham GE. 1988. Factors influencing survival and need for institutionalization following stroke: The Framingham study. *Arch Phys Med Rehabil* 69:415–418.

Lavsky-Shulan M, Wallace RB, Kohout FJ, Lemke JH, Morris MC, Smith IM. 1985. Prevalence and functional correlates of low back pain in the elderly: The Iowa 65+ Rural Health Study. *J Am Geriatr Soc* 33:23–28.

Lee P, Helewa A, Smythe HA, Bombardier C, Goldsmith CH. 1985. Epidemiology of musculoskeletal disorders (complaints) and related disability in Canada. *J Rheumatol* 12:1169–1173.

Lethbridge-Cejku M, Scott WW, Reichle R, Ettinger WH, Zonderman A, Costa P, Plato CC, Tobin JD, Hochberg MC. 1995. Association of radiographic features of osteoarthritis of the knee with knee pain: Data from the Baltimore Longitudinal Study of Aging. *Arthritis Care Res* 8:182–188.

Magaziner J, Simonsick EM, Kashner TM, Hebel JR, Kenzora JE. 1990. Predictors of functional recovery one year following hospital discharge for hip fracture: A prospective study. *J Gerontol* 45:M101–M107.

Mankin HJ. 1989. Clinical features of osteoarthritis. In: *Textbook of rheumatology,* edited by WN Kelley, ED Harris Jr., S Ruddy, CB Sledge. 2d ed. Pp. 1480–1500. Philadelphia: WB Saunders.

Mankin HJ, Brandt KD. 1989. Pathogenesis of osteoarthritis. In: *Textbook of rheumatology,* edited by WN Kelley, ED Harris Jr., S Ruddy, CB Sledge. 2d ed. Pp. 1469–1479. Philadelphia: WB Saunders.

Marks R. 1994. Reliability and validity of self-paced walking time measures for knee osteoarthritis. *Arthritis Care Res* 7:50–53.

Mattson E, Brostrom L-A. 1993. The physical and psychosocial effect of moderate osteoarthrosis of the knee. *Scand J Rehab Med* 23:215–218.

McAlindon TE, Snow S, Cooper C, Dieppe PA. 1992. Radiographic patterns of osteoarthritis of the knee joint in the community: The importance of the patellofemoral joint. *Ann Rheum Dis* 51: 844–849.

McAlindon TE, Cooper C, Kirwan JR, Dieppe PA. 1993. Determinants of disability in osteoarthritis of the knee. *Ann Rheum Dis* 52:258–262.

Meyers AM, Holliday PJ, Harvey KA, Hutchinson KS. 1993. Functional performance measures: Are they superior to self-assessments? *J Gerontol* 48:M196–M206.

Mor V, Murphy J, Masterson-Allen S, Willey C, Razmpour A, Jackson ME, Greer D, Katz S. 1989. Risk of functional decline among well elders. *J Clin Epidemiol* 42:895–904.

Morris WW, Boutelle S. 1985. Multidimensional functional assessment in two modes. *Gerontologist* 25:638–643.

Moskowitz RW. 1992. Osteoarthritis—symptoms and signs. In: *Osteoarthritis: Diagnosis and medical/surgical management,* edited by RW Moskowitz, DS Howell, VM Goldberg, HJ Mankin. 2d ed. Pp. 255–261. Philadelphia: WB Saunders.

Nagi SZ. 1976. An epidemiology of disability among adults in the United States. *Milbank Q* 54:439–467.

———. 1991. Disability concepts revisited: Implications for prevention. In: *Disability in America:*

Toward a national agenda for prevention, edited by AM Pope, AR Tarlov. Pp. 307–327. Washington, D.C.: National Academy Press.

Nickel JT, Chirikos TN. 1990. Functional disability of elderly patients with long-term coronary heart disease: A sex-stratified analysis. *J Gerontol* 45:S60-S68.

Philbin EF, Groff GD, Ries MD, Miller TE. 1995. Cardiovascular fitness and health in patients with end-stage osteoarthritis. *Arthritis Rheum* 38:799–805.

Pinsky JL, Branch LG, Jette AM, Haynes SG, Feinleib M, Cornoni-Huntley JC, Bailey KR. 1985. The Framingham Disability Study: Relationship of disability to cardiovascular risk factors among persons free of diagnosed cardiovascular disease. *Am J Epidemiol* 122:644–656.

Pinsky JL, Jette AM, Branch LG, Kannel WB, Feinleib M. 1990. The Framingham Disability Study: Relationship of various coronary heart disease manifestations to disability in older persons living in the community. *Am J Public Health* 80:1363–1368.

Satariano WA, Ragheb NE, Branch LG, Swanson GM. 1990. Difficulties in physical functioning reported by middle-aged and elderly women with breast cancer: A case control comparison. *J Gerontol* 45:M3–M11.

Scherr PA, Albert MS, Funkenstein HH, Cook NR, Hennekens CH, Branch LG, White LR, Taylor JO, Evans DA. 1988. Correlates of cognitive function in an elderly community population. *Am J Epidemiol* 128:1084–1101.

Summers MN, Haley WE, Reveille JD, Alarcon GS. 1988. Radiographic assessment and psychologic variables as predictors of pain and functional impairment in osteoarthritis of the knee or hip. *Arthritis Rheum* 31:204–209.

Verbrugge LM. 1992. Disability transitions for older persons with arthritis. *J Aging Health* 4:212–243.

Verbrugge LM, Patrick DL. 1995. Seven chronic conditions: Their impact on US adults' activity levels and use of medical services. *Am J Public Health* 85:173–182.

Verbrugge LM, Lepkowski JM, Imanaka Y. 1989. Comorbidity and its impact on disability. *Milbank Q* 67:450–484.

Verbrugge LM, Lepkowski JM, Konkol LL. 1991a. Levels of disability among U.S. adults with arthritis. *J Gerontol* 46:S71-S83.

Verbrugge LM, Gates DM, Ike RW. 1991b. Risk factors for disability among US adults with arthritis. *J Clin Epidemiol* 44:167–182.

Yelin EH, Spitz PP. 1990. Transitions in health status among community-dwelling elderly people with arthritis. *Arthritis Rheum* 33:1205–1215.

Yelin E, Lubeck D, Holman H, Epstein W. 1987. The impact of rheumatoid arthritis and osteoarthritis: The activities of patients with rheumatoid arthritis and osteoarthritis compared to controls. *J Rheumatol* 14:710–717.

Zimmer Z, Hickey T, Searle MS. 1995. Activity participation and well-being among older people with arthritis. *Gerontologist* 35:463–471.

7

The Aging Skeleton
Osteoarthritis and Osteoporosis

David Hamerman, M.D.

The Relationship between Osteoarthritis and Osteoporosis

Osteoarthritis (OA) and osteoporosis (OP) are similar in that they are age-associated conditions involving the skeleton and are more frequent in older women. Their differences with respect to bone density, however, have attracted a great deal of recent attention in the literature and justify the inclusion of OP in a book devoted to OA. Degradation and loss of the articular cartilage in involved joints are distinctive features of OA and until now have received the most attention in terms of the pathophysiologic processes involved (Woessner and Howell, 1993). However, clinically evident joint deformity in subjects with OA is associated with radiographic evidence of sclerosis and new bone formation in the subchondral bone beneath the articular cartilage, and in bony outgrowths, referred to as osteophytes, mostly near the joint margins (Hamerman, 1989; Spector and Cooper, 1993). The hallmark of OP, by contrast, is bone loss after the menopause. Densitometric techniques, which will be discussed in this chapter, identify a state of osteopenia when the findings are 1 standard deviation (SD) below the young normal mean. A diagnosis of OP can be made when bone mass is reduced 2.5 SD below the young normal mean, with the important potential implication of high risk of fracture (Nguyen et al., 1993; Kanis et al., 1994; Cooper, 1995). Fractures in the wrist (i.e., the Colles fracture) and vertebral bodies occur within a decade or so after the menopause, while fractures of the hip are observed later in life with growing frequency, approaching the magnitude of an "orthopaedic epidemic" (Wallace, 1983). Hip fracture is perhaps the defining public health concern in OP (Melton, 1993).

More than 20 years ago, Foss and Byers (1972) drew attention to the virtual absence of osteoarthritic changes in the fractured hips of subjects with OP. Since then, reports have suggested that "OA protects against hip fracture" (Dequeker et al., 1993a), and that there is an "inverse relationship" (Hart et al., 1994, p. 161) or "negative association" (Cooper et al., 1991, p. 541) between OA and OP with respect to bone density. The basis for the apparent lower incidence of hip fracture in subjects with hip OA has been attributed to greater bone density in the hip in OA than in OP, evidence for which will also be discussed in this chapter. Jones et al. (1995) also observed higher bone density in subjects with OA but found no difference in fracture incidence between those with self-reported OA and those not reporting OA. Increased postural sway among those with OA was thought to predispose to a greater frequency of falls. Thus, the issue of fracture frequency in OA and OP remains to be further defined, but the basis for bone density differences is perhaps the fundamental issue that needs to be explored.

Bone Density in Osteoarthritis and Osteoporosis

The predisposing environmental conditions, cellular interactions in bone, and genetic factors that contribute to bone loss are the central issues in OP research today. These efforts are spurred by the desire to identify those at risk, intervene therapeutically, and reduce late-life fracture incidence. The implications of subchondral sclerosis and increased bone density in OA have been less appreciated. Radin and Rose (1986) put forth the theory that dense subchondral bone fails to dissipate mechanical forces in the joint and contributes to cartilage matrix breakdown. Eckstein et al. (1995) considered that the "loading history" (p. 268), or the mechanical forces acting on the joint, trigger interaction of osteoblastic and osteoclastic functions in the bone, which are in turn reflected in the pattern of subchondral mineralization. Years ago, Harrison et al. (1953) linked cartilage degeneration with hyperemia of the subchondral bone and new bone formation. Whether increasing subchondral bone density predisposes to articular cartilage changes, or—as seems more likely—cartilage breakdown is the initial event, or both happen simultaneously remains to be elucidated. But the biochemical basis for increased subchondral bone density and osteophyte formation remains a key research challenge in OA, and the situation in OA research lags far behind the situation in OP research, in which our understanding of postmenopausal estrogen deficiency as the basis for bone loss has become increasingly defined (Manolagas, 1995).

For many years Dequeker (1985) highlighted anthropometric status and fracture risk differences in those with "advanced" manifestations of OP or OA, which he defined as follows: "All cases [of OP] had radiological evidence of multiple vertebral collapse or femoral neck fracture due to minimal trauma. Patients with thin bones (osteopenia) without structural failure are not included." "Cases [of OA] are primary, i.e., without known underlying cause; all cases had radiological evidence of degenerative joint disease of at least three or more joints and they had to have small hand joint involvement with Heberden's (distal joint) and/or Bouchard's (proximal interphalangeal joint) nodes" (p. 273). Table 7.1 summarizes his findings.

More recent studies have focused on community-dwelling postmenopausal subjects in whom clinical manifestations of OA were less florid, confined to the hip or knee, or manifest as so-called generalized OA (Kellgren and Moore, 1952). Bone density in these subjects was compared with that of age-matched controls without apparent OA.

Comparative studies of bone density in the axial or appendicular skeleton (the spine or the extremities, respectively) can be made by conventional radiographs, whole-body calcium determination, or densitometric techniques that measure bone mineral. As OP progresses, crystals of basic calcium phosphate as an apatite salt are lost from bone at a rate parallel to the rate of loss of the extracellular organic framework, called the matrix (Termine, 1988). Densitometric studies of mineral density thus reveal a reduced bone mass; the various methods of measurement are summarized in table 7.2.

Pelvic radiographs were reviewed in subjects admitted to a hospital for intravenous pyelograms or abdominal studies (Cooper et al., 1991), and the Singh index was used as an estimate of trabecular bone and hence bone density in the femoral head (Resnick and Niwayama, 1988). On the basis of the Singh index, those without radiographic evidence of OA had lower values for bone mass than did those with OA of the hip. Radiographs can provide a visual impression of higher bone density, as figure 7.1 shows in a study of the knee of an elderly woman with OA; however, loss of bone is less readily visualized, except in severe cases, as in the knee of a premenopausal woman on corticosteroid therapy for systemic lupus erythematosus—an illustration of "secondary," or steroid-induced, OP (fig. 7.2).

Using dual-energy x-ray absorptiometry (DEXA) (see table 7.2), Knight et al. (1992) observed an increase in bone density at the femoral neck in patients with OA of the hip "compared with predicted control values" (p. 1026). Hannan et al. (1993) investigated subjects in the Framingham study with and without knee OA. In early to moderate cases of knee OA with osteophyte formation,

Table 7.1.   Contrasts between Osteoarthritis and Osteoporosis

	Osteoarthritis	Osteoporosis
Vertebral fracture	rare	frequent
Hip fracture	rare	frequent
Anthropometric status		
Height	short	tall
Weight	heavier	lighter
Skinfold thickness	higher	lower
Muscle girth	greater	less
Body fat	increased	decreased

SOURCE: Data from Dequeker, 1985.

dual-photon absorptiometry showed greater bone mineral density in the femoral neck and the trochanter; however, single-photon absorptiometry of the distal radius showed no increase. Nevitt et al. (1995) found higher bone density in the hip, lumbar spine, radius, and calcaneus in elderly women with moderate to severe radiographic findings of hip OA strongly associated with hip osteophytes. They commented that the "possibility that regulators of bone metabolism might provide a link between skeletal status and OA is intriguing" (p. 914). Belmonte-Serrano et al. (1993) observed higher total body bone mineral density with knee and spine OA, especially when osteophytes were present.

Bone mineral density was studied by DEXA in middle-aged women in whom a more generalized form of OA involved various joints of the hand, such as the distal (DIP) and proximal (PIP) interphalangeal joints and the carpometacarpal (CMC) joints, as well as the knee and occasionally the hip. Greater bone density was observed in the lumbar spine, the distal forearm (Hordon et al., 1993) or the femoral neck (Hart et al., 1994) in subjects with OA than in those without OA. The greater the number of joints affected by OA, the greater the bone mineral density values measured by DEXA (Burger et al., 1996). In women with radiographic evidence of spinal OA, bone mineral density measured by DEXA was increased in the lumbar spine, the femoral neck, and the total body (Peel et al., 1995). A comment by Hart et al. (1994) deserves to be emphasized: "The clinical significance of a 5–7 percent increase in bone mineral density in the lumbar spine and femoral neck in OA . . . is equivalent to reducing age-related bone loss by five years, which becomes important in later life when hip and vertebral fractures can double in incidence over this time frame" (p. 161). However, other studies of the generalized form of OA with hand involvement (cited by Lane and Nevitt, 1994; Star and Hochberg, 1994) found no increase in bone density in the distal radius, or in total body calcium. Hochberg et al. (1994a) studied women participants in the Baltimore Longitudinal Study of Aging who had radiographic evidence of hand OA. Using the percentage of cortical area in the second metacarpal, and the bone mineral density of the distal radius measured by single-photon absorptiometry, no differences between the hand OA group and controls (those without hand OA) were observed when results were adjusted for age and body mass index. This will be commented upon later.

Thus, although the trend appears to be that OA of the spine, hip, or knee may be associated with both local joint increases in skeletal bone density and more widespread increases, the results are by no means clear for isolated hand OA. Little-understood variations in joint localization, risk factors, and the influence of systemic factors (Dieppe and Kirwan, 1994) exist for OA and are likely to create differences in the manifestations of subchondral bone density. But the type of bone may also be a factor.

There are two types of bone structure in the adult skeleton—cortical bone (or compacta), and trabecular bone (cancellous or spongiosa). Cortical

Table 7.2.   Techniques for Measuring Bone Density

Method	Site	Comments
Conventional radiography	lumbar spine, metacarpals	Insensitive to mineral loss < 20–40%.
Single-photon absorptiometry (SPA)	distal radius, calcaneus	Not for axial (spinal) skeleton, or for simultaneous measure of trabecular and cortical bone. See text for transition of cortical bone in distal radius.
Dual-photon absorptiometry (DPA)	lumbar spine, hip, total body	Long examination time. Examination is very dependent on reproducibility of postimaging analysis. Quantitates combined cortical and trabecular bone. Low radiation exposure. May be influenced by degenerative changes in spine.
Dual-energy x-ray absorptiometry (DEXA)	lumbar spine, hip, radius, total body	Better reproducibility. Short examination time. Low radiation dose. Combines trabecular and cortical bone densities. Aortic calcification and degenerative changes in spine may artificially increase density in PA views. Examination is very dependent on reproducibility of postimaging analysis.
Quantitative computed tomography (QCT)	spine	Quantitates trabecular bone. Higher radiation dose than DEXA. Changes in spine do not interfere.

SOURCE: Data from Genant, 1988; Johnston et al., 1991; Jergas and Genant, 1993; Belmonte-Serrano et al., 1993.

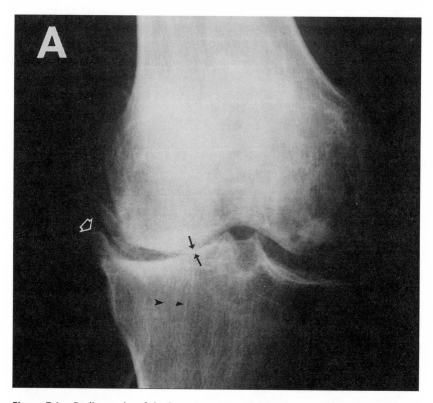

Figure 7.1.   Radiographs of the knee in osteoarthritis. These are frontal *(A)* and lateral *(B)* x-rays of the right knee of an 80-year-old woman, taken with the subject standing, and represent changes of severe osteoarthritis. In *A,* there is marked joint space narrowing at the lateral tibial plateau *(dark arrows)* owing to cartilage loss; osteophyte formation *(open arrow)* is present at the articular margin. The vertically

bone provides about three-quarters of the total skeletal mass but only one-third of the total surface, and forms principally the shafts of long bones of the appendicular skeleton. Trabecular bone provides one-quarter of the total skeletal mass but about two-thirds of the total surface. It consists of a three-dimensional network of plates and rods containing hematopoietic and fatty marrow and is found principally in the vertebrae and the ends of long bones (Parfitt, 1991). Large surface area and proximity to blood supply may account for the greater metabolic activity and higher turnover rate of trabecular bone (Woolf and Dixon, 1988): over a lifetime, women lose about 50 percent of their trabecular bone and about 35 percent of their cortical bone (Judd et al., 1995). This may explain the tendency for vertebral fractures to occur during the postmenopausal accelerated phase of trabecular bone loss, called type I, whereas in the later phase of age-

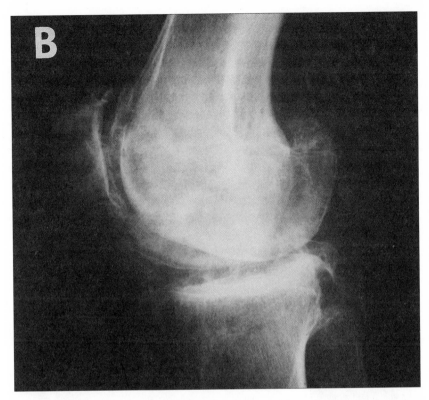

oriented weight-bearing trabeculae *(arrowheads)* in the subchondral bone are prominent and heavily mineralized. The lateral view *(B)* further reveals the loss of femorotibial joint space, dense subchondral bone with generalized increased bone density in the distal femur, and osteophyte formation.

related cortical bone loss, called type II, fractures occur in the femoral neck and intertrochanteric region as well.

While there are pitfalls in oversimplifying and treating each type of bone (trabecular or cortical) as a single compartment (Parfitt, 1991), it may nevertheless be appropriate to consider whether observed increases in bone density in OA occur primarily in the trabecular bone. Dual-photon or dual-energy x-ray absorptiometry usually detects increased density in trabecular bone in the femoral neck and the spine in subjects with large-joint OA. Single-photon absorptiometry localized to cortical bone in the distal radius may show no increased density. However, the cortical shell diminishes distally (toward the hand), and the proportion of trabecular bone increases, reaching 38 to 50 percent when the gap between the radius and the ulna measures 5 mm, and up to

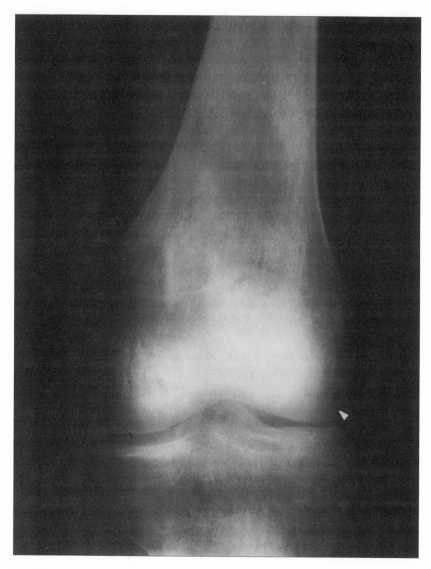

Figure 7.2.   Radiograph of a knee with steroid-induced bone loss. This is an x-ray of the knee of a premenopausal woman with longstanding systemic lupus erythematosus who is on corticosteroid therapy. The distal femur and proximal tibia are markedly osteopenic when compared to the knee in figure 7.1. The cortices are thinned *(white arrowhead)*. The region of increased bone density at the distal femoral articulation is caused by concomitant osteonecrosis. The effects of corticosteroid therapy as a cause of secondary osteoporosis are discussed by Formiga et al. (1995) and Dequeker and Westhovens (1995).

75 percent at the ultradistal site (Genant, 1988). Thus, Hannan et al. (1993) noted in their study of subjects with knee OA that density of cortical bone in the wrist showed no increase, although bone density was increased in the hip. Carlsson et al. (1979) studied cases of hip OA, and also observed no increase in density in the radius at a more proximal site (cortical bone); yet when the bone density of the radius was measured at a more distal site, corresponding to the tip of the ulnar styloid (trabecular bone), the density was greater in women with hip OA than in controls without hip OA. Thus, to return to the findings of Hochberg et al. (1994a) cited above, in subjects with hand OA it is possible that absorptiometry studies at a site more distal in the radius, involving trabecular bone, might have shown increased bone density.

Trabecular bone beneath the articular cartilage surface may show greater density in subjects with OA than in those without OA as a result of mechanical forces impacting on the cartilage and on the shaft (diaphysis) of the bone (Melton et al., 1988). These forces may differentially affect subchondral bone in subjects with OA and OP owing to differences in body habitus and obesity, as discussed above. The hyperemic response (Harrison et al., 1953) and microfractures in the trabecular plates (Termine, 1990) that occur in OA may promote new bone formation, as occurs in fracture repair, during which mesenchymal marrow cells differentiate into chondroblasts and osteoblasts, and vascular in-growth promotes new cartilage and bone formation (endochondral ossification) at the fracture site. Cooper et al. (1991) suggested that the variable response of subchondral bone to mechanical stress in OA and OP could be due to "accentuation" or "blunting," respectively, of the osteoblastic response (p. 542). Local and systemic growth-regulating factors are likely to influence cellular responses in subchondral bone. The remainder of this chapter presents evidence that growth factors and other mediators acting on bone cells may modify differentially the balance of bone deposition and resorption in OA and OP.

Regulatory Factors and Bone Remodeling

Although bone growth ceases in early adult life, bones continue to undergo the processes of resorption and deposition known as remodeling (for reviews, see Raisz, 1993; Mundy, 1994; Manolagas and Jilka, 1995; Parfitt, 1995). In healthy young premenopausal adults there is a balance, or coupling, between bone resorption by osteoclasts and bone formation by osteoblasts.

Mesenchymal/stromal cells in the bone marrow are the precursors for osteoblasts, while mononuclear phagocytes in the bone marrow are the lineage for osteoclasts. The osteoblast precursors influence osteoclast formation and proliferation within the marrow by release of mediators such as colony-stimulating factor (CSF-1), leukemia inhibitory factor (LIF), and interleukin-11 (IL-11). The maturing osteoblast—in response to interleukin-1 (IL-1), prostaglandins, and tumor necrosis factor (TNF) derived from circulating monocyte/macrophages—continues to influence osteoclast development. The outcome is the formation of the mature, multinucleate osteoclast, which, by way of its adhesion molecules, adheres to the bone site destined for excavation and resorption. These more mature osteoclasts with ruffled borders create an acidic milieu to remove calcium and then release lysosomal proteases to degrade the demineralized matrix (Judd et al., 1995). In normal remodeling conditions, osteoclasts discontinue the resorption process within 7–10 days and release signals (coupling factors) to promote osteoblast recruitment. When the osteoclasts have been removed, osteoblasts move into the site. Growth factors, released by proteolysis from their binding proteins in the bone, or brought to the bone site itself via the circulation, stimulate osteoblasts to lay down a matrix consisting of collagen type I and a number of noncollagenous proteins. The matrix is subsequently mineralized by calcium phosphate deposited as crystals of apatite.

In the premenopausal state, the presence of estrogen inhibits the effects of cytokines on the osteoblasts, which in turn limits the release of factors that promote osteoclastogenesis (Horowitz, 1993; Manolagas, 1995). After the menopause, estrogen deficiency appears principally to result in genetic up-regulation in the osteoblasts of the cytokine IL-6 and the soluble receptors of IL-6, which are potent stimulators of osteoclastogenesis. Loss of the remodeling balance occurs. Deeper resorption spaces develop, and the capacity for osteoblasts to fill them may be impaired (Turner et al., 1994). These deeper resorption spaces result in perforation of trabecular plates and loss of architectural elements, weakening the skeleton in regions that contain principally trabecular bone, hence the frequency of early vertebral fractures in OP. In mice subjected to "knockout" of the gene responsible for IL-6 production, ovariectomy did not lead to osteopenia and increased bone turnover, while ovariectomized littermates with intact capacity for IL-6 production lost 50 percent of their trabecular bone (Poli et al., 1994). One of the theories to explain greater bone density in individuals with OA relates to the frequent association of OA with obesity, identified as a risk factor for knee OA (see chapter 4). The adipose tissue in the obese subject is capable of aromatization of androgens to estrogens (Boyd, 1994), perhaps providing levels of estrogens that can sustain bone density for a longer period.

Growth factors need to be considered in relation to skeletal integrity (Canalis, 1993) because they are abundant in bone, and their effects on the remodeling process have received a great deal of attention (for a review, see Mundy, 1994). Parfitt (1991) noted that a "normal hormonal milieu is needed to sustain an appropriate level of bone turnover throughout the body" (p. 468). In considering growth factors in relation to aging and OP, Mundy (1991) wrote, "I wonder if during the aging process, and this may be relevant to other connective tissue systems as well, there is less accumulation or production of growth factors in the matrix. That would mean fewer regulatory factors were available during advancing age to regulate the cellular events which would ensure a balance between bone formation and resorption" (p. 150).

The growth factors present in bone, or brought to the bone via the circulation, share in common the feature of being bound to proteins or proteoglycans. Latency and binding proteins tend to protect growth factors from proteolytic degradation, promote their more gradual release, and thus finely control their action in situ. Transforming growth factor–β (TGF-β) is part of a large family of related growth factors, including bone morphogenetic proteins, that promote bone growth. TGF-β injected locally into sites of experimental fracture in animals stimulated mesenchymal cell proliferation, new cartilage and bone formation, and fracture repair (Joyce et al., 1990). TGF-β was localized by immunofluorescent staining at sites of cartilage degeneration and in the subchondral bone from subjects with OA, but joints uninvolved with OA were not available for comparison (D. Hamerman, M. Joyce, M. Bolander, unpublished observations, 1991). Estrogen appears to act on osteoblasts to promote TGF-β secretion; in ovariectomized rats, decreased content of TGF-β may contribute to osteopenia (Finkelman et al., 1992). Diminished synthesis or availability of TGF-β may retard osteoblast development and up-regulate osteoclast activity to account for diminished bone density in old mice (Kahn et al., 1995).

Acid and basic fibroblast growth factors (FGFs) are present in bone matrix bound to heparan sulfate proteoglycan. The biological roles of the FGFs include cell proliferation, migration, and angiogenesis, all of which occur in new cartilage and bone formation. Basic FGF infused into the joint of a rabbit with a surgical defect in the articular cartilage promoted repair of the cartilage lesion (Cuevas et al., 1988). Local injection of basic FGF into fracture sites induced repair (Joyce et al., 1990).

Insulin-like growth factors I and II (IGF-I and -II) are present in bone matrix; IGF-I is also brought to the bone via the circulation, primarily from the liver. These factors belong to a family called the somatomedins, which are under the control of pituitary-derived growth hormone (Inzucchi and Robbins, 1994). Under the influence of a hypothalamus-derived growth hormone–releasing hormone (GHRH) and somatostatin, growth hormone is released from the pituitary in pulsatile or episodic bursts; its variable levels and short half-life in blood make measurements of growth hormone difficult to interpret. IGF-I assays have been used as a more reliable means to assess growth hormone activity (Borst et al., 1994). The action of IGFs is also modulated by a number of binding proteins (Jones and Clemmons, 1995). Like growth hormone, estrogens and parathyroid hormone promote IGF-I-mediated osteoblast bone synthesis—which is one means by which parathyroid hormone exerts its anabolic effects (Delany et al., 1994).

In OP, aging, as well as estrogen deficiency after the menopause, may reduce the activity or availability of growth factors in bone and contribute to decreased bone density. The conditions contributing to increased bone density in OA are not understood. The factors predisposing to cartilage degradation, primarily by the actions of cytokines and proteases, have received more attention in the literature, but the mechanisms proposed for possible cartilage repair may be relevant to enhanced bone formation in OA (Hamerman, 1993; Hamerman and Taylor, 1993). A number of growth factors discussed here, including FGFs, TGF-β, and platelet-derived growth factor (PDGF), are present in synovial fluid from osteoarthritic joints (Hamerman et al., 1987), which is consistent with the view that they may play a role in the pathogenesis of increased bone density in OA.

Another growth factor that needs to be considered because of its profound influence on bone is colony-stimulating factor-1. Knowledge about the action of CSF-1 on bone has been derived in large part from studies on mice that develop osteopetrosis as a result of a spontaneously arising mutation *(op)* in the gene necessary for synthesis of CSF-1; because the CSF-1 produced is biologically inactive, osteoclasts fail to mature and are deficient in number, and bone produced cannot be resorbed (Pollard and Stanley, 1996). These osteopetrotic mice have virtually no marrow spaces, and their jaws are so dense that teeth cannot erupt. In human subjects with OA, assays of blood and knee joint fluids for CSF-1 have thus far not indicated diminished circulating levels of this growth factor, which might account for increased bone density in the involved joint (Hamerman and Stanley, 1996). However, other forms of CSF-1 may act locally: the proteoglycan form of CSF-1 binds to bone matrices; another form spans the cell membrane of osteoblasts and may act by cell-cell interaction (Pollard and Stanley, 1996). Thus, circulating levels may not reflect the local action of these forms of CSF-1. CSF-1 is also known to be a potent inducer of c-*fos*, an early response gene expressed through its receptor, the tyrosine kinase c-*fms*. "Knockout" mice lacking a functional c-*fos* gene develop severe osteopetrosis (Johnson et al., 1992). A targeted mutation in another tyrosine kinase, the c-*src* protooncogene, also results in osteopetrosis in mice (Soriano et al., 1991). In mice the insertion of a transgene that modifies a helix-loop-helix translational motif leads to micropthalmia *(mi)* and multiple other phenotypic abnormalities, including osteopetrosis (Hughes et al., 1993). Thus, different molecular genetic modifications in mice may ultimately lead to the osteopetrotic state through impaired osteoclastogenesis (i.e., failure of the progenitor cells in the bone marrow to mature to osteoclasts, and/or inability of multinucleate osteoclasts to resorb bone). Experimental animals such as the *op/op* mouse with osteopetrosis may be useful in providing a "model" in which to examine the relationship of dense subchondral bone to possible cartilage changes over time which may resemble human OA (Hamerman and Stanley, 1996). Subchondral bone thickness changes in OA developing spontaneously in cynomolgus monkeys and osteoarthritic changes induced in canine joints after transection of the cruciate ligament have recently been reviewed by Carlson et al. (1996).

The remainder of this chapter will be devoted to growth hormone—IGFs, which have been studied most intensively in relation to OP and have been investigated to some extent in OA.

Comparative Studies of Growth Hormone: Insulin-like Growth Factors

Aging is associated with changes in body composition: a decrease in bone density, an increase in the store of adipose tissue, and a loss of lean body mass (Lewis and Bell, 1990). With a more sedentary existence in old age there also occurs a decrease in muscle strength, which subjects with OA or OP may share. This may constitute a risk factor for knee OA, and in both OA and OP may predispose to falls and hip fracture, depending on the nature of the fall, the density of bone in the femur, and body mass index (Greenspan et al., 1994). Limb exercises that do not necessarily enhance cardiovascular status nevertheless may stabilize bone mineral content and preserve or even increase muscle mass, as discussed in chapters 8 and 9. Moreover, exercises involving treadmill walking, lower-limb resistance, or bicycle riding acutely elevate growth hormone levels (Borst et al., 1994; Hodes, 1994). Studies in the past 5 years have explored the premise that the age-associated decline in IGF-I levels, and changes in body composition as noted above, may be reversed, at least temporarily, during a period of growth hormone administration. Growth hormone administered for 6 months to men aged 60 to 80 years whose circulating levels of IGF-I were in the lower third for their age group resulted in reduced body fat, increased lean body mass, and increased lumbar vertebral bone mineral density (Rudman et al., 1990). Later reports by Holloway et al. (1994) and others indicated that results may not be so consistent when different populations are studied. It is generally agreed that growth hormone improves body composition (Papadakis et al., 1996) and also bone remodeling, largely through enhanced osteoblastic activity. However, the net effect on bone mass is not impressive, probably owing to physiologic coupling. That is, IGF-I induction from growth hormone administration leads to sustained bone formation but also to a corresponding enhancement of osteoclast precursors, resulting in bone resorption (Rosen et al., 1994). Caution is needed in the use of growth hormone for therapeutic purposes in view of the high incidence of side effects, including fluid retention and edema, carpal tunnel compression, arthralgias, hypertension, and glucose intolerance (de Boer et al., 1995).

Investigations of the use of IGF-I to treat OP are in a preliminary stage (Canalis, 1996; Ghiron et al., 1995). IGF-I injections result in an increase of serum markers for bone formation, such as bone-specific alkaline phosphatase, osteocalcin, and the carboxy-terminal peptide of procollagen type 1, but this is offset by a parallel increase in markers of bone resorption, such as the urinary calcium-to-creatinine ratio and hydroxyproline. Rosen et al. (1994) suggested that administration of IGF-I may have more direct effects on "senescent" osteoblasts and a less frequent occurrence of side effects than growth hormone. Lower levels of IGF-I were found in a group of men with OP at a younger age than is usually observed (mean 46 ± 8 years) (Ljunghall et al., 1992), but in most studies, when IGF-I serum levels were corrected for age no correlations were found in subjects with reduced bone mineral density. Bennett et al. (1984) note that "the possibility remains, however, that decreasing concentrations of serum IGF-I play a role in the more gradual loss of bone with aging (type II osteoporosis) in which impaired bone formation at the cellular level has been demonstrated" (p. 701).

No correlations between IGF-I levels and radiographic knee OA were found in some studies (McAlindon et al., 1993; Hochberg et al., 1994b); in one prospective study there was a relation between IGF-I concentrations and osteophytes, but no relation between IGF-I concentrations and joint space narrowing (Schouten et al., 1993). IGF-I levels were higher by 64 percent in women with radiographic evidence of bilateral moderate or severe knee joint space narrowing and osteophytosis than in subjects with no x-ray evidence of knee OA (Lloyd et al., 1996). IGF binding protein–3 appeared to be present in greater concentrations in subjects with OA (Wüster, 1992). The prevalence of radiographic OA was reported to be low in elderly subjects with growth hormone deficiency, while acromegalics with high levels of growth hormone had bone changes in their joints which were similar to OA (Bagge et al., 1993). Interestingly, bone mineral content in acromegalics was increased in the forearm but decreased in the spine, a finding that prompted Parfitt (1991) to comment that "growth hormone excess could not prevent the adverse effects of estrogen deficiency on the axial skeleton, even though the beneficial effects of IGF-I were apparently stronger in the appendicular skeleton" (p. 469).

In summary, when serum levels of IGF have been compared in subjects with OA or OP, consistent differences have not been found, perhaps because age-matched subjects with these conditions have not been studied simultaneously. Moreover, serum levels of IGF may not necessarily correlate with the content of this growth factor in bone and are dependent on the extent of growth hormone release from the pituitary and subsequent IGF-I production in the liver. The finding of Dequeker et al. (1993b) of increased IGF-I content in iliac bone biopsies from deceased subjects with hand OA should be extended to age-matched subjects with OP or OA, by means of carefully localized iliac bone biopsies taken at the time of open operative repair of hip fracture, or hip replacement, respectively.

Conclusions: A Public Health Perspective on Osteoarthritis and Osteoporosis

OA and OP intersect in many areas, although there are obvious divergences on the basis of bone density and the involvement of the joint in OA. Yet the points of comparison between OA and OP touch on aspects of OA discussed in virtually every other chapter in this book, and also justify the inclusion of OP in this chapter.

The primary consideration for both OA and OP is the influence of age itself (see chapter 4). The long "silent" period in OP ensues after the menopause, with the steady diminution of bone density from the peak bone mass. The manifestations of the long "silent" period in OA are unknown. To gain insight into this period, one may consider risk factors (i.e., environmental influences). The contributions of body habitus in relation to the development of OA and OP are noted above (table 7.1); in addition, early menopause, a diet low in calcium and vitamin D, smoking, and a sedentary life style are risk factors for the subsequent development of OP (Belmonte-Serrano et al., 1993; Christiansen, 1993). Congenital deformity of the hip appears to be a risk factor for hip OA, and joint calcification, reduced muscle mass, and meniscectomy may predispose to the development of knee OA (see chapter 10, and the review in Hamerman, 1995). Progression to overt clinical symptoms of OA and OP due to these presumed risk factors is not inevitable; weight loss and exercises for the limbs and back may slow or prevent the expression of OA (chapters 9 and 10), and exercises help to limit OP (Bouxsein and Marcus, 1994). In late adult life, the risk of falls enters the picture, bringing the dreaded potential for hip fracture, thought to be highly associated with low bone mineral density in OP (Nguyen et al., 1993) and therefore less prevalent in OA. However, OA, even with greater bone density, may not necessarily protect against hip fracture if individuals with OA are at greater risk for falls owing to muscle weakness and limb instability (Jones et al., 1995).

In addition to the environmental influences discussed above, insight into the long "silent" period of aging in relation to OP and OA could be gained if there was evidence of a genetic predisposition or serum "markers" for these conditions. Much interest has been raised by the demonstration that serum markers of bone turnover—osteocalcin and procollagen type 1 C-terminal propeptide—are more similar in identical (monozygotic) than in nonidentical (dizygotic) twins (Eisman, 1995). A candidate gene examined for osteocalcin regulation was the vitamin D receptor (VDR), and polymorphism appeared to be correlated with elevated markers of bone turnover and hence a predisposition to OP. While not all subsequent work has confirmed these findings (for reviews, see Eisman, 1995; Mundy, 1995), nevertheless they are a provocative approach to a clinical condition of enormous public health importance. Serum levels of bone markers may reveal those women who at the time of menopause are "fast losers" and at potential risk for OP (Delmas, 1993). Studies of the regulatory elements in the proximal part of the $5'$ upstream sequence of the collagenase gene revealed no consistent modifications in persons with OP that differentiated them from non-osteoporotic postmenopausal women (Thiry-Blaise et al., 1995). The association with a genetic indicator for type II collagen (specific for cartilage) has been made in a family with primary generalized OA and mild chondrodysplasia: a single base mutation results in the substitution of cysteine for arginine at position 519 of the $\alpha I(II)$ procollagen chain (Jiminez and Dharmavaram, 1994). There are also serum and synovial fluid markers related to cartilage degradation and bone turnover in OA, as reviewed in chapter 11.

In the pre-clinical, or incipient, period of OA, joint x-rays, imaging, and arthroscopy are not done for diagnostic purposes in asymptomatic individuals. Even in the presence of symptoms, arthroscopy, the presumed "gold standard" for demonstrating cartilage changes in early OA, may in fact fail to show lesions when standing radiographs of the knee appear to show joint space narrowing—a presumptive indicator of cartilage loss (Brandt et al., 1991) (fig. 7.1). There are pitfalls in the interpretation of standing radiographs for measuring joint space

in knee OA (Spector, 1995): perhaps in the twenty-first century the gold standard for OA may be newer imaging modalities (chapter 12), and the magnified
radiographic techniques developed by Buckland-Wright et al. (1995). Uncertainty in the assessment of early OA may lead to its being called something else:
Hadler (1992) suggested that "knee pain is the malady, not OA." There is at present no indication of what constitutes the preclinical or incipient condition
having the same relation to OA that osteopenia has to the overt expression of
OP and fractures (table 7.3). Lack of such information could mean delay in the
use of "chondroprotective drugs" when, as discussed in chapter 13, these become available for use early in the course of OA (Brandt, 1995). As for the contrast between aging and the expression of disease (chapter 1), reduction in bone
mass below 2.5 SD is one factor correlated with fracture risk in OP, and an overt
fracture may certainly be considered disease (Melton, 1995) because of the associated profound morbidity and significant mortality (Birge et al., 1994). The
interrelations of aging and disease in OA may depend on the extent of joint
pathology and clinical symptoms. Serum and synovial fluid markers may perhaps distinguish aging from disease (see chapter 11); we tend to consider OA as
disease when cartilage loss, joint space narrowing, osteophytes, and deformity
are associated with pain and with disability sufficient to bring the patient and
the orthopedic surgeon together to agree on joint replacement. (On disability
in OA, see chapter 6.)

The use of estrogens in women at the time of menopause and continued indefinitely (Cauley et al., 1995), "even in the elderly" (Ott, 1992), can be
justified empirically on the basis of prospects for maintaining bone mass at a
level that reduces OP and fracture risk. The potential for primary prevention
exists, although Hodes (1995) has cited concerns that by the "year 2024, calcium,
vitamin D, and sex steroids might only prevent about half of the problem" (p.
75). At present, therapeutic interventions for primary prevention of OA are not
available, although in the future it might be possible to achieve primary prevention by personal health practices, especially weight control and exercises,
started earlier in life (see chapter 10). Such life-long practices have salutary
effects on many organ functions as well (see chapter 8). Brandt (1995) has recently reviewed therapeutic approaches for OA, and no disease-modifying drug
for this condition in humans is as yet available. While attention has been focused on the primary preservation of cartilage (e.g., limiting the action of proteases or interleukins in the joint), perhaps means to reduce the density of subchondral bone—the exact opposite of OP therapy—may limit the progression
of cartilage changes if, as Radin and Rose postulated, cartilage degradation is
indeed secondary to the density and stiffness in the subchondral bone. It is not

Table 7.3. The Spectrum of "Aging" and "Disease" in Osteoarthritis and Osteoporosis

Condition	Risk Factor	"Aging" Incipient[a]	Primary Prevention	"Disease" Manifestations	Tertiary Prevention
Osteoporosis	thinness	osteopenia	estrogens	fractures	none
Osteoarthritis	obesity, low muscle mass in lower limbs, joint injury	not known	? maintenance of ideal body weight, ? knee exercises	deformity, limited mobility, pain	joint replacement

[a]Refers to a preclinical state with symptoms below threshold (see also text of this chapter, and fig. 1.1).

likely that therapy designed to reduce bone density could be administered selectively to affect the hip, knee, or facet joint of a vertebra, and indeed, even if it were possible, the therapy might reduce OA risk while increasing osteopenia and fracture risk. However, this is only one of the many potential therapeutic innovations that can be anticipated, including "gene therapy for arthritis" (Doherty, 1995). The widespread attention already focused on OP, and the growing interest in understanding OA as a dynamic process over time rather than as a merely degenerative process, raise expectations for imaginative new breakthroughs in diagnosis and therapy for these skeletal conditions that exact such a high toll in the aging population.

ACKNOWLEDGMENTS

The author is grateful to Dr. Jan Dequeker, Arthritis and Metabolic Bone Disease Research Unit, Leuven, Belgium, for helpful discussions; to Dr. Nogah Haramati, Head of Bone Radiology, Albert Einstein College of Medicine and Montefiore Medical Center, New York, for providing and interpreting the skeletal x-rays in figure 7.1 and 7.2, and for advice on table 7.2; and to Dawn Bowen-Jenkins for expert secretarial assistance.

REFERENCES

Bagge E, Eden S, Rosen T, Bengtsson BA. 1993. The prevalence of radiographic osteoarthritis is low in elderly patients with growth hormone deficiency. *Acta Endocrinol* 129:296–300.

Belmonte-Serrano MA, Bloch DA, Lane NE, Michel BE, Fries JF. 1993. The relationship between spinal and peripheral osteoarthritis and bone density measures. *J Rheumatol* 20:1005–1013.

Bennett AE, Wahner HW, Riggs L, Hintz RL. 1984. Insulin-like growth factors I and II: Aging and bone density in women. *J Clin Endocrinol Metab* 59:701–704.

Birge SJ, Morrow-Howell N, Proctor EK. 1994. Hip fracture. *Clin Geriatr Med* 10:589–610.

Borst SE, Millard WJ, Lowenthal DT. 1994. Growth hormone, exercise, and aging: The future of therapy for the frail elderly. *J Am Geriatr Soc* 42:528–535.

Bouxsein ML, Marcus R. 1994. Overview of exercise and bone mass. *Rheum Dis Clin North Am* 20:787–802.

Boyd J. 1994. Molecular genetics of human endometrial carcinoma. In: *Protooncogenes and growth factors in steroid hormone induced growth and differentiation,* edited by SA Khan, GM Stancel. Pp. 193–205. Boca Raton: CRC Press.

Brandt KD. 1995. Toward pharmacologic modification of joint damage in osteoarthritis. *Ann Intern Med* 122:874–875.

Brandt KD, Fife RS, Braunstein EM, Katz B. 1991. Radiographic grading of the severity of knee osteoarthritis: Relation of the Kellgren and Lawrence grade to a grade based on joint space narrowing, and correlation with arthroscopic evidence of articular cartilage degeneration. *Arthritis Rheum* 36:1381–1386.

Buckland-Wright JC, Macfarlane DG, Lynch JA, Jasani MK. 1995. Quantitative microfocal radiography detects changes in OA knee joint space width in patients with placebo controlled trial of NSAID therapy. *J Rheumatol* 22:937–943.

Burger H, van Daele PLA, Odding E, Valkenburg HA, Hofman A, Grobbee DE, Schütte HE, Birkenhäger JC, Pols HAP. 1996. Association of radiographically evident osteoarthritis with higher bone mineral density and increased bone loss with age. *Arthritis Rheum* 39:81–86.

Canalis E. 1993. Systemic and local factors and the maintenance of bone quality. *Calcif Tissue Int* 53(suppl. 1):S90-S93.

————. 1996. Insulin-like growth factors and their role in osteoporosis. *Calcif Tissue Int* 58:133–134.

Carlson CS, Loeser RF, Purser CB, Gardin JF, Jerome CP. 1996. Osteoarthritis in cynomolgus macaques: III. Effects of age, gender, and subchondral bone thickness on the severity of disease. *J Bone Miner Res* 11:1209–1217.

Carlsson A, Nilsson BE, Westlin NE. 1979. Bone mass in primary coxarthrosis. *Acta Orthop Scand* 50:540–542.

Cauley JA, Seeley DG, Ensrud K, Ettinger B, Black D, Cummings SR. 1995. Estrogen replacement therapy and fractures in older women. *Ann Intern Med* 122:9–16.

Christiansen C. 1993. Skeletal osteoporosis. *J Bone Miner Res* 8:S475-S480.

Cooper C. 1995. Osteoporosis in rheumatological practice: Questions to be answered. *Ann Rheum Dis* 54:1–2.

Cooper C, Cook PL, Osmond C, Fisher L, Cauley MID. 1991. Osteoarthritis of the hip and osteoporosis of the proximal femur. *Ann Rheum Dis* 50:540–542.

Cuevas P, Burgos J, Baird A. 1988. Basic fibroblast growth factor (FGF) promotes cartilage repair in vivo. *Biochem Biophys Res Commun* 156:611–618.

de Boer H, Blok G-J, Van der Veen EA. 1995. Clinical aspects of growth hormone deficiency in adults. *Endocr Rev* 16:63–86.

Delany AM, Pash JM, Canalis E. 1994. Cellular and clinical perspectives on skeletal insulin-like growth factor 1. *J Cell Biochem* 55:328–333.

Delmas PD. 1993. Biochemical markers of bone turnover. *J Bone Miner Res* 8:S549-S555.

Dequeker J. 1985. The relationship between osteoporosis and osteoarthritis. *Clin Rheum Dis* 11:271–296.

Dequeker J, Westhovens R. 1995. Low dose corticosteroid associated osteoporosis in rheumatoid arthritis and its prophylaxis and treatment: Bones of contention. *J Rheumatol* 22:1013–1019.

Dequeker J, Johnell O, the MEDOS Study Group. 1993a. Osteoarthritis protects against femoral neck fracture: The MEDOS study experience. *Bone* 14:S51-S56.

Dequeker J, Mohan S, Finkelman RD, Aerssens J, Baylink DJ. 1993b. Generalized osteoarthritis associated with increased insulin-like growth factor types I and II and transforming growth factor β in cortical bone from the iliac crest. *Arthritis Rheum* 36:1702–1708.

Dieppe P, Kirwan J. 1994. The localization of osteoarthritis. *Br J Rheumatol* 33:201–204.

Doherty PJ. 1995. Gene therapy and arthritis. *J Rheumatol* 22:1220–1223.

Eckstein F, Müller-Gerbl M, Steinlechner M, Kierse R, Putz R. 1995. Subchondral bone density in the human elbow assessed by computed tomography osteo-absorptiometry: A reflection of the loading history of the joint surfaces. *J Orthop Res* 13:268–278.

Eisman JA. 1995. Vitamin D receptor gene alleles and osteoporosis: An affirmative view. *J Bone Min Res* 10:1289–1293.

Finkelman RD, Bell NH, Strong DD, Demers LM, Baylink DJ. 1992. Ovariectomy selectively reduces the concentration of transforming growth factor beta in rat bone: Implications for estrogen deficiency–associated bone loss. *Proc Natl Acad Sci USA* 89:12190–12193.

Formiga F, Moga I, Nolla JM, Pac M, Mitjavila F, Roig-Escofet D. 1995. Loss of bone mineral density in premenopausal women with systemic lupus erythematosus. *Ann Rheum Dis* 54:274–276.

Foss M, Byers PD. 1972. Bone density, osteoarthrosis of the hip, and fracture of the upper end of the femur. *Ann Rheum Dis* 31:259–264.

Genant HK. 1988. Quantitative bone mineral analysis. In: *Diagnosis of bone and joint disorders*, edited by D Resnick, G Niwayama. 2d ed. Vol. 4, pp. 1998–2020. Philadelphia: WB Saunders.

Ghiron LJ, Thompson JL, Holloway L, Hintz RL, Butterfield GE, Hoffman AR, Marcus R. 1995. Effects of recombinant insulin-like growth factor–1 and growth hormone on bone turnover in elderly women. *J Bone Miner Res* 10:1844–1852.

Greenspan SL, Myers ER, Maitland LA, Resnick NM, Hayes WC. 1994. Fall severity and bone mineral density as risk factors for hip fracture in ambulatory elderly. *JAMA* 271:128–133.

Hadler NM. 1992. Knee pain is the malady—not osteoarthritis. *Ann Rheum Dis* 53:143–146.

Hamerman D. 1989. The biology of osteoarthritis. *N Engl J Med* 320:1322–1330.

———. 1993. Prospects for medical intervention in cartilage repair. In: *Joint cartilage degradation: Basic and clinical aspects,* edited by JF Woessner Jr., DS Howell. Pp. 529–546, New York: Marcel Dekker.

———. 1995. Clinical implications of osteoarthritis and ageing. *Ann Rheum Dis* 54:82–85.

Hamerman D, Stanley ER. 1996. Perspective: Implications of increased bone density in osteoarthritis. *J Bone Miner Res* 11:1205–1208.

Hamerman D, Taylor S. 1993. Humoral factors in the pathogenesis of osteoarthritis. In: *Humoral factors in the regulation of tissue growth,* edited by PP Foa. Pp. 267–285. New York: Springer Verlag.

Hamerman D, Taylor S, Kirschenbaum I, Klagsbrun M, Raines EW, Ross R, Thomas KA. 1987. Growth factors with heparin binding affinity in human synovial fluid. *Proc Soc Exp Biol Med* 186:384–389.

Hannan MT, Anderson JJ, Zhang Y, Levy D, Felson DT. 1993. Bone mineral density and knee osteoarthritis in elderly men and women. *Arthritis Rheum* 36:1671–1689.

Harrison MHM, Schajowicz F, Trueta J. 1953. Osteoarthritis of the hip: A study of the nature and the evolution of the disease. *J Bone Joint Surg* 35B:598–626.

Hart DJ, Mootoosamy I, Doyle DV, Spector TD. 1994. The relationship between osteoarthritis and osteoporosis in the general population: The Chingford Study. *Ann Rheum Dis* 53:158–162.

Hochberg MC, Lethbridge-Cejku M, Scott WW Jr., Plato CC, Tobin JD. 1994a. Appendicular bone mass and osteoarthritis of the hands in women: Data from the Baltimore Longitudinal Study of Aging. *J Rheumatol* 21:1532–1536.

Hochberg MC, Lethbridge-Cejku M, Scott WW Jr., Reichle R, Plato CC, Tobin JD. 1994b. Serum levels of insulin-like growth factor 1 in subjects with osteoarthritis of the knee. *Arthritis Rheum* 37:1177–1180.

Hodes RJ. 1994. Frailty and disability: Can growth hormone or other trophic agents make a difference? *J Am Geriatr Soc* 42:1208–1211.

———. 1995. Osteoporosis: Emerging research strategies aim at bone biology, risk factors, interventions. *J Am Geriatr Soc* 43:75–77.

Holloway L, Butterfield G, Hintz RL, Gesundheit N, Marcus R. 1994. Effects of recombinant human growth hormone on metabolic indices, body composition, and bone turnover in healthy elderly women. *J Clin Endocrinol Metab* 79:470–479.

Hordon LD, Stewart SP, Troughton PR, Wright V, Horsman A, Smith MA. 1993. Primary generalized osteoarthritis and bone mass. *Br J Rheumatol* 32:1059–1061.

Horowitz MC. 1993. Cytokines and estrogen in bone: Anti-osteoporotic effects. *Science* 260:626–627.

Hughes MJ, Lingrel JB, Krakowsky JM, Anderson KP. 1993. A helix-loop-helix transcription factor-like gene is located at the mi locus. *J Biol Chem* 268:20687–20690.

Inzucchi SE, Robbins RJ. 1994. Effects of growth hormone on human bone biology. *J Clin Endocrinol Metab* 79:691–684.

Jergas M, Genant HK. 1993. Current methods and recent advances in the diagnosis of osteoporosis. *Arthritis Rheum* 36:1649–1662.

Jiminez SA, Dharmavaram RM. 1994. Genetic aspects of familial osteoarthritis. *Ann Rheum Dis* 53:789–797.

Johnson RS, Spiegelman BM, Papaioannou V. 1992. Pleiotropic effects of a null mutation in the c-fos proto-oncogene. *Cell* 71:577–586.

Johnston CC Jr., Slemenda CW, Melton LJ III. 1991. Clinical use of bone densitometry. *N Engl J Med* 324:1105–1109.

Jones G, Nguyen T, Sambrook PN, Lord SR, Kelly PJ, Eisman JA. 1995. Osteoarthritis, bone density, postural stability, and osteoporotic fractures: A population based study. *J Rheumatol* 22:921–925.

Jones JI, Clemmons DR. 1995. Insulin-like growth factors and their binding proteins: Biological actions. *Endocr Rev* 16:3–34.

Joyce ME, Roberts AB, Sporn MB, Bolander ME. 1990. Transforming growth factor-β and the initiation of chondrogenesis and osteogenesis in the rat femur. *J Cell Biol* 110:2195–2207.

Judd J, Kremer M, Oursler MJ. 1995. Age dependence of estrogen responsiveness. *Calcif Tissue Int* 56:S25-S26.

Kahn A, Gibbons R, Perkins S, Gazit D. 1995. Age-related bone loss. *Clin Orthop Rel Res* 313:69–75.

Kanis JA, Melton LJ III, Christiansen C, Johnston CC, Khaltaev N. 1994. The diagnosis of osteoporosis. *J Bone Miner Res* 9:1137–1141.

Kellgren JH, Moore R. 1952. Generalized osteoarthritis and Heberden's nodes. *Br Med J* 1:181–187.

Knight SM, Ring EFJ, Bhalla AK. 1992. Bone mineral density and osteoarthritis. *Ann Rheum Dis* 51:1025–1026.

Lane NE, Nevitt MC. 1994. Osteoarthritis and bone mass. *J Rheumatol* 21:1393–1396.

Lewis LJ, Bell SJ. 1990. Nutritional assessment of the elderly. In: *Geriatric nutrition,* edited by JE Morley, Z Glick, LZ Rubenstein. Pp. 73–87. New York: Raven Press.

Ljunghall S, Johansson AG, Burman P, Kämpe O, Lindh E, Karlsson FA. 1992. Low plasma levels of insulin-like growth factor 1 (IGF-1) in male patients with idiopathic osteoporosis. *J Intern Med* 232:59–64.

Lloyd ME, Hart DJ, Nandra D, McAlindon TE, Wheeler M, Doyle DV, Spector TD. 1996. The relationship between insulin like growth factor–1 levels, knee osteoarthritis, bone density, and fracture in the general population: The Chingford Study. *Ann Rheum Dis* 55:870–874.

Manolagas SC. 1995. Role of cytokines in bone resorption. *Bone* 17:63S-76S.

Manolagas SC, Jilka RL. 1995. Bone marrow, cytokines, and bone remodeling. *N Engl J Med* 332:305–311.

McAlindon RE, Teale JD, Dieppe P. 1993. Levels of insulin related growth factor 1 in osteoarthritis of the knee. *Ann Rheum Dis* 52:229–231.

Melton LJ III. 1993. Hip fractures: A worldwide problem today and tomorrow. *Bone* 14:S1-S8.

———. 1995. How many women have osteoporosis now? *J Bone Miner Res* 10:175–177.

Melton LJ III, Chao EYS, Lane J. 1988. Biomechanical aspects of fractures. In: *Osteoporosis: Etiology, diagnosis, and management,* edited by BL Riggs, LJ Melton III. Pp. 111–131. New York: Raven Press.

Mundy GR. 1991. The effects of TGF-β on bone. In: *Clinical applications of TGF-β,* edited by GR Bock, J Marsh. Pp. 137–151. Ciba Foundation Symposium 157. Chichester, U.K.: John Wiley and Sons.

———. 1994. Peptides and growth regulatory factors in bone. *Rheum Dis Clin North Am* 20:577–588.

———. 1995. The genetics of osteoporosis. *Endocrinologist* 5:176–179.

Nevitt MC, Lane NE, Scott JC, Hochberg MC, Pressman AR, Genant HK, Cummings SR. 1995. Radiographic osteoarthritis of the hip and bone mineral density. *Arthritis Rheum* 38:907–916.

Nguyen T, Sambrook P, Kelly PJ, Jones G, Lord S, Freund J, Eisman J. 1993. Prediction of osteoporotic fractures by postural instability and bone density. *Br Med J* 307:1111–1115.

Ott SM. 1992. Estrogen therapy for osteoporosis—even in the elderly. *Ann Intern Med* 117:85–86.

Papadakis MA, Grady D, Black D, Tierney MJ, Gooding GAW, Schambelan M, Grunfeld C. 1996. Growth hormone replacement in healthy older men improves body composition but not functional ability. *Ann Intern Med* 124:708–716.

Parfitt AM. 1991. Growth hormone and adult bone remodelling. *Clin Endocrinol* 35:467–470.

———. 1995. Problems in the application of *in vitro* systems to the study of human bone remodelling. *Calcif Tissue Int* 56(suppl. 1):S5-S7.

Peel NFA, Barrington NA, Blumsohn A, Colwell A, Hannon R, Eastell R. 1995. Bone mineral density and bone turnover in spinal osteoarthrosis. *Ann Rheum Dis* 54:867–871.

Poli V, Balena R, Fattori E, Markatos A, Yamamoto M, Tanaka H, Ciliberto G, Rodan GA, Costantini F. 1994. Interleukin-6 deficient mice are protected from bone loss caused by estrogen depletion. *EMBO J* 13:1189–1196.

Pollard JW, Stanley ER. 1996. Pleiotropic roles for CSF-1 in development defined by the mouse mutation osteopetrotic *(op)*. *Adv Develop Biochem* 4:153–196.

Radin EL, Rose RM. 1986. Role of subchondral bone in the initiation and progression of cartilage damage. *Clin Orthop* 213:34–40.

Raisz LG. 1993. Bone cell biology: Approaches and unanswered questions. *J Bone Min Res* 8(suppl. 2):S457-S465.

Resnick D, Niwayama G. 1988. Osteoporosis. In: *Diagnosis of bone and joint disorders,* edited by D Resnick, G Niwayama. 2d ed. Vol. 14, pp. 2022–2085. Philadelphia: WB Saunders.

Rosen CJ, Donahue LR, Hunter SJ. 1994. Insulin-like growth factors and bone: The osteoporosis connection. *Proc Soc Exp Biol Med* 206:83–102.

Rudman D, Feller AG, Nagraj HS, Gergans GA, Lalitha PY, Goldberg AF, Schlenker RA, et al. 1990. Effect of human growth hormone in men over 60 years old. *N Engl J Med* 323:1–6.

Schouten JSAG, van den Ouweland FA, Valkenburg HA, Lamberts SWJ. 1993. Insulin-like growth factor–1: A prognostic factor of knee osteoarthritis. *Br J Rheumatol* 32:274–280.

Soriano P, Montgomery C, Geske R, Bradley A. 1991. Targeted disruption of the c-src proto-oncogene leads to osteopetrosis in mice. *Cell* 64:693–702.

Spector TD. 1995. Measuring joint space in knee osteoarthritis: Position or precision? *J Rheumatol* 22:807–808.

Spector TD, Cooper C. 1993. Radiographic assessment of osteoarthritis in population studies: Whither Kellgren and Lawrence? *Osteoarthritis Cartilage* 1:203–206.

Star VL, Hochberg MC. 1994. Osteoporosis in patients with rheumatic diseases. *Rheum Dis Clin North Am* 20:561–576.

Termine JD. 1988. Non-collagenous proteins in bone. In: *Cell and molecular biology of vertebrate hard tissues,* edited by D Evered, S Harnett. Pp. 178–190. Ciba Foundation Symposium 136. Chichester, U.K.: John Wiley and Sons.

————. 1990. Cellular activity, matrix proteins, and aging bone. *Exp Gerontol* 25:217–221.

Thiry-Blaise LM, Taquet A-N, Reginster JY, Nusgens B, Franchimont P, Lapière ChM. 1995. Investigation of the relationship between osteoporosis and the collagenase gene by means of polymorphism of the 5′ upstream region of this gene. *Calcif Tissue Int* 56:88–91.

Turner RT, Riggs BL, Spelsberg TC. 1994. Skeletal effects of estrogen. *Endocr Rev* 15:275–300.

Wallace WA. 1983. The increasing incidence of fractures of the proximal femur: An orthopaedic epidemic. *Lancet* 1:1413–1414.

Woessner JF Jr., Howell DS, eds. 1993. *Joint and cartilage degradation: Basic and clinical aspects.* New York: Marcel Dekker.

Woolf AD, Dixon ASJ. 1988. *Osteoporosis: A clinical guide.* Philadelphia: JB Lippincott.

Wüster C. 1992. Growth hormone and bone metabolism. *Acta Endocrinol* 128:14–18.

PART III

Exercise as a Therapeutic Modality in Aging and Osteoarthritis

8

The Principles and Prescription of Exercise for Frail Older Persons

James Oat Judge, M.D.

This chapter discusses the importance of physical activity and exercise as a primary and secondary preventive strategy to maintain independent functioning for older persons. Maintaining independence is a primary clinical goal for all health professionals who work with older persons. Physical activity and regular exercise may be the most effective preventive strategy to increase the proportion of older persons who are independent into their ninth and tenth decades. This chapter will also review prospective epidemiologic studies and clinical research findings that support the recommendations for physical activity and exercise, and the components of a complete exercise program.

Current Physical Activity Recommendations

The Centers for Disease Control and Prevention (CDC-P) and the American College of Sports Medicine (ACSM) developed a consensus recommendation for physical activity for adults in 1995. The recommendation is that adults engage in 180 minutes or more of physical activity every week, and the activity should occur on most, if not all, days (Pate et al., 1995). This translates into about 25 minutes of physical activity per day. Normal everyday activities such as walking to the store to get a newspaper, carrying laundry, carrying the trash, and doing certain types of gardening would be considered physical activity by the consensus panel.

The benefits of a physically active lifestyle accrue from direct effects on muscle strength, endurance and flexibility, maintenance of body composition

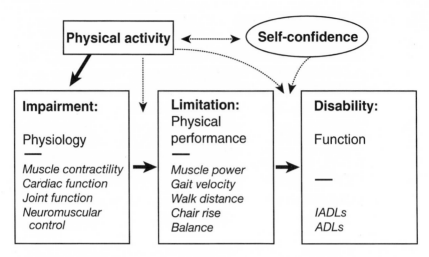

Figure 8.1.   Postulated model of the influence of physical activity on function. The model of disability is adapted from Nagi (1976). The thick *solid lines* represent associations that have been found in prospective and cross-sectional studies. The *dotted lines* represent plausible relationships between physical activity, self-confidence, performance, and function.

(bone mineral density, muscle mass, and percentage of body fat), and possibly balance. An active lifestyle maintains independence indirectly—physical activity lowers the incidence of conditions such as cardiovascular disease, stroke, and diabetes mellitus, which are important causes of disability (Fried et al., 1994). Heart disease, stroke, arthritis, and dementia are the four leading medical conditions that are responsible for disability in older persons. Physical activity prevents vascular diseases and may slow bone loss (primary prevention), and exercise programs improve functional status in persons with knee arthritis and coronary artery disease (secondary or tertiary prevention). Chapter 10 discusses aspects of exercise in the primary prevention of knee osteoarthritis.

In the population over age 75, the prevalence of dependence is greatest with regard to activities that require combinations of endurance, strength, and balance (e.g., shopping, traveling, walking more than one-half mile, and doing heavy housework). For such activities, there are 0.67 Instrumental Activities of Daily Living (IADL) dependencies per person in the population over age 75 (USDHHS, 1992). Activities that require balance and joint flexibility (e.g., dressing, grooming oneself, and eating) have much lower rates of dependency. Incidence rates of dependence declined significantly over the years 1982–89 (Manton et al., 1993). Figure 8.1 illustrates the documented and theoretical relationships between physical activity and disability. The model of disability in this figure was developed by Nagi (1976). The Nagi disability model distinguishes between impairment in physiology (at the organ level), limitations (at the organism level), and social roles (activities of daily living [ADL]). This is also discussed in chapter 5. Physical activity and disease help determine the degree of physiologic impairment. However, in persons with disease and known physiologic impairment, physical activity can also prevent limitation in physical performance and dependence in ADL (Mor et al., 1989; Young et al., 1995).

A strategy that combines primary prevention efforts to increase the physical activity levels of healthy older adults with secondary prevention efforts to increase activity in persons at high risk for disability is likely to be most effective. While the trials that will determine the efficacy of increasing physical activity in persons with early impairments in function are only beginning, there is sufficient epidemiologic and intervention data to prescribe physical activity for nearly all older persons (Buchner et al., 1992; Wagner et al., 1992).

The Role of Physical Activity in Primary Prevention of Mobility Defects

In prospective studies, physically active older persons, free of chronic diseases, have a risk of developing mobility deficits which is only 40 to 70 percent as great as the risk found among inactive older persons (Mor et al., 1989; LaCroix et al., 1993; Young et al., 1995). However, almost half of the older population engages in no regular physical activity. For the majority of older adults, a sedentary lifestyle precedes and predicts disability (Simonsick et al., 1993).

Some physical activities that are not considered "exercise" reduce overall mortality and cardiovascular mortality. Low levels of physical activity or reduced cardiovascular endurance are independent risk factors for all-cause and cardiovascular mortality (Blair et al., 1989). A study of Harvard alumni found that beginning exercise or increasing physical activity late in life (after age 60) was still effective in prolonging life (Lee et al., 1995). The Harvard alumni study also reported that vigorous physical activity (activities of 6 METs or greater) is required to prolong life (Lee et al., 1995). (A MET is equal to 3.5 mL $\times$ kg^{-1} $\times$ min^{-1} of oxygen consumption and represents a person's metabolic rate.) This level of activity can be achieved with brisk walking, jogging, or walking up hills (American College of Sports Medicine, 1993).

Physical activity (exercise at least once per week) also reduced the incidence of diabetes mellitus about 40 percent in males as a group, and 60 percent in overweight men (Helmrich et al., 1991). High levels of physical activity are also associated with significantly lower rates of colon cancer (Giovannucci et al., 1995).

While there are many strategies to increase physical activity and fitness levels, one model suggests that the greatest reduction in death and disability will be achieved by increasing individuals' usual activity to the "next higher level"— that is, by getting sedentary persons to be occasionally active, occasionally active persons to be regularly active, and regularly active persons to become regular exercisers (Pate et al., 1995). This strategy makes sense from a behavioral perspective: it is reasonable to encourage persons to increase the frequency or intensity of their physical activities but it is probably unrealistic to expect a large proportion of older sedentary persons to become senior Olympians, or master athletes.

Maintenance of Body Composition and Muscle Power

Body composition is dependent on long-term patterns of usual activity, energy (food) intake, and status of anabolic and catabolic hormones. Muscle mass is lost at a rate of 0.5 percent to 1.0 percent annually after the age of 60 years. As body weight is stable or increases, the percentage of body mass made up by fat increases substantially (Flynn et al., 1989). Muscle strength declines by 20 to 40 percent between the third and the eighth decade (Stalberg et al., 1989; Overend et al., 1992). This decline is due to loss of muscle mass and contractility (force per square centimeter of muscle cross-section). Vigorous physical activity is associated with maintaining muscle strength, mass, and contractility (Klitgaard et al., 1990).

Maintenance of bone mineral density is also related to one's lifetime pattern of usual physical activity, and fracture rates are inversely related to lifetime physical activity. A lifetime of a high level of physical activity was associated with greater femoral bone density, a prime protector against hip fracture (Greendale et al., 1995). A sedentary lifestyle (spending less than 4 hours a day standing) and low levels of physical activity were independent risk factors for hip fractures for older white women, after adjusting for age and bone density (Cummings et al., 1995). Intense endurance or resistance training in post-menopausal women increases spinal and femoral bone mineral density modestly (Dalsky et al., 1988; Nelson, 1995).

Physical Activity and Confidence

Confidence is an important factor in maintaining independence in ADL (see fig. 8.1). Confidence in performing activities safely is strongly associated with independence in IADL and affects the relationship between physical performance capability and functional independence (Tinetti et al., 1994b). An older person with muscle weakness, lower endurance, or impaired balance must decide which activities can be performed safely. Many older persons stop performing activities because they are concerned that they cannot complete the activities safely. Curtailing physical activity decreases strength and endurance and may possibly worsen balance. The vicious cycle of declining activity, performance, and self-confidence may be interrupted by interventions that improve components of function (e.g., strength, flexibility, endurance) and performance (e.g., walking, challenging balance activities).

The Role of Physical Activity in Secondary Prevention of Mobility Defects

Maintaining Independence in the Face of Disease

Older persons with chronic disease benefit from physical activity because it helps them to maintain functional independence (Kaplan et al., 1987; Young et al., 1995). There is strong evidence that physical impairments are associated with prevalent difficulty in IADL, as well as with risk of future loss of mobility and nursing home admission (Guralnik et al., 1994, 1995). There is some controversy about whether loss of mobility is disease specific (Fried et al., 1994) or whether loss of function is part of a syndrome of failing function (Tinetti et al., 1995). The disease-based model will suggest that interventions targeted at the disease process will be most effective in preventing disability. The syndrome approach suggests that a multifaceted intervention to prevent disability will be most effective.

Interventions in Frail Elderly Persons

Tinetti et al. (1994a) used a multifaceted intervention (syndrome approach) in older persons at risk for falls, and succeeded in reducing fall rates by 31 percent, as well as improving clinical measures of poor balance and muscle weakness. Standard interventions were given to subjects on the basis of the deficits present during baseline testing. For example, subjects with impaired balance received balance exercises, and subjects with lower-extremity muscle weakness performed muscle strengthening with resistance supplied by thick rubber bands. Kovar et al. (1992) used a disease-specific approach to test the effects of exercise training in subjects with knee osteoarthritis (OA), as discussed in chapter 9.

Many frail elderly persons have more than one chronic condition or illness, and thus, for the majority, interventions must take a syndrome approach. For example, slow gait velocity may be due to a combination of cardiac disease that limits cardiac output, and OA, which makes walking less efficient (more energy consuming). The combination of two diseases may result in greater disability than the sum of both diseases separately, as is also noted in chapter 6. That is, there may be a synergy in the effect of chronic diseases on performance and function.

Components of Function

Muscle Strength

Muscle weakness is associated with declines in gait, with IADL dependence, and with increased risk of falls (Tinetti et al., 1989). Knee extension (quadriceps) and ankle plantar flexor (gastrocnemius/soleus) strength are associated with gait velocity and step length (Bassey et al., 1988). However, the association between strength and gait may be due to two pathways: a direct causal link between muscle strength and gait; and a direct causal link between a high level of physical activity and gait. Physical activity can maintain muscle strength and balance (Judge et al., 1995).

Effects of Strength (Resistance) Training

Short-term supervised resistance training can increase strength substantially and is well tolerated by both independent and frail elderly persons. A 12-week resistance training program of knee flexion and extension in older men (aged 60–72 years) increased isokinetic knee moments (torque or strength) 10.0–18.5 percent, doubled the 1-repetition maximum weight lifted (1 RM), and increased mid-thigh muscle area 11 percent (Frontera et al., 1988). Older women (64–86 years) can increase lower-extremity strength (1 RM) substantially with short-term intense resistance training (Charette et al., 1991; Nichols et al., 1993). Comparable results occur with upper-extremity training (Brown and Holloszy, 1993). Nursing home residents had greater percentage improvements in 1 RM compared to studies of healthy elderly persons, but the absolute gains (in numbers of kilograms lifted) are similar or lower in nursing home subjects (Fiatarone et al., 1994).

Resistance training improves muscle contractility—a given cross-sectional area of muscle can generate more force during maximal voluntary effort, or can shorten faster under a given load and develop greater power (Sale, 1988). The increase in muscle power is due predominantly to increased neural drive of muscles, not to muscle hypertrophy (Moritani and DeVries, 1979). Resistance training had little or no effect on muscle mass in nursing home subjects in a short-term study (Fiatarone et al., 1994), but it maintained or increased muscle mass in medium-term and long-term studies (Nelson et al., 1995; Sipila and Suominen, 1995).

Functional Benefits of Resistance Training

Resistance training results are most impressive when the outcome is 1 RM (maximum lift on the training machine). The gains are much smaller when the outcome is the maximum lift on another machine, or force or joint movement at a different speed of contraction—for example, when strength is measured during fast movement when slow movements were trained, or when a different mode of contraction (e.g., isokinetic rather than isotonic) is measured (Moffroid and Whipple, 1970; Fleck and Kraemer, 1987). The specificity of resistance training effects suggests that to improve functional status, resistance training exercises should resemble challenging functional tasks in joint speed, range of motion (ROM), and the type of force generated (shortening or lengthening). For example, a sitting leg press exercise trains multiple muscle groups (quadriceps, hamstrings, gluteus, gastrocnemius, and soleus) to generate force in a coordinated fashion. This exercise is similar to getting out of a chair without using one's arms, or rising from a crouch position. This would theoretically be a better exercise than isolated muscle group resistance training, but no studies have compared the effects of different modes of resistance training on function.

In nursing home residents, intense resistance training that included leg press training increased gait velocity 12 percent (an increase of 0.05 m/sec) and increased stair-climbing power 23–38 percent (Fiatarone et al., 1994). Combined resistance-balance training in life-care community residents increased gait velocity 8 percent (0.08 m/sec) (Judge et al., 1993). Resistance training in relatively healthy community-dwelling older subjects did not increase gait velocity (Brown and Holloszy, 1993; Judge et al., 1994).

Endurance

Endurance, or fitness, usually expressed as vO_2 max or oxygen uptake (in milliliters of O_2 per kilogram per minute) declines with aging in sedentary people and athletes, but the rate of decline is about twice as great in sedentary persons. This results in older athletes having fitness levels comparable to sedentary persons 20–30 years younger. Fitness declines in parallel with reduction in skeletal mass, and about half the decline in fitness with age can be explained by the loss of muscle mass (Fleg and Lakatta, 1988). The other half is due to reduced maximum heart rate, reduced maximum stroke volume, and reduced oxygen extraction by working muscle. Endurance exercise can improve all of the factors that contribute to fitness except maximum heart rate. Endurance training improves cardiac output primarily by increasing stroke volume. Endurance exercise increases blood volume in older persons, which improves blood flow back to the heart during exercise (Carroll et al., 1995).

Increased oxygen extraction (atrioventricular O_2 difference) by working muscle is responsible for much of the improvement in fitness which results from endurance training (Spina et al., 1993). The response to endurance training, when measured as a percentage improvement in fitness (oxygen uptake), is similar in young and old persons. The improvement in fitness measures is related to the intensity of the endurance training. Vigorous training, at about 75 percent of maximum heart rate, four times weekly for 45 minutes (3 hours total exercise per week) for 9 or more months will increase maximum oxygen uptake about 20 percent (Coggan et al., 1992; Spina et al., 1993). Lower-intensity endurance training increases oxygen uptake about 10–15 percent, but there are no definitive studies in frail older subjects. While walking programs, including walking uphill on a treadmill, are generally well tolerated (Carroll et al., 1995), running and jogging are associated with high rates of musculoskeletal injuries (Pollock et al., 1991).

Interactions of Endurance and Strength Training

The association of muscle mass and fitness noted above provides an opportunity for training in either domain (strength or fitness) to improve physiologic reserve in the other. For example, while resistance training does not improve endurance function in young subjects, 10 weeks of heavy resistance training in older men increased aerobic power of the leg (as measured by oxygen consumption on a bicycle ergometer) (Frontera et al., 1988). Two recent studies have found that endurance programs improve strength, maximal work, and muscle cross-sectional area. A long-term program of aerobic training and low-resistance exercise in older women (with a mean age of 72) improved oxygen uptake 16 percent, isokinetic strength 6.5 percent, and muscle cross-sectional area (Cress et al., 1991). Other endurance training studies have failed to improve muscle cross-sectional area (Sipila and Suominen, 1995). Prolonged endurance training in older sedentary subjects aged 60–75 years reduced body fat and maintained or increased muscle mass (Kohrt et al., 1992). Combined endurance and light resistance training improved fitness and strength measures in older men (Morey et al., 1991).

Functional Benefits of Endurance Training

One trial of sequential training—3 months of resistance training followed by endurance exercises for 12 months (a combination of walking, uphill treadmill walking, bicycling, and jogging) at 75–85 percent of maximum heart rate—had striking results. Three months of resistance training increased plantar flexor strength between 17 and 23 percent, and knee extension between 7 and 12 percent, but gait velocity (which was 1.09 m/sec) did not improve. The 12-month endurance program increased gait velocity 8 percent and increased isometric plantar flexor strength 16 percent above the resistance training level but did not improve knee extension strength (Brown and Holloszy, 1993). This study suggests that vigorous endurance programs can maintain or increase the strength gains achieved by resistance training and that performance gains are training specific—endurance training will improve walking more than will resistance training.

Flexibility

Restrictions in joint ROM are very common in older persons and are due more frequently to muscle/tendon tightness than to joint contractures. Tight calf muscles are also very common and may limit dorsiflexor power to prevent backward falls. Tight hip flexors and adductors are frequently found in persons with thoracic kyphosis. Tightness in hip adductors and hip abductors is also frequent.

Balance

The balance function depends on the processing of sensory data, the generation of appropriate motor responses, and the generation of joint moments (muscle force or power) to control the movement of the body while moving or turning, and to prevent a fall after a perturbation of the body's center of mass. The decline in balance measures which occurs with advancing age is related to muscle weakness, but muscle weakness explains only a portion of the decline in balance (Judge et al., 1995). Older persons improve balance measures with repeated attempts (Wolfson et al., 1992; Judge et al., 1995). The acute improvement in laboratory-based measures suggests that balance performance is "plastic" and that balance performance can improve with training. Laboratory measures of balance can improve with a combination of high-tech performance systems (visual biofeedback of center of pressure position, and tilt exercises). Several balance training trials have improved laboratory measures of balance, and a meta-analysis of the Frailties and Injuries: Cooperative Studies of Intervention Techniques (FICSIT) trial found that balance training reduced fall rates 17 percent in a wide range of older subjects (Province et al., 1995). Older persons at high risk for falls who performed a combination of balance, strength, and flexibility exercises (in combination with adjustments in medication) reduced the risk of falls substantially over 12 months (Tinetti et al., 1994a).

Training in specific challenging activities such as reaching, leaning, turning, and lifting may improve balance performance. This training strategy may reduce the frequency of losses of balance. Components of Tai Chi, a traditional part of Chinese martial arts training which employs the practice of slow, deliberate movements, have been used in several studies (Judge et al., 1993; Wolfson et al., 1996). A large trial using Tai Chi as the primary intervention is in progress (Wolf et al., 1996), but the effects of Tai Chi training on falls has been included in a meta-analysis that found that balance training decreases the fall rate (Province et al., 1995).

Prescribing Exercise and Physical Activity

Exercise programs can reduce physiologic limitations over the short term (2–3 months), but long-lasting improvement in performance and functional status will probably require a long-term change in lifestyle involving a higher level of physical activity. There are no conclusive data on why people adapt and maintain an increased level of physical activity (Garcia and King, 1991; King, in American College of Sports Medicine, 1993). An exercise program should be designed to achieve the personal goals of the older person and to incorporate activities that are enjoyable, or at least not unpleasant to perform. Individual performance goals vary widely—for example, they may range from becoming able to get in and out of the bathtub independently, to becoming able to walk briskly up hills through the woods. Our current recommendation is that the older person should set specific performance goals that have personal meaning or value. These self-selected performance goals will serve as yardsticks (metrics), which will demonstrate improvement in performance and function due to increased physical activity.

The exercise components listed in table 8.1 can serve as a checklist in prescribing exercise. The use of an exercise prescription form with a checklist of items listed in table 8.1 will also demonstrate the importance the physician attaches to increased physical activity.

Resistance (Strength) Training

Resistance training has immediate benefits in terms of muscle strength; these benefits occur within 6–8 weeks and are a result of improvements in muscle contractility. Gains in strength (as a percentage of baseline strength) have been greatest in subjects in nursing home studies (Fiatarone et al., 1994). Functional activities require generating static force, generating power, and absorbing power. For example, holding a laundry basket or a quart of milk requires static muscle force (isometric muscle contraction), rising from a chair or climbing stairs requires power generation (concentric muscle contraction), and walking briskly or descending stairs requires substantial power absorption (eccentric muscle contraction).

Intensity

To increase muscle force (strength) substantially, exercising the muscle at a high percentage of its maximal force until it reaches a state of fatigue is recommended. Muscle fatigue occurs when the muscle can no longer generate force despite maximal voluntary neural drive. The higher the resistance (as a proportion of maximal force), the lower the number of lifts that can be performed before muscle fatigue occurs. Resistance training to fatigue involves performing a series of lifts (a "set") until a lift cannot be completed with correct form. A set is defined as a number of lifts performed with little or no rest between lifts. Some protocols prescribe a fixed number of lifts (e.g., 12–15) per set and do not train to muscle fatigue. Most training protocols adjust the resistance so that fatigue occurs after 8–14 lifts. The intensity of resistance training varies between studies, but most studies that have found substantial strength improvements trained muscles at 70–80 percent of the maximum single lift the person could perform (i.e., the one-repetition maximum, or 1 RM). However, a recent study in healthy older women found that low-intensity (40% of 1 RM) resistance training achieved an improvement in 1 RM similar to that achieved by high-intensity resistance training (80% of 1 RM), in hip abduction and adduction, knee flexion, leg press, biceps curl, and back extension. Only knee extension improved significantly more in the high-intensity group than in the low-intensity group (79% and 39%, respectively) (Taaffe et al., 1995). More studies are needed to determine the dose/response curve of resistance training

Table 8.1. Exercise Prescription

Component	Mode	Frequency	Intensity	Duration
Flexibility and posture	static stretch calf hamstrings hip abductors shoulders thoracic/cervical spine extension ("Attention!")	daily	should elicit feeling of stretch, not pain	15 sec per muscle group
Endurance	walking walking up hills and/or stairs climbing and/or step-ups cycling (recumbent or upright) swimming walking in water	> 4 times per week	moderate perceived exertion: Borg RPE scale 3–5; "moderate to strong," or 50–75% of maximum (age-predicted) heart rate	20–30 min/day (activity not necessarily continuous); increase duration, then increase intensity
Resistance	isolated muscle group contractions multiple joint motions (unilateral and bilateral) chair rises step-ups, step-downs water resistance	2–3 times per week	for rapid gains: high intensity (75–80% of 1 RM), increase resistance weekly; for slower gains or maintenance: moderate intensity (40–70% of 1 RM)	2 or 3 sets of each motion, limited by fatigue
Balance	concentration—postural awareness while standing, leaning, and turning torso control (pelvic tilt exercise) Tai Chi mobility: dance movements, walking over obstacles, vertical transfers, turns	1–3 times per week	depends on supervision and individual balance function; safety is primary concern	variable; can be incorporated into flexibility exercises

in older subjects. In very elderly frail subjects, the best study suggests that high-intensity training will achieve better results (Fiatarone et al., 1994). Hemo-dynamic responses are greater if resistance is set at more than 80 percent of the maximum lift. There is no additional benefit, only risk for cardiovascular and musculoskeletal injury, with training at an intensity setting greater than 80 percent of 1 RM. Nearly every "high-intensity" training study has started with several weeks of lower-intensity (50–70% of 1 RM) training before beginning high-intensity training. Two or three sets of each exercise are performed during a training session.

Frequency and Duration

Most training studies that achieved substantial strength gains in older persons trained three times a week. It is possible that training muscle groups twice a week may be sufficient to increase strength. The duration of the resistance session probably should not exceed 45 minutes unless substantial rest periods are included. Most protocols have trained five or fewer muscle groups during a session.

Substantial strength gains commonly occur within 8–12 weeks but may not plateau until training has continued for at least 24 weeks (McCartney et al., 1995). It is reasonable to prescribe resistance training for muscle groups with identified weakness for at least 12 weeks, or for several weeks after a plateau in strength is reached. Maintaining strength gains probably requires one or two training sessions per week at the final training resistance, but there are few data to support this claim (Pollock et al., 1991).

Exercises for Improving Strength

Frail persons are more likely to improve their performance of functional tasks if the resistance exercises train movement and patterns of muscle contraction which are similar to the patterns of muscle contraction during functional tasks. Nearly all machine and free weight exercises provide combined concentric (shortening) and eccentric (lengthening) muscle training. There is insufficient information on whether isolated muscle group training (e.g., unilateral knee extension or flexion) is superior to multiple-joint resistance training (some types of which are termed "closed-chain exercise"). The sitting leg press is an example of a multiple-joint exercise that combines hip, knee, and ankle extension during a single movement. Repeated chair rises and step-ups are closed-chain motions: training these motions directly trains performance of functional tasks. The military press and seated row exercises are multiple-joint upper-extremity exercises that involve movement at elbow, shoulder, and scapula, and stabilization of the wrist. While awaiting definitive trials, it is reasonable to prescribe both isolated muscle group training and multiple-joint (and closed-chain) training.

Sandbags can provide a sufficient load for resistance training for weak individuals in certain movements (hip extension and abduction, knee extension and flexion). For example, frail persons with weak quadriceps can benefit from sandbag resistance training, but stronger persons, to have a training stimulus, need more resistance than can be attached at the ankle. Wide elastic tubing (attached to furniture, heavy boards, or door handles), available through physical therapists, provides sufficient resistance training for older persons. Elastic bands, which are available from physical therapists and rehabilitation centers, are available to provide several levels of resistance and can be used in parallel to double or triple the resistance. Elastic bands have been used successfully in a home-based intervention with frail subjects; the subjects were initially taught how to use the elastic bands but performed most of the exercises on their own, with occasional supervision for technique (Tinetti et al., 1995).

A person's body weight or extremity weight can also provide a resistance stimulus. For example, a step-up exercise (using body weight as "resistance") provides a training stimulus for frail persons who cannot perform more than 15 or more step-ups without fatigue. The "step-up" is a closed-chain, multiple-joint exercise that is part of many mobility tasks, such as climbing and descending stairs and curbs. The difficulty of the exercise can be adjusted by varying the height of the step from 5 to 20 cm (about 2–8 in.). Arm supports or guardrails can stabilize a person with poor balance, and permit arm strength to assist the step-up in persons with leg weakness. Heel rises (moving from normal stance to standing on toes and metatarsals) use body weight to provide resistance training for the plantar flexors. To increase the work, the range of the lift can be increased by placing the metatarsals near the edge of a board about 2–3 cm in thickness, with the heel on the floor at the beginning of the lift (about 10 degrees of dorsiflexion). To increase the intensity, raises using a single leg are performed, and weighted vests or waist belts can increase resistance. Heel rise exercises increased plantar flexor moment in a trial of relatively healthy elderly subjects (Judge et al., 1994).

Chair rises are a functional activity that can also be a form of closed-chain resistance training. Progression in these exercises can involve (1) increasing the number of repetitions (up to a maximum of about 15); (2) decreasing seat height; (3) using a soft seat; (4) adding a waist belt or weighted vest (up to 10 kilograms added resistance).

Supervision and Setting

An exercise specialist or physical therapist should provide encouragement and guidance at the start of resistance training for frail elderly persons. The training can take place in an adult center or in the home. The advantage of a center is that better equipment and supervision are available. The disadvantage is that the people who have the greatest need may not be able to get to a center. Therefore, the setting of resistance exercise will be related more to travel logistics and to support systems than to physiologic limitations of the potential exerciser.

Endurance Training and Physical Activity

The benefits from increased sustained physical activity include improved endurance (the time one can perform an activity without fatigue), maintenance of body composition, and probably stimulation of balance control in walking programs. If endurance training reduces the perceived difficulty of a specific activity, such as shopping, the activity is more likely to be performed.

Intensity

The general recommendation is to begin the activity at a moderate pace. Endurance prescriptions have been revised to reflect the fact that health benefits have been found to result from lower-intensity activities (Pate et al., 1995). Pulse rate prescriptions, using predictions based on nomograms of estimated maximum heart rate, are being de-emphasized by many exercise leaders. Pulse rate nomograms have wide confidence ranges because of the physiologic variability of maximum heart rate in older persons. Also, many older people have difficulty measuring and calculating their pulse rate. Some exercise leaders now use the Borg "Rating of Perceived Exertion Scale" (RPE scale) (table 8.2) to monitor the exercise intensity. This rating scale reflects the exerciser's subjective rating of exertion and is a reliable predictor of the heart rate response during training. Rather than stopping to take a pulse, the exerciser focuses on the perceived difficulty of the activity. The rating scale is from "very, very weak" (RPE = 0.5) to "maximal" (RPE = 10). Exercisers can be taught to exercise in the "moderate" (RPE = 3), to "strong" (RPE = 5) range, which corresponds to an exercise intensity of about 55–70 percent of maximal oxygen uptake.

Frequency and Duration

The initial recommendation for duration of endurance activity is based on the person's baseline endurance. If persons cannot maintain their preferred

Table 8.2.   Rating of Perceived Exertion (RPE) Scale

RPE Rating	Verbal Equivalent
0	nothing at all
0.5	very, very weak
1	very weak
2	weak
3	moderate
4	somewhat strong
5	strong
6	
7	very strong
8	
9	very, very strong
10	maximal

SOURCE: Reprinted from G. V. Borg, Psychophysical bases of perceived exertion. *Medicine and Science in Sports and Exercise* 14:377–381 (1982), with permission.

walking pace for 6 minutes, the initial goal is to increase the duration before increasing the intensity. A goal is to be able to sustain the endurance activity for 10 minutes. In a person who is regularly active, a persistent inability to be active for 10 sustained minutes suggests either that the person is at an intensity that is too high, or that he or she may have clinically significant cardiac, pulmonary, or musculoskeletal disease.

Current physical activity goals are 25 minutes or more of physical activity (not specifically exercise) daily. The activities do not need to be sustained— that is, two 10-minute walks a day are similar (not identical) to one sustained walk for 20 minutes, or one 40-minute walk every other day.

Estimating Endurance and Walking Capacity

Some researchers and practitioners use the 6-minute walk distance to estimate endurance function (Guyatt et al., 1985). The 6-minute walk measures the maximal distance a person can walk in 6 minutes, and is usually measured in a long hallway or a large room by recording the number of laps completed. While there are no population-based standards for the test, a 6-minute walk distance of less than 360 meters (average velocity of 1 m/sec) would imply an impairment in endurance or a gait problem. It may be difficult to determine if a low 6-minute walk distance is due to poor balance, musculoskeletal problems, poor endurance, or some combination of all three factors. An alternative measure is maximal gait velocity over a short course (8 or 12 meters). A maximal

velocity of < 1.3 m/sec or a usual velocity of < 1.0 m/sec would also be suggestive of impaired gait (Hageman and Blanke, 1986; Hinman et al., 1988).

Exercises for Improving Endurance

Activities that are likely to increase endurance include walking, golf (not
using a cart), bicycling, dancing, and swimming and other water-based activities. Of the endurance activities, walking can be considered the preferred exercise for primary prevention because it provides both endurance and balance
stimuli, and walking is a primary performance on which many IADL depend.
Endurance walking carries the risk of falls, which are less likely to occur during
stationary bicycle or water-based exercise.

Bicycles with reciprocal moving rowing arms are commonly used in
cardiac rehabilitation programs and are well tolerated. Water-based exercises
have been recommended for persons with knee or hip OA or foot problems,
who do not tolerate or enjoy land-based endurance exercise (chapter 9). Water-
based exercises include swimming, walking in the water, and performing resistance exercises using paddles attached to arms and legs to increase resistance to
movement.

Rowing machines and cross-country ski machines are also used by some
older persons. These machines require good control of the torso by abdominal
and lumbar muscles and can lead to lower back complaints if not performed
correctly. Correct form is essential to prevent injury, and intensity should be
gradually increased only after reliable form at low intensity is mastered. Generally, these machines will require supervision at the onset of training to prevent
injury. Stair climbing, treadmill walking on an incline, and walking up hills can
increase in intensity when an exerciser reaches a plateau with brisk walking.
Running or jogging is not recommended, because of the high incidence of musculoskeletal complaints.

Flexibility Training

Flexibility exercises are an important component of an exercise program. Stretching begins most programs, to reduce the risk of musculo-tendonous injuries from exercise and to increase the ROM of joints. Flexibility exercises usually include static stretching (for > 15 seconds) of individual muscle
groups. The posterior calf muscle group (gastrocnemius-soleus) is commonly
tight and can be stretched using several techniques: one technique is to lean for-
ward against a wall with knees fully extended (to stretch the gastrocnemius and

soleus), and then to lean with the knee flexed slightly (to stretch predominantly the soleus). The hip flexors can be stretched in a prone or a lunge position, and the hip abductors can be stretched in a side-lying or standing position. Neck restrictions in ROM are common, particularly in extension and lateral rotation, and caution should be used in any neck motions to reduce the risk of pain and muscle spasm. A forward-leaning posture in those with kyphosis will probably benefit from postural exercises designed to maximize thoracic extension and neck extension. One such exercise is the military "attention" posture, in which the chin is tucked (head posterior but not tilted), the thoracic spine is extended, and the shoulders are back. Shoulder circles, and slow, gentle, limited torso (lumbar spine) rotation exercises are commonly performed as part of a warm-up. Flexion exercises (of lumbar and thoracic spine) are not encouraged because of the theoretical risk of compression fracture. Although there is very limited data on their efficacy, these exercises are sensible ones to include in an exercise program.

Balance Training

Balance helps control the motion of the body during the performance of regular daily activities such as reaching, picking up objects, turning, stepping into a bathtub, and walking over uneven surfaces. Balance is similar to other complex motor tasks in that performance is dependent on regular practice as well as natural agility or ability. Repeated performance of movements that stress postural control may be very important in maintaining balance performance during everyday activities.

Many types of balance exercises are performed in exercise classes for older persons. Several interventions have improved laboratory or clinical balance measures, but there is insufficient information to determine what type of training is most effective in improving mobility (Judge et al., 1993; Wolfson et al., 1996). Balance training can reduce the rate of falls by 17 percent (Province et al., 1995). The specificity of training effects demonstrated in other modes of exercise leads to the recommendation that training should include movements that are similar to challenging functional activities (such as reaching, turning, and going up and down steps).

Many balance training programs try to increase awareness of posture and awareness of the location of the center of mass (COM) relative to the feet. Increased awareness of sensory input (both visual input and pressure and proprioception at the foot and ankle) is also stressed. Biofeedback of the position of center of pressure (which is similar to the position of the COM) has been used to magnify sensory input (Wolfson et al., 1996). Most training programs stress attention to the task, and avoidance of distractions when performing challenging tasks. Tai Chi, a traditional Chinese exercise practice, stresses concentration and controlled, slow movements. Tai Chi exercise classes are popular, and a definitive trial is in progress (Wolf et al., 1996).

Appropriate supervision is critical when training individuals for balance. Exercise mats and balance aids—such as sturdy chairs and bars attached to hallway walls—are needed. An alternative is practicing in a corner (with two walls or kitchen counters for support). The principle is that the risk of injury should be low if a loss of balance should occur during training. Individual assistance is required for some movements.

Pre-exercise Evaluation

Musculoskeletal Problems

Many patients who have been sedentary for many years will have reduced flexibility, muscle weakness, poor endurance, and limited balance performance. Joint motion restriction due to musculo-tendonous tightness or joint pain may increase the risk that sudden changes in activity will produce soreness or injury. The screening musculoskeletal examination should identify muscle weakness, as well as restrictions in activities or in ROM which are painful. In our experience, tightness of the calf muscles is expected, particularly in women who have worn high-heeled shoes.

The musculoskeletal evaluation for an exercise program must include an evaluation of the foot. Foot abnormalities are extremely common in older persons and can become symptomatic with increased activity, particularly walking. Examination of the plantar surface of the foot will disclose callus or corns, which are usually evidence of increased pressure or shear forces during walking. Examination in the standing position will demonstrate changes in the longitudinal arch, but loss of the transverse arch is probably easier to notice by a pattern of callus over the second and third metatarsal heads. Bunions and hammer toes are common, particularly in women.

In patients with knee complaints, assessment of joint stability (collateral ligaments, cruciate ligaments) is important, and persons who develop genu varus or valgus during gait should be seen by an orthopedist before a walking program is instituted. Identified musculoskeletal problems are best addressed by consulting with a physical therapist or an exercise leader experienced in working with older persons. Several sessions with a therapist to develop an individualized stretching and strengthening program will permit many persons with musculoskeletal limitations to participate in group-based or individually paced exercise programs.

Cardiac Disease and Cardiac Risk Factors

Regular physical activity is recommended for most patients with stable cardiac disease (American Heart Association Consensus Panel, 1995). However, there is uncertainty regarding pre-exercise testing for older persons. In asymptomatic persons with two or more risk factors for coronary artery disease, a stress test is recommended by most authorities before a vigorous exercise program is started. There is no consensus on the use of stress testing before starting a program of increased physical activity such as sustained walking (US Preventive Services Task Force, 1989; American College of Sports Medicine, 1993). If a person increases the duration of physical activity without increasing intensity, there should be a modest increase in rate-pressure product (pulse × systolic blood pressure), which is a primary determinant of cardiac oxygen consumption. The present recommendation for sedentary persons is to increase physical activity and not to perform strenuous exercise. Activities that do not raise the rate-pressure product substantially are less likely to induce cardiac ischemia due to fixed coronary artery lesions than are strenuous activities. Two large case-control studies found that heavy physical exertion in persons who do not exercise regularly is risky. The risk of a myocardial infarction within 24 hours following heavy exertion was more than 10-fold higher in persons who exercised infrequently than in persons who were frequent exercisers (Mittleman et al., 1993; Willich et al., 1993).

Balance

Persons who show impaired balance on simple clinical testing—who are unable to perform tandem stance or semitandem stance, who have a poor response to a sternal nudge, or who have poor turning ability (or later path deviations while walking)—are at high risk for falls during exercise. Pre-exercise identification of poor balance is especially important for those who are about to join exercise classes with a high participant-to-teacher ratio.

Settings for Exercise Programs

The location where the exercise is performed is much less important than the frequency and duration of the exercise. Compliance and endurance improvements are similar in group-based and solo exercise programs (King et al., 1991). Many older persons enjoy the socializing that is part of a group exercise program, and socialization may help long-term maintenance of increased physical activity. Others have difficulty attending a center-based program because transportation is costly or inconvenient, and some older persons simply prefer to exercise on their own. A home-based exercise and fall risk amelioration program in persons at high risk for falls reduced fall risk by 31 percent (Tinetti et al., 1994a). However, exercise compliance declined sharply when study personnel visited subjects only once a month. The most cost-effective strategy to prevent loss of independence has not yet been determined.

Many shopping malls encourage people to use the mall for walking programs before the stores open. Many congregate living centers and town-based senior services provide van service to a mall. The potential advantages of mall walking are a climate-controlled setting and a fairly safe (obstacle-free) walking surface. However, the hard, noncompliant surfaces of most malls are likely to increase foot or knee complaints if appropriate shoes are not worn.

Potential Problems Associated with Increased Activity

Increasing physical activity in sedentary persons may exacerbate arthritis symptoms, back problems, and foot problems. Extreme exertion in inactive persons increases the rate of myocardial infarction for about 24 hours, as noted, but the risk is substantially reduced by regular exercise (Mittleman et al., 1993). The recommendation to "start low, go slow" is important to assure that inactive persons do not perform extreme exertion during the first sessions of exercise training.

In persons with poor balance, increasing physical activity, especially brisk walking, may increase the risk of falls and injury unless balance improves at the same rate as gait velocity. Persons with clinically apparent impairments in gait and balance (Tinetti et al., 1989) are likely to benefit from a supervised exercise program and walking in a safe environment (on dense carpet or compliant floor, with good lighting and no confusing changes in floor levels).

Conclusions

Regular physical activity prolongs life and independence. Most persons, even those with significant joint disease and poor mobility, should be able to tolerate a well-designed program to increase physical activity. While waiting for the results of definitive intervention studies which will determine the effects of changes in physical activity and exercise patterns begun late in life, it is reasonable to recommend a primary prevention program of stretching and walking for independent persons without cardiovascular or musculoskeletal disease. For frail older persons with impaired muscle strength, endurance, or balance, an exercise program should be designed and initially supervised by an exercise specialist or physical therapist. The exercise prescription should be designed to eventually require minimal ongoing supervision. Most frail persons will be able to exercise independently after a period of observation and coaching. It is possible that continued encouragement from family members and health professionals will help sustain a higher level of physical activity. Health professionals may also play a crucial role in an older person's return to physical activity following an acute illness.

REFERENCES

American College of Sports Medicine. 1993. *ACSM resource manual for guidelines for exercise testing and prescription.* Philadelphia: Lea and Febiger.

American Heart Association Consensus Panel. 1995. Preventing heart attack and death in patients with coronary artery disease. *J Am Coll Cardiol* 26:292–294.

Bassey EJ, Bendal MJ, Pearson M. 1988. Muscle strength in the triceps surae and objectively measured customary walking activity in men and women over 65 years of age. *Clin Sci* 74:85–89.

Blair SN, Kohl HW, Paffenbarger RS, Clark DG, Cooper KH, Gibbons LW. 1989. Physical fitness and all-cause mortality. *JAMA* 262:2395–2401.

Borg GV. 1982. Psychophysical bases of perceived exertion. *Med Sci Sports Exerc* 14:377–381.

Brown MB, Holloszy JO. 1993. Effects of walking, jogging, and cycling on strength, flexibility, speed, and balance in 60- to 72-year olds. *Aging Clin Exp Res* 5:427–434.

Buchner DM, Beresford SAA, Larson EB, LaCroix AZ, Wagner EH. 1992. Effects of physical activity on health status in older adults: II. Intervention studies. *Ann Rev Public Health* 13:469–488.

Carroll JF, Convertino VA, Wood CE, Graves JE, Lowenthal DT, Pollock ML. 1995. Effect of training on blood volume and plasma hormone concentrations in the elderly. *Med Sci Sports Exerc* 27:79–84.

Charette SL, McEvoy L, Pyka G, Snow-Harter C, Guido D, Wiswell RA, Marcus R. 1991. Muscle hypertrophy response to resistance training in older women. *J Appl Physiol* 70:1912–1916.

Coggan AR, Spina RJ, King DS, Rogers MA, Brown MB, Nemeth PM, Holloszy JO. 1992. Skeletal muscle adaptations to endurance training in 60 to 70 yr-old men and women. *J Appl Physiol* 72:1780–1786.

Cress ME, Thomas DP, Johnson J, Kasch FW, Cassens RG, Smith EL, Agre JC. 1991. Effects of training on VO₂ max, thigh strength, and muscle morphology in septuagenarian women. *Med Sci Sports Exer* 23:752–758.

Cummings SR, Nevitt MC, Browner WS, Stone K, Fox KM, Ensrud KE, Cauley J, Black D, Vogt TM. 1995. Risk factors for hip fracture in white women. *N Engl J Med* 332:767–773.

Dalsky GP, Stocke KS, Ehsani AA, Slatopolsky E, Lee WC, Birge SJ Jr. 1988. Weight-bearing exercise training and lumbar bone mineral content in post-menopausal women. *Ann Intern Med* 108:824–828.

Ettinger WH, Davis MA, Neuhaus JM, Mallon KP. 1994. Long-term physical functioning in persons with knee osteoarthritis from NHANES 1: Effects of comorbid medical conditions. *J Clin Epidemiol* 47:809–815.

Fiatarone MA, O'Neill EF, Ryan ND, Clements KM, Solares GR, Nelson ME, Roberts SB, Kehayias

JJ, Lipsitz LA, Evans WJ. 1994. Exercise training and nutritional supplementation for physical frailty in very elderly people. *N Engl J Med* 330:1769–1775.

Fleck SJ, Kraemer WJ. 1987. *Designing resistance training programs.* Champaign, Ill.: Human Kinetics Books.

Fleg JL, Lakatta EG. 1988. Role of muscle loss in the age-associated reduction in vO$_2$ max. *J Appl Physiol* 65:1147–1151.

Flynn MA, Nolph GB, Baker AS, Martin WM, Krause G. 1989. Total body potassium in aging humans: A longitudinal study. *Am J Clin Nutr* 50:713–717.

Fried LP, Ettinger WH, Lind B, Newman AB, Gardin J. 1994. Physical disability in older adults: A physiological approach. *J Clin Epidemiol* 47:747–760.

Frontera WR, Meredith CN, O'Reilly KP, Knuttgen HG, Evans WJ. 1988. Strength conditioning in older men: Skeletal muscle hypertrophy and improved function. *J Appl Physiol* 64:1038–1044.

Frontera WR, Hughes VA, Lutz KJ, Evans WJ. 1991. A cross-sectional study of muscle strength and mass in 45- to 78-yr-old men and women. *J Appl Physiol* 71:644–650.

Garcia AW, King AC. 1991. Predicting long-term adherence to aerobic exercise: A comparison of two models. *J Sport Exer Psych* 13:394–411.

Giovannucci E, Ascherio A, Rimm EB, Colditz GA, Stampfer MJ, Willett WC. 1995. Physical activity, obesity, and risk for colon cancer and adenoma in men. *Ann Intern Med* 122:327–334.

Greendale GA, Barrett-Connor E, Edelstein S, Ingles S, Haile R. 1995. Lifetime leisure exercise and osteoporosis: The Rancho Bernardo study. *Am J Epidemiol* 141:951–959.

Guralnik JM, Simonsick EM, Ferrucci L, Glynn RJ, Berkman LF, Blazer DG, Scherr PA, Wallace RB. 1994. A short physical performance battery assessing lower extremity function: Association with self-reported disability and prediction of mortality and nursing home admission. *J Gerontol* 49:M85–M94.

Guralnik JM, Ferrucci L, Simonsick EM, Salive ME. 1995. Lower extremity function in persons over the age of 70 years as a predictor of subsequent disability. *N Engl J Med* 332:556–561.

Guyatt GH, Thompson PJ, Berman LB, Sullivan MJ, Townsend M, Jones NL, Pugsley SO. 1985. How should we measure function in patients with chronic heart and lung disease? *J Chronic Dis* 38:517–524.

Hageman PA, Blanke DJ. 1986. Comparison of gait of young women and elderly women. *Phys Ther* 66:1383–1387.

Helmrich SP, Ragland DR, Leung RW, Paffenbarger RS Jr. 1991. Physical activity and reduced occurrence of non-insulin-dependent diabetes mellitus. *N Engl J Med* 325:147–152.

Hinman JE, Cunningham DA, Rechnitzer PA, Paterson DH. 1988. Age-related changes in speed of walking. *Med Sci Sports Exerc* 20:161–166.

Judge JO, Lindsey C, Underwood M, Winsemius D. 1993. Balance improvements in older women: Effects of exercise training. *Phys Ther* 73:254–265.

Judge JO, Whipple RH, Wolfson LI. 1994. Effects of resistance training and balance exercises on isokinetic strength in older persons. *J Am Geriatr Soc* 42:937–946.

Judge JO, King MB, Whipple RH, Clive J, Wolfson LI. 1995. Dynamic balance in older persons: Effects of reduced visual and proprioceptive input. *J Gerontol* 50A:M263–M270.

Kaplan GA, Seeman TE, Cohen RD, Knudsen LP, Guralnik J. 1987. Mortality among the elderly in the Alameda County Study: Behavioral and demographic risk factors. *Am J Public Health* 77:307–12.

King AC, Haskell WL, Taylor CB, Kraemer HC, DeBusk RF. 1991. Group versus home-based exercise training in healthy older adults. *JAMA* 266:1535–1542.

Klitgaard H, Mantoni M, Schiaffino S, Ausoni S, Gorza L, Laurent-Winter C, Schnohr P, Saltin B. 1990. Function, morphology, and protein expression of ageing skeletal muscle: A cross-sectional study of elderly men with different training backgrounds. *Acta Physiol Scand* 140:41–54.

Kohrt WM, Obert KA, Holloszy JO. 1992. Exercise training improves fat distribution patterns in 60–70 year old men and women. *J Gerontol* 47:M99-M105.

Kovar PA, Allegrante JP, MacKenzie CR, Peterson MGE, Gutin B, Charlson ME. 1992. Supervised fitness walking in patients with osteoarthritis of the knee. *Ann Intern Med* 116:529–534.

LaCroix AZ, Guralnik JM, Berkman LF, Wallace RB, Satterfield S. 1993. Maintaining mobility in late life: II. Smoking, alcohol consumption, physical activity, and body mass index. *Am J Epidemiol* 137:858–869.

Lee I-Min, Hsieh CC, Paffenbarger RS. 1995. Exercise intensity and longevity in men. *JAMA* 273: 1179–1184.

Manton KG, Corder LS, Stallard E. 1993. Estimates of change in chronic disability and institutional incidence and prevalence rates in the U.S. elderly population from the 1982, 1984, and 1989 National Long Term Care Survey. *J Gerontol* 48:S153–S166.

McCartney N, Hicks AL, Martin J, Webber CE. 1995. Long term resistance training in the elderly: Effects on dynamic strength, exercise capacity, muscle, and bone. *J Gerontol* 50A:B97–B104.

Mittleman MA, Maclure M, Tofler GH, Sherwood JB, Goldberg RJ, Muller JE. 1993. Triggering of acute myocardial infarction by heavy physical exertion. *N Engl J Med* 329:1677–1683.

Moffroid MT, Whipple RH. 1970. Specificity of speed of exercise. *Phys Ther* 50:1693–1699.

Mor V, Murphy J, Masterson-Allen S, Willey C, Razmpour A, Jackson ME, Greer D, Katz S. 1989. Risk of functional decline among well elders. *J Clin Epidemiol* 42:895–904.

Morey MC, Cowper PA, Feussner JR, DiPasquale RC, Crowley GM, Sullivan RJ. 1991. Two-year trends in physical performance following supervised exercise among community-dwelling older veterans. *J Am Geriatr Soc* 39:549–554.

Moritani T, DeVries HA. 1979. Neural factors versus hypertrophy in the time course of muscle strength gain. *Am J Phys Med* 58:115–129.

Nagi SZ. 1976. An epidemiology of disability among adults in the United States. *Milbank Mem Fund Q* 54:439–468.

Nelson ME, Fiatarone MA, Morganti CM, Trice I, Greenber RA, Evans WJ. 1995. Effects of high-intensity strength training on multiple risk factors for osteoporotic fractures: A randomized control trial. *JAMA* 272:1901–1914.

Nichols JF, Omizo DK, Peterson KK, Nelson KP. 1993. Efficacy of heavy-resistance training for active women over sixty: Muscular strength, body composition, and program adherence. *J Am Geriatr Soc* 41:205–210.

Overend TJ, Cunningham DA, Kramer JF, Lefcoe MS, Paterson DH. 1992. Knee extensor and knee flexor strength: Cross-sectional area ratios in young and elderly men. *J Gerontol* 47:M204–M210.

Pate RR, Pratt M, Blair SN, Hakell WL, Macera CA, Bouchard C, Buchner D, Ettinger W, Heath GW, King AC, et al. 1995. Physical activity and public health: A recommendation from the Centers for Disease Control and Prevention and the American College of Sports Medicine. *JAMA* 273:402–407.

Pollock ML, Carrol JF, Graves JE, Leggett SH, Braith RW, Limacher M, Hagberg JM. 1991. Injuries and adherence to walk/jog and resistance training programs in the elderly. *Med Sci Sports Exer* 23:1194–1200.

Province M, Hadley EC, Hornbrook MC, Lipsitz LA, Miller JP, Mulrow CD, Ory MG, Sannin RW, Tinetti ME, Wolf SL. 1995. The effect of exercise on falls in elderly patients: A preplanned meta-analysis of the FICSIT trials. *JAMA* 273:1341–1347.

Sale DG. 1988. Neural adaptations to resistance training. *Med Sci Sports Exerc* 20:S135-S145.

Simonsick EM, Lafferty ME, Phillips CL, Mendes de Leon CF, Kasl SV, Seeman TE, Fillenbaum G, Hebert P, Lemke JH. 1993. Risk due to physical inactivity in physically capable older adults. *Am J Public Health* 83:1443–1450.

Sipila S, Suominen H. 1995. Effects of strength and endurance training on thigh and leg muscle mass and composition in elderly women. *J Appl Physiol* 78:334–340.

Spina RJ, Ogawa T, Kohrt WM, Martin WH III, Holloszy JO, Ehsani AA. 1993. Difference in cardio-vascular adaptation to endurance training between older men and women. *J Appl Physiol* 75: 849–855.

Stalberg E, Borges O, Ericsson M, Essen-Gustavsson B, Fawcett PR, Nordesjo LO, Nordgren B, Uhlin R. 1989. The quadriceps femoris muscle in 20–70-year-old subjects: Relationship between knee extension torque, electrophysiologic parameters, and muscle fiber characteristics. *Muscle Nerve* 12:382–389.

Taaffe DR, Pruitt L, Reim J, Butterfield G, Marcus R. 1995. Effect of sustained resistance training on basal metabolic rate in older women. *J Am Geriatr Soc* 43:465–471.

Tinetti ME, Speechle M, Ginter SF. 1989. Risk factors for falls among elderly persons living in the community. *N Engl J Med* 320:1055–1059.

Tinetti ME, Baker DI, McAvay G, Claus EB, Garret P, Gottschalk M, Koch ML, Trainor K, Horwitz RL. 1994a. A multifactorial intervention to reduce the risk of falling among elderly people living in the community. *N Engl J Med* 331:821–827.

Tinetti M, Mendes de Leon CF, Doucette JT, Baker DI. 1994b. Fear of falling and fall-related efficacy in relationship to functioning among community-living elders. *J Gerontol* 49:M140–M147.

Tinetti ME, Inouye SK, Gill TM, Doucette JT. 1995. Shared risk factors for falls, incontinence, and functional dependence: Unifying the approach to geriatric syndromes. *JAMA* 273:1348–1353.

US Department of Health and Human Services (USDHHS). 1992. *Health data on older Americans.* DHHS Publication no. (PHS) 93-1411. Vital and Health Statistics, ser. 3, no. 27, pp. 32–34.

US Preventive Services Task Force. 1989. *Guide to clinical preventive services: An assessment of the effectiveness of 169 interventions.* Baltimore: Williams and Wilkins.

Wagner EH, LaCroix AZ, Buchner DM, Larson EB. 1992. Effects of physical activity on health status in older adults: I. Observational studies. *Ann Rev Public Health* 13:451–468.

Willich SN, Lewis M, Lowël H, Arntz H-R, Schubert F, Schröder R. 1993. Physical exertion as a trigger of acute myocardial infarction. *N Engl J Med* 329:1684–1689.

Wolf SL, Barnhart HX, Kutner NG, McNeely E, Coogler C, Xu T, and the Atlanta FICSIT Group. 1996. Reducing frailty and falls in older persons: An investigation of Tai Chi and computerized balance training. *J Am Geriatr Soc* 44:489–497.

Wolfson L, Whipple R, Derby C, Amerman P, Murphy T, Tobin JN, Nashner L. 1992. A dynamic posturography study in healthy elderly. *Neurology* 42:2069–2075.

Wolfson L, Whipple R, Derby C, Judge J, King M, Amerman P, Schmidt J, Smyers D. 1996. Balance and strength training in older adults: Intervention gains and Tai Chi maintenance. *J Am Geriatr Soc* 44:498–506.

Young DR, Masaki KH, Curb JD. 1995. Associations of physical activity with performance-based and self-reported physical functioning in older men: The Honolulu Heart Program. *J Am Geriatr Soc* 43:845–854.

9

Osteoarthritis and Exercise

Marian A. Minor, P.T., Ph.D., and John P. Allegrante, Ph.D.

Osteoarthritis (OA) is a disease of aging. Although the disease process of OA typically confines itself to the affected joint, physical impairment, functional limitation, and progressive disability related to OA can reach far beyond the perimeters of articular cartilage and subchondral bone. Osteoarthritis often is compared to other arthritides and defined by what it is not: it is not a disease with systemic manifestations, it is not primarily an inflammatory disease, and it is not life threatening. Too often OA has also been considered uninteresting, unimportant, and unresponsive to conservative treatment. However, reports documenting the personal and socioeconomic impact of OA increasingly recognize its importance (Yelin and Felts, 1990). Moreover, recent scientific advances in understanding the pathogenesis of OA have stimulated research (Mankin et al., 1986) and new approaches to its clinical management (e.g., see Baker and Brandt, 1993).

This chapter summarizes briefly what is known about OA as a pathogenic entity and discusses in greater length the role of exercise in its management. Recommendations are provided for exercise to reduce impairment and improve function, protect joints, prevent disability, and improve overall health status in older persons.

Osteoarthritis as a Pathogenic Entity

Osteoarthritis is a complex pathogenic entity and is characterized by specific changes in articular cartilage and subchondral bone. Typically, cartilage

This chapter is adapted, with permission of the publisher, from M. A. Minor, "Exercise in the management of osteoarthritis of the hip and knee," *Arthritis Care Res* 7(1994):169–175.

shows fibrillations, increased water content, and loss of integrity. Underlying bone is less compliant and may show evidence of microfractures, sclerosis, and osteophytes at the joint margins (Ghosh, 1988). These changes result in increased friction, decreased shock absorption, and greater impact loading of the joint. The traditional view of OA is that the disease process starts with an unrepaired injury to articular cartilage. There is also evidence, however, that reduced compliance in bone and periarticular structures may initiate pathologic processes (Radin and Paul, 1970, 1971).

Although radiographic features of joint space narrowing and osteophytes may help to confirm a diagnosis of OA, the accepted clinical criteria for hip and knee OA are described in terms of pain and limitation of motion (Moskowitz and Goldberg, 1988; Altman et al., 1991) (see table 9.1). Radiography may or may not add to the accuracy of the clinical diagnosis. Moreover, there is no clear association between radiographic findings and function or pain. In fact, in knee OA, muscular weakness and pain are more explanatory of functional loss than are radiographic findings (McAlindon et al., 1993). Thus, it is critical that clinical evaluation of the patient with OA include a thorough assessment of functional status.

Osteoarthritis is classified as either idiopathic, or secondary to trauma or pathology (Mankin et al., 1986). The most common sites of OA are the hands, feet, knees, and hips, as well as the cervical and lumbar spine. The disease is considered generalized if three or more sites are involved. Moderate to severe hip OA occurs in 3.1 percent of persons 55 to 74 years of age, while knee OA affects 13.8 percent of persons 65 to 74 (Mankin et al., 1986). Osteoarthritis in the weight-bearing joints produces the greatest disability and thus has the greatest potential for limiting functional status in elderly persons.

Exercise and the Management of Osteoarthritis

Range of motion exercises and isometric strengthening exercises for involved joints are commonly recommended by clinicians in the management of hip and knee OA (Brandt, 1988). Recommendations are usually based on clinical assessment of flexibility, strength, and pain at the affected joint and include the essential components of a comprehensive exercise program designed to address impairment at the disease site. However, in OA—a disease that can result in severe functional limitation and disability—effective clinical management must be attentive to more than the localized joint impairment if the goal of improved overall functioning is to be achieved.

Exercise in OA should be considered in terms of treatment goals and

Table 9.1. Clinical Classification Criteria for Osteoarthritis

Knee osteoarthritis
    Age of 50 and at least three of the following:
    1. knee pain
    2. joint stiffness < 30 min
    3. crepitus
    4. bony enlargement
    5. bony tenderness
    6. no palpable warmth
Hip osteoarthritis
    Presence of hip pain in combination with *either*
    1. hip internal rotation ≥ 15° with pain, morning stiffness ≤
       60 min, and age > 50 years, *or*
    2. hip internal rotation < 15°, and hip flexion ≤ 155°

SOURCE: Classification criteria for knee osteoarthritis from Schumacher, 1993; criteria for hip osteoarthritis from Altman et al., 1991.

outcome measures that address impairment, functional limitation, and disability. Thus, the treatment goals of exercise in OA are to (1) reduce impairment and improve function (i.e., decrease pain, increase range of motion (ROM) and strength, normalize gait, and facilitate activities of daily living); (2) protect vulnerable joints from further damage (i.e., reduce joint stress, attenuate joint forces, and improve biomechanics); and (3) prevent disability and improve overall health status (i.e., increase daily physical activity levels and improve strength and overall physical fitness). These goals are achieved through therapeutic exercise and regular participation in health-promoting levels of physical activity.

Exercise to Reduce Impairment and Improve Function

The older person with OA seeks care when pain is severe or when his or her ability to perform functional activity is compromised. Joint pain that appears during a rehabilitation exercise program or some other medically supervised exercise program usually attracts professional attention to an osteoarthritic joint. Range of motion and strengthening exercise directed at the affected joint can reduce pain (Minor and Sanford, 1993); however, similar improvements in function are not as well documented. Reports of muscle performance and motion analysis of older persons with OA provide helpful information to guide exercise prescription toward better functional outcomes.

A number of studies demonstrate that OA in only one joint is a multiple-joint problem. A consistent finding regarding lower-extremity ROM in the presence of OA of the knee is decreased ROM in the hip, knee, and ankle of the involved side, as well as significantly limited motion in all three joints of the uninvolved limb. When older persons with knee OA are compared to non-arthritic controls, ROM in both limbs, at all joints, is diminished (Messier et al., 1992; Jesevar et al., 1993).

A study investigating knee joint motion, strength, and gait in older persons who had undergone unilateral total knee replacement 1 year previously and who were considered to be "rehabilitation successes" found significant differences between the postoperative OA subjects and controls in lower-extremity ROM, muscle performance, and gait. When the postoperative group was compared with the control group without OA, the results showed that during walking, the active knee ROM, push-off (bilaterally), gait velocity, and stride length were significantly lower in subjects who had undergone total knee replacement. Furthermore, in the knee replacement subjects, ROM and angular velocity of the knee and hip were less on the side that had undergone joint replacement and greater on the unaffected side; joint loading was less at heel strike on the operated side and greater and more rapid on the unaffected side (Jesevar et al., 1993).

Osteoarthritis of the hip commonly results in decreased ROM, with a tendency for the hip to be held in a somewhat flexed, abducted, and externally rotated position and the knee to be held in flexion. Decreased hip ROM is clearly associated with decreased walking speed, decreased stride length, and increased energy expenditure. A maximum walking speed of 3 kph (1.8 mph) is not uncommon in older persons with hip OA and decreased hip motion (Gussoni et al., 1990). Moreover, decreased hip ROM is commonly associated with pain, loss of function, and limitations in physical activity (Mankin, 1989).

When there is OA in a hip or knee, active motion in functional positions should be assessed in all joints of both lower extremities. To evaluate the motions actually used during gait, stair climbing, and arising from a chair, it is important to observe these locomotor activities for symmetry and smoothness. Ascending stairs requires the greatest amount and velocity of knee flexion (Jesevar et al., 1993) and may be one of the best activities to evaluate when assessing knee function. Available ROM in excess of that required for daily tasks is protective and may decrease the risk of injury and falls. The need to recover from a tumble during walking may increase the need for hip and knee flexion to almost 50 and 90 degrees, respectively (Grabiner et al., 1993). The functional requirements for lower-extremity joint ROM should be kept clearly in mind when setting treatment goals (see table 9.2).

In the presence of knee OA, knee extension strength declines in both the affected and the unaffected knee. Static and dynamic strength deficits of up to

Table 9.2.   Lower Extremity Functional Ranges of Motion

Joint	Motion	Range (degrees)
Hip	extension	15
	flexion	120
	abduction	20
	adduction	5
	internal rotation	20
	external rotation	20
Knee	extension	0
	flexion	110
Ankle	dorsiflexion	10
	plantarflexion	20

SOURCE: Data from Goldstein, 1991; Norkin and Levangie, 1992.

60 percent have been demonstrated (Lankhorst et al., 1982, 1985; Fisher et al., 1991). Therapeutic programs to strengthen knee extension have shown that significant strength gains can be achieved and that these gains are associated with decreased pain (Chamberlain et al., 1982) and improved gait (Judge et al., 1993). A study investigating the relationship of muscle strength to function reported strong positive correlations between isometric and isokinetic strength measures; however, these strength measures were able to explain no more than 25 percent of the improvement in function and gait (Lankhorst et al., 1985). In contrast, a controlled trial of progressive knee extension strengthening, including training to increase contraction velocity and endurance as well as isometric and isotonic strength, demonstrated significant improvements in function, pain, and independence. Together, strength, endurance, and speed explained 75 percent of the functional improvement in older persons with knee OA (Fisher et al., 1991). A comprehensive program of resistive strengthening of hip, knee, and ankle and postural control exercises resulted in significant improvements in both strength and gait in older subjects, many of whom had OA (Judge et al., 1993).

The functional threshold for lower-extremity strength has yet to be determined. However, reports from studies that have assessed knee strength as a percentage of body weight suggested that isokinetic strength measured at velocities between 60 and 180 degrees per second should be 20–30 percent of body weight for knee extension, and 20–25 percent for knee flexion (Messier et al., 1992; Jesevar et al., 1993). Isometric knee extension below 10 kilograms of force (measured with the hip at neutral and the knee at 90 degrees) corresponded to marked disability in a study of persons with OA of the knee (McAlindon et al., 1993).

Despite the fact that the ankle is rarely a site of OA, limitations in ankle motion and strength are common in persons with OA. Lower-extremity pain and decreased motion result in gait deviations that include diminished push-off, decreased limb loading at heel strike, and less ankle ROM (Messier et al., 1992; Jesevar et al., 1993). Such gait deviations lead to deconditioning of calf musculature and loss of motion at the ankle. Adequate motion, strength, endurance, and power at the ankle are crucial for gait, balance, stair climbing, and arising from a chair. These attributes are quickly lost with the onset of hip or knee pain and stiffness. The increased postural sway that accompanies aging (Lord et al., 1991), and the use of a hip strategy rather than an ankle strategy for controlling balance, may be due in part to decreased ankle motion and strength.

Thus, we recommend that the physician consider collaboration with a physical therapist to

1. assess ROM, strength, and endurance in a comprehensive manner;
2. determine functional capacity and needs;
3. prescribe exercise, therapeutic and recreational, to reduce impairment and improve function;
4. monitor progress and revise exercise recommendations as necessary.

Exercise to Protect Vulnerable Joints from Further Damage

The overall goal of exercise related to joint protection in OA is to provide a healthful environment in which joint structures are stimulated adequately for remodeling and repair and in which the risk of musculoskeletal injury is minimized. The objectives are (1) to reduce joint stress, (2) to improve shock attenuation during exercise and activities of daily living, and (3) to maintain or improve active joint motion and alignment. Joints affected by OA should be considered to be at high risk for injury and activity-induced trauma owing to the high probability of joint laxity, poor alignment, increased biomechanical stress, weak or stiff periarticular tissues, disturbed motion patterns, and diminished proprioception. The combination of neural deficits and joint instability can lead to rapid and marked joint damage (Slowman-Kovacs et al., 1990).

Reducing Joint Stress

Joint stress is reduced by lessening the weight load imposed on the joint. This can be achieved by maintenance of proper body weight, exercise in a gravity-reduced environment (e.g., in water or on a bicycle), and reduction in the weight of the loads carried. Neumann (1989) showed that carrying a load weighing as little as 10 percent of body weight can significantly increase hip joint compressive force. This can be minimized by dividing the load between the two hands, carrying the load on the same side as the affected hip, or carrying the load close to the center of gravity. Although the mechanisms through which body weight affects the severity of knee OA in women are not fully understood, Felson et al. (1992) found significant positive relationships between body weight in middle age and knee OA in later life (see chapter 4). It also appears that reduction in current body weight is related to a reduction in severity of symptoms (see chapter 10).

Joint stress also can be reduced by decreasing joint reaction forces. In hip OA, proper use of a cane on the contralateral side can reduce joint reaction forces at the hip by as much as 50 percent (Neumann, 1989). Joint reaction force at the hip and knee can be reduced by avoiding stairs. Maximum joint loading and impact forces occur during stair climbing and descent (Krebs et al., 1990; Minor and Sanford, 1993). Although using the stairs is often recommended to incorporate aerobic exercise into the daily routine, it may not be wise for persons with hip or knee OA.

Another method to reduce joint reaction force at the knee is to walk at a speed that does not increase biomechanical stress. Faster walking speeds and running increase knee joint stress and can result in activity-induced injury. Older persons with knee OA should walk at speeds that do not produce increased pain or swelling. Two studies of walking as aerobic activity for persons with OA in hips or knees included knee ROM exercises and strengthening exercises as warm-up activities in a gradually progressive aerobic walking program (Minor et al., 1989; Kovar et al., 1992). Both studies reported significant increases in fitness and endurance with no exacerbation of joint symptoms and no dropouts due to joint pain. In the study by Kovar and colleagues, functional status was improved substantially without an increase in medication. In addition, gait characteristics such as stride length were improved (Peterson et al., 1993).

Decreased walking speed is common in arthritis, and there is general agreement that increased walking speed is a meaningful measure of functional improvement. For example, a person's ability to walk fast enough to cross the street with the timing of the traffic light is important for functional community locomotion (Robinett and Vondran, 1988). However, without attention to joint biomechanics, increased walking speed may be undesirable. In a clinical trial of a nonsteroidal drug for persons with knee OA, all with a varus deformity, gait variables were included as outcome measures. The investigators found that self-reported pain diminished and walking speed increased in the active therapy group. At the same time, kinetic analysis of joint forces showed that the increased speed was accompanied by increased adductor moment at the knee and greater loading of the medial compartment (Schnitzer et al., 1993). This additional loading of the joint and increased stress on lateral supporting tissue may not be worth the gains of increased speed. Attention to biomechanical factors thus should be considered in comprehensive management, even when drug therapy decreases pain and improves gait speed.

Improving Shock Attenuation

The importance of shock attenuation to protect cartilage from peak forces of impact loading is supported by animal studies (Radin et al., 1991), in which sudden impact loading, not motion with loading, led to cartilage damage. A sudden impact significantly increased joint friction, and this friction stayed elevated and cartilage was severely damaged after no more than 2–3 days of continuous motion. However, motion even under large loads resulted in only a transient increase in joint friction, and no cartilage damage occurred when the motion was stopped after 20 days.

The primary mechanisms that attenuate shock are neuromuscular responsiveness (Radin et al., 1991) and tissue compliance (Radin and Paul, 1971). The importance of neuromuscular readiness in attenuating impact was demonstrated by an experiment that measured the timing of muscular response and the force of impact when a research subject had varying amounts of time to prepare for a feet-first landing (Jones and Watt, 1971). The findings clearly showed that inadequate neuromuscular readiness was consistently related to greater impact and reported discomfort. In this experiment, the subjects were healthy young men and the experimental results only measured neuromuscular readiness for impact. Shock attenuation by persons with a healthy locomotor system is about 30 percent greater than shock attenuation by persons with joint disease (Voloshin and Wosk, 1981).

The other crucial requirements for neuromuscular attenuation of impact are adequately conditioned muscle mass and the ability to generate force quickly for an eccentric contraction. The necessary components—muscle mass, contractile velocity, force production, endurance for repetitive motions, and motor skill—are often compromised by the consequences of pain and inactivity. To optimize an older person's neuromuscular capacity to protect joints from sudden impact loading, and to attenuate impact loading, it is necessary to include muscular conditioning (to promote concentric and eccentric strength and endurance at functional speeds) and motor skill learning in any exercise program.

In a series of studies designed to determine the relative shock-attenuating properties of articular cartilage, synovial fluid, periarticular soft tissue, and bone, it was demonstrated that compliance within this joint system decreased peak impact. The components that contributed significantly to this attenuation were joint capsule, ligament, synovial tissue, and bone. Although it is often assumed that cartilage is the most important shock absorber, distributor of joint forces, or both, these studies showed that articular cartilage and synovial fluid had little effect on shock attenuation (Radin and Paul, 1971). Thus, it appears that joints could be protected to some degree from damaging peak forces by maintaining or improving the compliance of periarticular soft tissue (i.e., joint capsule and ligaments).

Finally, impact forces also can be attenuated and impact reduced by the use of viscoelastic materials in shoe soles and insoles (Light et al., 1980; Voloshin and Wosk, 1981). Viscoelastic insoles were shown to decrease the shock measured at the proximal tibia by 42 percent in a sample of 10 subjects walking at 4 kph (2.4 mph) (Voloshin and Wosk, 1981). This suggests the importance of counseling the older person about the use of proper athletic footwear during exercise.

Maintaining Active Joint Motion and Alignment

The third joint protection consideration related to exercise and physical activity concerns ROM and weight-bearing activities. Cartilage is avascular and aneural, requiring regular motion with compression and decompression for adequate nutrition and stimulation of remodeling and repair (Bland and Cooper, 1984; Ghosh, 1988; Houlbrooke et al., 1990). It has been shown repeatedly that immobilization and lack of weight-bearing cause cartilage changes similar to those found in OA. Daily exercise that includes the complete active ROM and periods of weight-bearing and non-weight-bearing is the optimal prescription to maintain cartilage viability (Bland and Cooper, 1984; Bunning and Materson, 1991). During periods when weight-bearing is temporarily contraindicated or joint immobilization is necessary, there is evidence that maintenance of either intermittent weight-bearing or regular motion will help to maintain cartilage health (Houlbrooke et al., 1990). An interesting relationship between regular joint motion and osteophyte development was suggested by a study in which more osteophyte formation in knee joints was observed in persons who stopped running than in those who continued to do so. Those who stopped running did so for reasons other than joint pain or stiffness (Michel et al., 1992).

Comprehensive management should include recommendations to

1. reduce weight load on joints by attaining and maintaining proper body weight, or by exercising in water, or on a bicycle, or on a rowing machine;

2. reduce compressive forces by using a cane on the contralateral side, avoid carrying loads over 10 percent of body weight, carry loads on the same side as the affected hip, and reduce stair climbing;
3. select a walking speed that does not exacerbate knee joint symptoms;
4. maintain ROM and flexibility;
5. condition lower-extremity musculature for strength, endurance, and neuromuscular readiness;
6. perform neuromuscular warm-up before walking;
7. alternate weight-bearing and non-weight-bearing activities throughout the day;
8. select shoes and insoles for shock attenuation; and
9. use semirigid or rigid orthoses for biomechanical correction at ankle and knee if necessary.

Exercise to Prevent Disability and Improve Overall Health Status

The problem list for the older person with arthritis can be considerable. Historically, many of these problems were accepted either as the natural progression of arthritis or as unavoidable consequences of therapy. Recently, medical science has recognized that prolonged inactivity also produces many of these same problems, including muscle atrophy, weakness, decreased flexibility, cardiovascular deficit, fatigue, poor endurance, problems of coordination, falls, osteoporosis, depression, sleep disturbance, and low pain threshold.

Arthritis restricts physical activity both directly and indirectly. Direct consequences of the disease process, indirect consequences of therapy, and the psychosocial impact of the disease encourage prolonged inactivity. Inactivity, in turn, contributes to illness and dysfunction as individuals age. In a national health survey, nearly 12 percent of persons over 65 reported limitation of activity due to arthritis (Epstein et al., 1986). Arthritis is the major reason for activity limitation in this age group, and is reported slightly more frequently than heart disease. People with arthritis are less active and tend to be less fit, in both musculoskeletal and cardiovascular status, than their nonarthritic peers (Lankhorst et al., 1985; Minor et al., 1988; Fisher et al., 1991; Philbin et al., 1995).

In contrast to the traditional belief that older persons with hip or knee OA should avoid vigorous and weight-bearing exercise, studies have reported that many older persons with symptomatic joints can safely participate in appropriate conditioning exercise programs to improve their physical fitness and overall health status without exacerbation of disease symptoms (Chamberlain et al., 1982; Minor et al., 1989; Fisher et al., 1991; Kovar et al., 1992; Judge et al., 1993). These studies also have reported good retention and maintenance of exercise behaviors by subjects. In a randomized, controlled trial of aerobic exercise, 80 persons with symptomatic OA of the hip or knee participated in 12 weeks of

Table 9.3.   Exercise Prescription for Health

Exercise mode	activities that involve large muscle groups, entire body if possible, in dynamic, repetitive motion (e.g., walking, swimming, dancing, bicycling, rowing, and calisthenics)
Frequency	3–4 times per week for moderate intensity; daily for low intensity
Duration	accumulation of 30 min per exercise day
Intensity	low to moderate intensity: 50–75% of age-predicted heart rate; 3–5 METs; 1,100–3,000 kcal/wk
Self-monitoring strategies	exercise heart rate per exercise prescription; scale of perceived exertion (0–10): 3–5 exercise exertion; talk-test (i.e., ability to converse comfortably during exercise)

SOURCE: Data from Blair et al., 1992.

aerobic walking, aerobic pool exercise, or nonaerobic ROM exercise. The aerobic exercise groups showed significant improvement over the control group in aerobic capacity. All groups showed similar clinical improvements in joint pain and tenderness and self-reported pain. Medication use was similar between groups and remained stable through the study period (Minor et al., 1989).

A randomized, controlled trial of fitness walking in patients with OA of the knee evaluated functional status, pain, and medication use in more than 100 persons. The 8-week walking program included flexibility and strengthening exercises as a warm-up, and gradual progression of walking from 5 minutes to 30 minutes three times a week in a supervised setting, along with a socially supportive program of patient education designed to facilitate coping with the disease (Allegrante, 1993; Allegrante et al., 1993). The walking group showed significant improvements over the controls in walking distance, self-reported physical activity, and pain (Kovar et al., 1992), with no increase in the use of medication. Moreover, evidence from a recent study showed that a 3-month resistance training program also improved significantly the leg strength and submaximal walking endurance of healthy, community-dwelling elderly persons (Ades et al., 1996).

Impressive evidence from a series of studies by Blair et al. (1989, 1992) showed that regular physical activity is important for people of all ages. People who exercise regularly live longer and have better health status than do people who are sedentary (Blair et al., 1989; Philbin et al., 1995). Recent epidemiologic studies indicate that exercise for improved health does not need to be as intense as was previously thought (Blair et al., 1992) (see table 9.3). This is good news for many older persons with arthritis who are not able to engage safely in long-duration or high-intensity physical activities. This is also important information for health care providers, who can now recommend safe and effective exercise to improve health and prevent unnecessary disability for almost everyone.

In the beginning stage of an exercise program, it is important to encourage the patient to

1. perform flexibility, strengthening, and neuromuscular conditioning exercises as necessary to prepare for more vigorous, aerobic activity;

2. choose non-weight-bearing (bicycle, rowing machine, restorator) or partial weight-bearing (aquatic) exercises for the initial aerobic exercise mode when pain or joint vulnerability limits weight-bearing activity; and proceed to weight-bearing activity as safety and tolerance permit;

3. increase the duration of aerobic activity gradually, starting with as little as 2 minutes of continuous activity, and accumulating the exercise dose in short bouts throughout the day, if necessary;

4. consider postexercise joint pain or swelling as an activity-related or overuse injury, and treat accordingly by modifying the current program to avoid reinjury and adding conditioning exercises as injury-prevention measures;

5. learn the skills for exercise self-management and long-term maintenance, as well as how to respond appropriately to joint pain and flare-ups in disease activity, and how to recognize and avoid physical demands that may aggravate symptoms.

Conclusions

There is converging evidence from several large epidemiologic studies which demonstrates the importance of regular physical activity in the promotion of health and the prevention of premature disease and disability. Physical activity is an important element in the treatment of the older person with OA (Ettinger and Afable, 1994). Evidence from multiple trials of nonmedicinal and noninvasive therapies shows that strengthening exercises, in particular, appear to help patients with OA to reduce pain while increasing the patients' capacity for functioning (Puett and Griffin, 1994). With the accumulation of evidence that prolonged inactivity is a risk factor for a number of chronic and degenerative diseases, as well as for traumatic falls and hip fracture in older people, the importance of exercise in the management of patients with OA is becoming increasingly recognized. Recent studies have shown that older persons and even physically frail elderly persons can safely participate in conditioning exercise programs designed to prevent falls (Fiatarone et al., 1994; Tinetti et al., 1994), and that such exercise reduces the incidence of falls (Province et al., 1995). Although protection of the vulnerable joint from pathologic stress and further damage remains a central tenet of OA management, there is much evidence that older persons with OA can remain physically active without exacerbating their disease or its symptoms. Weight-bearing and resistive exercise of a recreational nature are now viewed as essential for joint health and stability in patients with relatively stable joints and little pain (Minor, 1994). Additionally, strength training also appears to have a positive effect on walking endurance in healthy elderly persons (Ades et al., 1996).

In spite of the knowledge that regular exercise is an important component in the comprehensive management of OA, and the fact that opportunities to exercise are increasing, most people with arthritis are not active and do not participate regularly in exercise programs. The Arthritis Foundation estimates that less than 1 percent of the 37 million people with arthritis participate in the programs sponsored by the foundation. Studies of exercise habits indicate that less than 30 percent of persons with arthritis perform any kind of exercise on a regular basis (Dexter, 1992; Jensen and Lorish, 1994). The most common reasons given for not exercising include lack of belief in its effectiveness, lack of confidence in one's ability to exercise, and the belief that pain and stiffness are reasons not to exercise (Gecht et al., 1996). In a study of exercise behavior in older persons with OA, few of the subjects could remember being encouraged by a health care provider to exercise, and even fewer could remember ever being asked about their exercise habits or given written material about exercise. Of those who could remember receiving advice, written materials, and reinforcement by a physician, nearly two-thirds were performing some type of exercise (Dexter, 1992). Thus, the challenge to health professionals and older persons with OA is to undertake exercise programs that allow adaptation to changing needs and at the same time contain elements necessary for promoting health and improving outcomes. To meet this challenge it is necessary to understand the requirements of health and fitness, the principles of exercise, including behavioral strategies designed to help older persons to maintain physically active lives, and the biomechanics of locomotion, as well as the disease process of OA.

REFERENCES

Ades PA, Ballor DL, Ashikaga T, Utton JR, Sreekumaran NK. 1996. Weight training improves walking endurance in healthy elderly persons. *Ann Intern Med* 124:568–572.

Allegrante JP. 1993. The role of physical activity and patient education in the management of osteoarthritis. In: *Reappraisal of the management of patients with osteoarthritis,* edited by JR Baker, K Brandt. Pp. 31–34. Springfield, N.J.: Scientific Therapeutics Information.

Allegrante JP, Kovar PA, MacKenzie CR, Peterson MGE, Gutin B. 1993. A walking education program for patients with osteoarthritis of the knee: Theory and intervention strategies. *Health Educ Q* 20:63–81.

Altman R, Alarcon G, Appelrouth D, et al. 1991. The American College of Rheumatology criteria for the classification and reporting of osteoarthritis of the hip. *Arthritis Rheum* 34:505–514.

Baker JR, Brandt K, eds. 1993. *Reappraisal of the management of patients with osteoarthritis.* Springfield, N.J.: Scientific Therapeutics Information.

Blair SN, Kohl HW, Paffenbarger RS, Clark DG, Cooper KH. 1989. Physical fitness and all-cause mortality: A prospective study of healthy men and women. *JAMA* 262:2395–2401.

Blair SN, Kohl HW, Gordon NF, Paffenbarger RS. 1992. How much physical activity is good for health? *Ann Rev Public Health* 13:99–126.

Bland JH, Cooper SM. 1984. Osteoarthritis: A review of the cell biology involved and evidence for reversibility. Management rationally related to known genesis and pathophysiology. *Semin Arthritis Rheum* 14:106–132.

Brandt KD. 1988. Management of osteoarthritis. In: *Textbook of Rheumatology,* edited by WN Kelley, ED Harris, S Ruddy, CB Sledge. 3d ed. Pp. 1501–1512. Philadelphia: WB Saunders.

Bunning RD, Materson RS. 1991. A rational program of exercise for patients with osteoarthritis. *Semin Arthritis Rheum* 21:33–43.

Chamberlain MA, Care G, Harfield B. 1982. Physiotherapy in osteoarthrosis of the knees: A controlled trial of hospital versus home exercises. *Int Rehab Med* 4:101–106.

Dexter PA. 1992. Joint exercise in elderly persons with symptomatic osteoarthritis of the hip or knee: Performance patterns, medical support patterns, and relationships between exercising and medical care. *Arthritis Care Res* 5:36–41.

Epstein WV, Yelin EH, Nevitt M, Kramer JS. 1986. Arthritis: A major health problem in the elderly. In: *Arthritis and the elderly,* edited by RW Moskowitz, MR Haug. Pp. 5–17. New York: Springer.

Ettinger WH Jr., Afable RF. 1994. Physical disability from knee osteoarthritis: The role of exercise as an intervention. *Med Sci Sports Exerc* 26:1435–1440.

Felson DT, Zhang Y, Anthony JM, Naimark A, Anderson JJ. 1992. Weight loss reduces the risk for symptomatic knee osteoarthritis in women: The Framingham study. *Ann Intern Med* 116:535–539.

Fiatarone MA, O'Neill EF, Ryan ND, Clements KM, Solares GR, Nelson ME, Roberts SB, Kehayias JJ, Lipsitz LA, Evans WJ. 1994. Exercise training and nutritional supplementation for physical frailty in very elderly people. *N Engl J Med* 330:1769–1775.

Fisher NM, Pendergast DR, Gresham GE, Calkins E. 1991. Muscle rehabilitation: Its effect on muscular and functional performance of patients with knee osteoarthritis. *Arch Phys Med Rehabil* 72:367–374.

Gecht MR, Connell KJ, Sinacore JM, Prohaska TR. 1996. A survey of exercise beliefs and exercise habits among people with arthritis. *Arthritis Care Res* 9:82–88.

Ghosh P. 1988. Articular cartilage: What it is, why it fails in osteoarthritis, and what can be done about it. *Arthritis Care Res* 1:211–221.

Goldstein TS. 1991. *Geriatric orthopedics.* Gaithersburg, Md.: Aspen Publications.

Grabiner MD, Koh TJ, Lundin TM, Jahnigen DW. 1993. Kinematics of recovery from a stumble. *J Gerontol* 48:M97–M102.

Gussoni M, Margonata V, Ventura R, Veicsteinas A. 1990. Energy cost of walking with hip joint impairment. *Phys Ther* 70:295–301.

Houlbrooke K, Vause K, Merrilees MJ. 1990. Effects of movement and weightbearing on the glycosamineglycan content of sheep articular cartilage. *Australian Physiotherapy* 36:88–91.

Jensen GM, Lorish CD. 1994. Promoting patient cooperation with exercise programs: Linking research, theory, and practice. *Arthritis Care Res* 7:181–189.

Jesevar DS, Riley PO, Hodge WA, Krebs DE. 1993. Knee kinematics and kinetics during locomotor activities of daily living in subjects with knee arthroplasty and in healthy controls. *Phys Ther* 73:229–242.

Jones GM, Watt DG. 1971. Muscular control of landing from unexpected falls in man. *J Physiol* 219:729–737.

Judge JO, Underwood M, Genosa T. 1993. Exercise to improve gait velocity in older persons. *Arch Phys Med Rehabil* 74:400–406.

Kovar PA, Allegrante JP, MacKenzie CR, Peterson MGE, Gutin B, Charlson ME. 1992. Supervised fitness walking in patients with osteoarthritis of the knee: A randomized, controlled trial. *Ann Intern Med* 116:529–534.

Krebs DE, Elbaum L, Riley PO, Hodge WA, Mann RW. 1990. Exercise and gait effects on in vivo hip contact pressures. *Phys Ther* 71:301–309.

Lankhorst GJ, van de Stadt RJ, van der Korst JK, Hinlopen-Bonrath E, Griffioen FMM, deBoer W. 1982. Relationship of isometric knee extension torque and functional variables in osteoarthrosis of the knee. *Scand J Rehabil Med* 14:7–10.

Lankhorst GJ, van de Stadt RJ, van der Korst JK. 1985. The relationships of functional capacity, pain, and isometric and isokinetic torque in osteoarthritis of the knee. *Scan J Rehab Med* 17:167–172.

Light LH, McLellan GF, Klenerman L. 1980. Skeletal transients on heelstrike in normal walking with different footwear. *J Biomech* 13:477–480.

Lord SR, Clark RD, Webster IW. 1991. Postural stability and associated physiological factors in a population of aged persons. *J Gerontol* 46:M69–M76.

Mankin HJ. 1989. Clinical features of osteoarthritis. In: *Textbook of Rheumatology,* edited by WN Kelley, ED Harris, S Ruddy, CB Sledge. 3d ed. Pp. 1480–1500. Philadelphia: WB Saunders.

Mankin HJ, Brandt KD, Shulman LE. 1986. Workshop on etiopathogenesis of osteoarthritis. *J Rheumatol* 13:1130–1160.

McAlindon TE, Cooper C, Kirwan JR, Dieppe PA. 1993. Determinants of disability in osteoarthritis of the knee. *Ann Rheum Dis* 52:258–262.

Messier SP, Loeser RF, Hoover EL, Semble EL, Wise CM. 1992. Osteoarthritis of the knee: Effects on gait, strength, and flexibility. *Arch Phys Med Rehabil* 73:29–36.

Michel BA, Fries JF, Bloch DA, Lane NE, Jones HH. 1992. Osteophytosis of the knee: Association with changes in weight-bearing exercise. *Clin Rheumatol* 11:235–238.

Minor MA. 1994. Exercise in the management of osteoarthritis of the hip and knee. *Arthritis Care Res* 32:1396–1405.

Minor MA, Sanford MK. 1993. Physical interventions in the management of pain in arthritis. *Arthritis Care Res* 6:197–206.

Minor MA, Hewett JE, Webel RR, Dreisinger TE, Kay D. 1988. Exercise tolerance and disease related measures in patients with rheumatoid arthritis and osteoarthritis. *J Rheumatol* 15:905–911.

Minor MA, Hewett JE, Webel RR, Anderson SK, Kay DR. 1989. Efficacy of physical conditioning exercise in patients with rheumatoid arthritis and osteoarthritis. *Arthritis Rheum* 32:1396–1405.

Moskowitz RW, Goldberg VM. 1988. Osteoarthritis. In: *Primer on the rheumatic diseases,* edited by HR Schumacher. 9th ed. P. 172. Atlanta: Arthritis Foundation.

Neumann DA. 1989. Biomechanical analysis of selected principles of hip joint protection. *Arthritis Care Res* 2:146–155.

Norkin CC, Levangie PK. 1992. *Joint structure and function.* 2d ed. Philadelphia: FA Davis.

Peterson MGE, Kovar PA, Otis JC, Allegrante JP, MacKenzie CR, Gutin B, Kroll M. 1993. Effect of a walking program on gait characteristics in patients with osteoarthritis. *Arthritis Care Res* 6:11–16.

Philbin EF, Groff GD, Ries MD, Miller TE. 1995. Cardiovascular fitness and health in patients with end-stage osteoarthritis. *Arthritis Rheum* 38:799–805.

Province MA, Hadley EC, Hornbrook MC, Lipsitz LA, Miller JP, Mulrow CD, Ory MG, Sannin RW, Tinetti ME, Wolf SL. 1995. The effects of exercise on falls in elderly patients: A preplanned meta-analysis of the FICSIT trials. *JAMA* 273:1341–1347.

Puett DW, Griffin MR. 1994. Published trials of nonmedicinal and noninvasive therapies for hip and knee osteoarthritis. *Ann Intern Med* 121:133–140.

Radin EL, Paul IL. 1970. Does cartilage compliance reduce skeletal impact loads? The relative force-attenuating properties of articular cartilage, synovial fluid, periarticular soft tissues, and bone. *Arthritis Rheum* 13:139–144.

Radin EL, Paul IL. 1971. Response of joints to impact loading: I. In vitro wear. *Arthritis Rheum* 14:356–362.

Radin EL, Yang KH, Riegger C, Kish VL, O'Connor JJ. 1991. Relationship between lower limb dynamics and knee joint pain. *J Orthop Res* 9:398–405.

Robinett CS, Vondran MA. 1988. Functional ambulation velocity and distance requirements in rural and urban communities. *Phys Ther* 68:1371–1373.

Schnitzer TJ, Popovich JM, Andersson GBJ, Andriacchi TP. 1993. Effect of piroxicam on gait in patients with osteoarthritis of the knee. *Arthritis Rheum* 36:1207–1213.

Schumacher HR, ed. 1993. *Primer on the rheumatic diseases.* 10th ed. Pp. 331–332. Atlanta: Arthritis Foundation.

Slowman-Kovacs SD, Braunstein EM, Brandt KD. 1990. Rapidly progressive charcot arthropathy following minor joint trauma in patients with diabetic neuropathy. *Arthritis Rheum* 33:412–417.

Tinetti ME, Baker DI, McAvay G, Claus EB, Garrett P, Gottschalk M, Koch ML, Trainor K, Horwitz RL. 1994. A multifactorial intervention to reduce the risk of falling among elderly people living in the community. *N Engl J Med* 331:821–827.

Voloshin D, Wosk J. 1981. Influence of artificial shock absorbers on human gait. *Clin Orthop Rel Res* 160:52–56.

Yelin EH, Felts WR. 1990. A summary of the impact of musculoskeletal conditions in the United States. *Arthritis Rheum* 33:750–755.

PART IV

Prospects for the Prevention of Osteoarthritis

10

Epidemiologic Considerations in the Primary Prevention of Osteoarthritis

Marc C. Hochberg, M.D., M.P.H.,
and Margaret Lethbridge-Cejku, M.Sc.

Osteoarthritis, also referred to as osteoarthrosis and degenerative joint disease, is the most common form of arthritis (Kelsey and Hochberg, 1988; Scott and Hochberg, 1993). Most epidemiologic studies have used the presence of radiographic features of osteoarthritis (OA) in selected joints for case definition (Department of Rheumatology and Medical Illustration, 1973). Thus, knowledge of the descriptive and analytic epidemiology of OA is primarily based on studies of the prevalence and incidence of radiographic features of the disorder, and analytic studies have focused on factors associated with radiographic features of the disorder. Few epidemiologic studies, however, have used the presence of symptomatic OA as the outcome of interest (Hochberg et al., 1989; Felson et al., 1992; Cooper et al., 1994a).

Several reviews of the epidemiology of OA have been published in the past decade (Scott and Hochberg, 1987; Felson, 1988; Silman and Hochberg, 1993). These authors have discussed the classification and definition of OA, the prevalence and incidence of OA and its variation across regions and among ethnic/racial groups, and factors associated with the presence of OA. These factors include genetic and nongenetic host factors, and environmental factors (table 10.1). This chapter focuses on three potentially modifiable factors associated with OA of the knee and hip: overweight, occupation and physical activity, and joint injury and trauma, in the context of a discussion of opportunities for primary prevention of OA of the knee and hip. The reader is referred to the above-cited reviews for a detailed discussion of the role of other factors in the devel-

Table 10.1.   Factors Associated with the Presence of Osteoarthritis

Genetic host factors
  Gender
  Inherited disorders of type II collagen gene (e.g., Stickler syndrome)
  Other inherited disorders of bones and joints
  Race/ethnicity
Nongenetic host factors
  Increasing age
  Overweight
  Depletion of female sex hormones (e.g., postmenopausal state) (?)
  Developmental and acquired bone and joint diseases
  Previous joint surgery (e.g., meniscectomy)
Environmental factors
  Occupations and physical demands of work
  Major trauma to joints
  Leisure and/or sports activities

opment of OA at these joint groups as well as at other sites, including the hand and the spine.

Overweight

Overweight is clearly the most important modifiable risk factor for the development of knee OA in both sexes; however, its role as a risk factor for the development of OA of the hip remains controversial (Felson, 1995). Many epidemiologic studies have found a cross-sectional association between obesity and radiographically defined knee OA (Acheson and Collart 1975; Lawrence, 1977; Hartz et al., 1986; Anderson and Felson 1988; van Saase et al., 1988; Davis et al. 1988a, 1988b, 1989, 1990; Bagge et al., 1991; Hart and Spector, 1993; Hochberg et al., 1995) (see table 10.2).

Anderson and Felson (1988) studied the association between overweight and radiographic OA of the knee in 5,193 subjects aged 35 to 74 years who participated in the First National Health and Nutrition Examination Survey (NHANES I). Of these, 315 had definite OA of one or both knees. In age-adjusted multiple logistic regression models, there was a significant direct association between body mass index and OA of the knee in both sexes: for each 5-unit increase in body mass index, the odds ratio (95% confidence intervals [CI]) for the association with OA of the knee was 2.10 (1.70, 2.58) in men and 2.20 (1.95, 2.50) in women. After adjustment for other covariates including race, socioeconomic status, serum uric acid level, and number of packs of cigarettes smoked per day, the odds ratio increased in men to 2.53 (1.75, 3.68) but remained constant in women at 2.17 (1.74, 2.77). Finally, using a comparison or referent group of subjects with normal weight (body mass index < 25 kg/m²), Anderson and Felson (1988) demonstrated a dose-response relationship between overweight and OA in both sexes: in models adjusted for age and race, subjects who were categorized as obese (i.e., who had a body mass index of 30–35 kg/m²) and those who were very obese (whose body mass index was > 35 kg/m²) had higher odds of knee OA than subjects who were only overweight (whose body mass index was 25–30 kg/m²).

Davis and colleagues (1989) studied the association between overweight and unilateral and bilateral radiographic OA of the knee in 3,885 subjects aged 45 to 74 years who participated in NHANES I. Of these, 226 (5.8%) had bilateral OA, and 75 (1.9%) had unilateral OA. Overall, 65.0 percent of subjects with bilateral knee OA had a body mass index above 30 kg/m², compared to 37.4 percent of 37 subjects with right knee OA, 43.3 percent of 38 subjects with left knee OA, and 17.7 percent of 3,584 with normal radiographs. In multiple polychotomous logistic regression analysis adjusting for age, sex, and history of knee injury, the odds ratio (95% CI) for the association of overweight with bilateral knee OA was 6.58 (4.71, 9.18), as compared with right knee OA and left knee OA of 3.26 (1.55, 7.29) and 2.35 (0.96, 5.75), respectively.

Is the association of overweight with OA of the knee related to the distribution of body weight and/or the amount of body fat? Davis and colleagues (1990) examined the relationship between body fat distribution and OA of the knees in subjects aged 45 to 74 years in NHANES I. Central fat distribution was measured as subscapular skinfold thickness, while peripheral fat distribution was measured as triceps skinfold thickness. There was no association of subscapular skinfold thickness or triceps skinfold thickness with either unilateral or bilateral osteoarthritis of the knees in men or women after adjustment for age, race, and body mass index. Body mass index remained significantly associated with bilateral knee OA in both sexes, and with unilateral knee OA in men only.

Hochberg and colleagues (1995) examined the relationship between body fat distribution and percentage of body fat in 465 white men and 275 white women participating in the Baltimore Longitudinal Study of Aging; 169 men and 99 women in this study had radiographic features of definite knee OA. Body fat distribution was measured using the ratio of waist and hip girth, while percentage of body fat was estimated from standard equations using the subscapular, triceps, and abdominal skinfold thicknesses. As expected, body mass index was significantly associated with the presence of knee OA in both sexes. A central body fat distribution, defined as a higher waist-hip ratio, was weakly

Table 10.2. Obesity as a Risk Factor for Osteoarthritis of the Knee and/or Hip

Site and Study	Age (years)	Measure of Association	Results	
			Males	Females
Knee				
Lawrence, 1977	45+	OR (95% CI) for obesity	1.6 (1.0, 2.4)	2.7 (2.0, 3.6)
Hartz et al., 1986	40–69	relative weight (observed/ideal)	OA 124, normal 114	OA 144, normal 115
Davis et al., 1988a, 1988b	45–74	OR (95% CI) for BMI > 30 kg/m^2	2.4 (1.3, 3.4)	6.5 (5.7, 7.6)
van Saase et al., 1988	45–64	OR for BMI quintile V versus I	right 3.7, left 1.8	right 1.9, left 1.8
Anderson and Felson, 1988	35–74	OR (95% CI) per 5-unit BMI increase	2.1 (1.8, 3.7)	2.2 (1.7, 2.8)
Felson et al., 1988	37+	RR (95% CI) of quintile BMI V versus I	1.5 (1.2, 2.0)	2.1 (1.7, 2.6)
Spector et al., 1994	45–64	OR (95% CI) tertile BMI III versus I	n/a	4.7 (0.6, 34.8)
Hip				
Lawrence, 1977	50+	OR (95% CI) for obesity	2.1 (1.0, 4.0)	n/a
Hartz et al., 1986	40–69	relative weight (observed/ideal)	OA 118, normal 114	OA 126, normal 115
van Saase et al., 1988	45–64	OR for quintile BMI V versus I	right 3.2, left 2.2	right 0.4, left 0.7
Vingard, 1991	40–70	OR (95% CI) tertiles BMI highest versus lowest	age 30: 1.8 (1.0, 3.2) age 40: 2.5 (1.4, 4.5) age 50: 2.3 (1.2, 4.4)	n/a
Croft et al., 1992a	60–76	OR (95% CI) tertile BMI highest versus lowest	2.0 (0.7, 5.5)	n/a
Heliovaara et al., 1993	30–75	OR (95% CI) quartile BMI highest versus lowest	bilateral 2.8 (1.4, 5.7)	both sexes
Tepper and Hochberg, 1933	55–74	OR (95% CI) BMI ≥ 27.3	1.0 (0.4, 2.3)	1.2 (0.6, 2.4)

[a]ABBREVIATIONS: OR = odds ratio, CI = confidence intervals, BMI = body mass index, RR = relative risk, OA = osteoarthritis, n/a = not applicable.

associated with bilateral knee OA in both sexes; however, after adjustment for body mass index, body fat distribution was no longer significantly related to the presence of knee OA. A higher percentage of body fat was significantly related to knee OA in women but not men; similarly, however, after adjustment for body mass index, the percentage of body fat was no longer significantly related to the presence of knee OA. Thus, on the basis of these two studies, it appears that being overweight—not whether the weight is predominantly fat or lean body weight, or where the weight is distributed—is the important factor related to the presence of knee OA.

Is the relationship between overweight and knee OA mediated by biomechanical factors or by metabolic factors related to obesity? Davis and colleagues (1988a) examined the role of metabolic factors in subjects participating in NHANES I. They found that the strength of the association between overweight and the presence of knee OA was not diminished by adjustment for potential confounding variables including blood pressure, serum cholesterol, serum uric acid, body fat distribution, and history of diabetes. Similar results have been demonstrated in analyses from the Baltimore Longitudinal Study of Aging, which failed to show that blood pressure, fasting and 2-hour serum glucose and insulin levels, or fasting serum lipid levels, including cholesterol, triglycerides, and HDL-cholesterol, produced significant confounding or effect modification of the association of body mass index with definite knee OA (Martin et al., 1995); and in the population study "70-Year-Old People in Goteborg" (Bagge et al., 1991).

These cross-sectional data demonstrating an association between overweight and OA of the knee were confirmed in an analysis of longitudinal data from the Framingham study (Felson et al., 1988). Felson and colleagues examined the relationship between weight measured at examination 1, which was conducted between 1948 and 1952, and the presence of radiographic knee OA measured 36 years later, at the 18th biennial examination, in 1983–85. When subjects were grouped into quintiles on the basis of their sex- and height-adjusted weight at baseline, both men and women in the highest quintiles were significantly more likely to have developed knee OA; the relative risks (95% CI) were 1.51 (1.14, 1.98) and 2.07 (1.67, 2.55) in men and women, respectively. Furthermore, women in the fourth quintile also had an elevated relative risk of developing knee OA: 1.44 (1.11, 1.86).

Further evidence for a causal role of overweight in knee OA comes from data from the Chingford study (Spector et al., 1994). Of a cohort of 1,003 women aged 45 to 64 years living in East London, 58 of 67 with unilateral knee OA on their initial radiograph in 1988 returned for a follow-up radiograph 24 months later. Fifteen (47%) of 32 women whose body mass index was 26 kg/m^2 or higher at baseline developed incident OA in the originally unaffected knee, compared to only 1 (10%) of the 10 whose body mass index at baseline was less than 23 kg/m^2; for each 5 kg increase in body weight at baseline, the risk of incident knee OA was 6.5 percent. Thus, these data confirm that overweight is a risk factor for the development of knee OA.

Does weight loss or prevention of weight gain among overweight persons result in a decreased risk of developing knee OA? Felson and colleagues (1992) analyzed data from the Framingham study to examine the effect of weight change from the baseline examination on the incidence of symptomatic knee OA in women. The outcome in this analysis was the recalled year of onset of knee symptoms in those who had had radiographic knee OA at the 18th biennial examination and also had current knee symptoms. After adjusting for baseline body mass index, Felson et al. showed a relationship between weight change between 6 and 12 years prior to radiographic examination, and symptomatic knee OA: the risk of having current symptomatic knee OA was 25 to 35 percent greater among women whose body mass index had increased by 2 kg/m^2 than among women without weight change, while those whose body mass index had decreased by 2 kg/m^2 had a reduced risk of developing current symptomatic knee OA. Focusing on the 10-year interval before the radiographic examination, the authors showed that the odds of having current symptomatic knee OA were reduced by 50 percent for a loss of every 2 kg/m^2. Thus, these data suggest that weight loss during adulthood can reduce the risk of developing symptomatic knee OA.

As noted above, the results of cross-sectional studies examining the association of obesity with hip OA are inconsistent, although the majority suggest a relationship that is of lower strength than the relationship of overweight with OA of the knee (Saville and Dickson, 1968; Lawrence, 1977; Hartz et al., 1986; van Saase et al., 1988; Vingard, 1991; Croft et al., 1992b; Heliovaara et al., 1993; Tepper and Hochberg, 1993).

Tepper and Hochberg (1993) studied the association between overweight and radiographic OA of the hip in 2,358 subjects aged 55 to 74 years who participated in NHANES I, of whom only 73 (3.1%) had definite OA of one or both hips. In multiple logistic regression models adjusted for age, race, and education, there was not a significant association between overweight—defined as a body mass index exceeding 27.3 kg/m^2 and 27.8 kg/m^2 in women and men, respectively—and OA of the hip in either sex. When the analysis was performed examining the relationship between overweight and either unilateral or bilateral hip OA, however, the odds ratio (95% CI) for the association of over-weight with bilateral hip OA was 2.00 (0.97, 4.15); the corresponding figure for unilateral hip OA was 0.54 (0.26, 1.16).

Heliovaara and colleagues (1993) studied the relation between over-weight and clinically diagnosed hip OA in a population study in Finland. In mul-tiple logistic regression models adjusted for age, gender, history of lower-limb injury, and physical stress at work, and using a body mass index of less than 25 kg/m² to define the referent group with normal weight, these authors demon-strated a dose-response relationship between overweight and OA in both sexes: subjects who were obese, defined as having a body mass index of 30 kg/m² or greater, had higher odds of hip OA than did subjects who were only overweight, defined as having a body mass index between 25 kg/m² and 30 kg/m². Interest-ingly, the association of overweight was stronger with bilateral than with uni-lateral hip OA; an analysis for trend demonstrated a highly significant relation-ship between increasing weight and bilateral hip OA, but only a marginally significant relationship between increasing weight and unilateral hip OA. Thus, these data suggest that overweight may be a more important risk factor for bi-lateral than for unilateral hip OA. Studies examining the effect of confounding or effect modification by metabolic correlates of overweight, or examining the effect of weight change on the incidence of hip OA, have not been reported.

Occupation and Physical Activity

Certain occupations that require repetitive use of particular joints over long periods of time have been associated with the development of site-specific OA. Specific occupational groups with increased risks of OA include miners, who have an excess of knee and lumbar spine disease (Kellgren and Lawrence, 1952); dockers and shipyard workers, who have an excess of hand and knee OA (Partridge and Duthie, 1968; Lindberg and Montgomery, 1987); cotton and mill workers, who have an excess of hand OA involving specific finger joints (Law-rence, 1961; Hadler et al., 1978); pneumatic tool operators, who have an excess of elbow and wrist OA (Copeman, 1940; Hunter et al., 1945; Bovenzi et al., 1980, 1987); concrete workers and painters, who have an excess of knee OA (Wick-strom et al., 1983); and farmers, who have an excess of hip OA (Lougot and Savin, 1966; Typpo, 1985; Jacobson et al., 1987; Axmacher and Lindberg, 1993; Thelin, 1990; Vingard et al., 1991a; Croft et al., 1992a) (see table 10.3). The rela-tionship between occupation and OA has been the subject of several reviews (Genti, 1989; Felson, 1994; Cooper, 1995). In addition, Buckwalter (1995) has

Table 10.3.   Occupation as a Risk Factor for Osteoarthritis of the Knee and/or Hip

Study	Site	Occupational Group or Type of Activity	Odds Ratio
Kellgren and Lawrence, 1952	knee or spine	miners	2.0
Partridge and Duthie, 1968	knee or hand	dockers	2.0
Wickstrom et al., 1983	knee	concrete workers	1.0
Lindberg and Montgomery, 1987	knee	shipyard workers	2.8
Anderson and Felson, 1988	knee	high knee-bending	males: 2.5
Cooper et al., 1994a	knee	prolonged squatting	6.9
		prolonged kneeling	3.4
		climbing ≥ 10 flights	2.7
		heavy lifting	1.4
Vingard et al., 1991b	hip	high work load (lifting)	2.4
		heavy lifting, ages 30–49	3.3
Croft et al., 1992a	hip	farmers (1–9 years)[a]	4.5
		farmers (≥ 10 years)[a]	9.3 (1.9, 44.5)
Axmacher and Lindberg, 1993	hip	farmers (n = 565)	12.0 (6.7, 21.4)

[a]Duration of occupation or activity.

reviewed the biomechanical mechanisms underlying the relationship between abuse of joints and development of OA.

Anderson and Felson (1988) examined data from NHANES I to study the relationship between occupation and knee OA in the general population. Occupations were grouped into seven broad categories, and the physical demand and the knee-bending requirement for each occupational category were characterized by three-level variables: low/moderate/high and none/some/much, respectively. The workers whose jobs demanded high levels of strength included laborers and service workers; those who had to do much knee bending included laborers, service workers, and craftsmen. In multiple logistic regression models adjusted for race, body mass index, and education levels, male and female subjects aged 55 to 64 years who worked in jobs with increasing strength demands had greater odds of radiographic knee OA, and men and women who worked in jobs with increasing knee-bending demands also had greater odds of radiographic knee OA.

Cooper and colleagues (1994a) tested the hypothesis that specific occupational physical activities were risk factors for knee OA in a population-based case-control study in Bristol, England. Subjects with moderate-to-severe knee OA were significantly more likely than controls to report occupations that required at least 30 minutes per day of squatting or kneeling, or climbing more than 10 flights of stairs. Furthermore, subjects employed in occupations requiring these types of physical activities who also regularly lifted more than 25 kg had greater odds of knee OA than those who didn't regularly lift heavy weights. There was no interaction between occupational physical demands and history of knee injury in increasing the odds of knee OA.

The association between occupational physical demands and knee OA has been confirmed in men in the longitudinal Framingham study (Felson et al., 1991). Occupational status was assessed between examinations 1 and 6 (which took place in 1948–51 and 1958–61, respectively), and the presence of radiographic knee OA was determined at examination 18, in 1983–85. The workers whose jobs involved at least a medium level of physical demand and knee bending included craftsmen, operators and transporters, and laborers and service workers. Men who were employed in jobs requiring knee bending and medium, heavy, or very heavy physical demands had a twofold greater risk of developing radiographic knee OA than did men employed in jobs not requiring knee bending and making minimal or light physical demands. Furthermore, Felson and colleagues estimated that the proportion of radiographic knee OA in men attributable to these occupational factors was 15 percent. Thus, certain occupations that repetitively stress apparently normal knee joints through repeated use appear to predispose to the development of knee OA.

Occupational physical activity has also shown to be associated with hip OA in several studies (Thelin, 1990; Vingard et al., 1991b; Croft et al., 1992a, 1992b; Axmacher and Lindberg, 1993; Heliovaara et al., 1993; Roach et al., 1994). The association of farming with hip OA was noted above.

Vingard and colleagues (1991b) studied the relationship between physical work loads and the risk of hip OA in a study of 233 Swedish men aged 50 to 70 years who had undergone total hip arthroplasty, and 302 population-based controls. In multiple logistic regression models, adjusting for age, body mass index, smoking, and sports activities up to the age of 29 years, men who worked in occupations requiring medium and high static and/or dynamic forces or who frequently lifted weights heavier than 40 kg or performed jumps between different levels had significantly higher odds of undergoing total hip arthroplasty for hip osteoarthritis than did men without these types of high occupational exposures. On the basis of these data, Olsen and colleagues (1994) estimated that 40 percent of hip OA resulting in total joint arthroplasty could be attributed to physical work load.

Roach and colleagues (1994) compared occupational work load, defined by estimated joint compression forces produced by an occupational activity, in 99 men with primary hip OA and 233 male controls known to be free of radiographic hip OA. The work load was categorized as light, intermediate, or heavy on the basis of the type and duration of exposure to different amounts of sitting, standing, walking, or lifting in the subjects' jobs. In multiple logistic regression models, adjusting for obesity and history of sports activities, men with hip OA had 2.5-fold greater odds of having performed heavy work than did controls. Furthermore, the duration of performance of heavy work also appeared to be significantly related to increasing the odds of hip OA.

Heliovaara and colleagues (1993) examined the relationship between physical stress at work and clinically diagnosed hip OA in a population-based study in Finland. Physical stress was defined as lifting or carrying heavy objects, working in a stooped, twisted, or otherwise awkward position, using vibrating equipment, continuously repeating a series of movements, or having one's working speed determined by machine. In multiple logistic regression models adjusted for age, gender, body mass index, and history of lower-limb injury, there was a significant dose-response relationship between the presence and number of physical stressors at work and increased odds of clinically diagnosed hip OA, both unilateral and bilateral. Subjects with two of these stressors were twice as likely to have hip OA, while those with three or more stressors were almost three times as likely to have hip OA.

Given these findings of an association between occupational factors and both hip and knee OA, the most effective form of primary prevention would be modification of working conditions (Genti, 1989).

Sports and Exercise

Many studies have been conducted to examine the relationship between regular physical activity and OA (table 10.4). Most of the recent studies have included elite athletes, particularly football players, runners, and soccer players (Puranen et al., 1975; Lane et al., 1993; Lindberg et al., 1993; Neyret et al., 1993; Vingard et al., 1993; Kujala et al., 1994, 1995; Roos et al., 1994). Panush and Lane (1994) and Lane et al. (1993) recently reviewed these and older studies (e.g., Klunder et al., 1980; Sohn and Micheli, 1985) and concluded that individuals who participate in sports at a highly competitive level (i.e., elite athletes) or who have abnormal or injured joints appear to be at increased risk of developing OA by comparison with persons with normal joints who participate in low-impact activities.

Kujala and colleagues (1994) studied the incidence of hospital admission for OA affecting the hip or knee from 1970 to 1990 among a cohort of 2,049 male athletes who had represented Finland in international events between 1920

Table 10.4. Sports and Leisure Physical Activity as a Risk Factor for Osteoarthritis

Study	Site	Group Studied	Odds Ratio Estimate
Klunder et al., 1980	hip or knee	former professional soccer players	1.9
Puranen et al., 1975	hip	former champion runners	0.5
Sohn and Micheli, 1985	hip or knee	runners	0.8
Lane et al., 1986	knee	long-distance runners	1.0
Panush et al., 1986	knee	runners	1.0
Marti et al., 1989	knee	former long-distance runners	4.0
Vingard, 1991	hip	persons with medium exposure to sports at < 49 yrs of age	2.6
		persons with high exposure to sports at < 49 yrs of age	4.5
Croft 1992a, 1992b	hip	persons with any exposure to sports after school	1.0

and 1965 and a cohort of 1,403 healthy controls. During a 21-year followup period, the risk for an OA hospitalization was twice as great among the athletes as among the controls. The excess risk was predominantly found in those athletes who participated in mixed sports (soccer, ice hockey, basketball, and track and field) and power sports (boxing, wrestling, weight lifting, and throwing). After adjusting for age and body mass index, however, the authors found a significantly elevated risk of being hospitalized for OA of the hip or knee even among athletes who participated in endurance sports (long-distance running and cross-country skiing).

Kujala and colleagues (1995) extended these observations in a study of a sample of 117 of these male athletes who had responded to a questionnaire in 1985 and were alive in 1992. Radiographic changes indicative of knee OA were present in almost one-third of soccer players and weight lifters, as compared to one-sixth of long-distance runners. The factors related to radiographic knee OA included knee injuries (among soccer players), and higher body mass index and number of years in kneeling and squatting work (among weight lifters).

The increased prevalence of knee OA and the role of knee injury in soccer players as a risk factor for development of knee OA was also studied by Roos and colleagues (1994) and Neyret and colleagues (1993). Elite soccer players had significantly increased odds of knee OA compared to controls; furthermore, meniscectomies and known anterior cruciate ligament injuries were common among the elite players with knee OA (Roos et al., 1994). Among a group of elite soccer players who had all undergone rim-preserving meniscectomy for knee injuries, a ruptured anterior cruciate ligament noted at the time of meniscectomy was associated with significantly greater risk of developing radiographic knee OA and requiring further knee surgery (Neyret et al., 1993).

In the absence of knee injury, running as a recreational activity does not appear to be a risk factor for the development of OA of the knee (Lane et al., 1986, 1990, 1993; Panush et al., 1986; Konradsen et al., 1990).

Hip OA is also more common among elite soccer players (Lindberg et al., 1993). In addition, in a case-control study of Swedish men undergoing total hip arthroplasty, Vingard and colleagues (1993) found increased odds of hip OA among individuals participating in sports at either a medium or a high level before age 50. Furthermore, these authors demonstrated an interaction between the level of sport exposure and the level of occupational physical demands. Compared with those who had low levels of both sport exposure and occupational physical activity, subjects with high levels of both had 8.5-fold greater odds of hip OA; those with a high level of sports activity and a low level of occupational physical activity had 2-fold greater odds of hip OA; and those with a low level of sports activity and a high level of occupational physical activity had 3-fold greater odds of hip OA.

Joint Injury and Trauma

As noted above, in the absence of joint injury leisure physical activity does not appear to be associated with an increased risk of either knee or hip OA. Furthermore, knee injury, especially rupture of the anterior cruciate ligament, is associated with an increased risk of knee OA in elite soccer players. Is joint injury associated with knee and hip OA in the general population?

Davis and colleagues (1989) studied the association between knee injury and unilateral and bilateral radiographic OA of the knee in 3,885 subjects aged 45 to 74 years who participated in NHANES I. Overall, a history of right knee injury was present in 5.8 percent of subjects with bilateral knee OA, 15.8 percent of 37 subjects with right knee OA, and 1.5 percent of controls, while a history of left knee injury was present in 4.6 percent of those with bilateral knee OA, 27.0 percent of subjects with left knee OA, and 1.8 percent of controls. In multiple polychotomous logistic regression analysis adjusting for age, sex, and body mass index, the odds ratio (95% CI) for the association of knee injury with bilateral knee OA was 3.51 (1.80, 6.83) as compared with an odds ratio of 16.30 (6.50, 40.9) for right knee OA and an odds ratio of 10.90 (3.72, 31.93) for left knee OA.

Cooper and colleagues (1994b) examined the relationship of knee injury to symptomatic knee OA involving the tibiofemoral and/or patellofemoral compartment. In multiple logistic regression models adjusted for age, body mass index, family history of knee arthritis, and presence of Heberden nodes, knee injury was associated with significantly higher odds of radiographic knee OA in both sexes: an odds ratio (95% CI) of 3.4 (1.7, 6.7). The strength of the association was comparable for men and women, and for subjects with tibiofemoral compartment and patellofemoral compartment OA.

Two studies have examined the relationship between a history of hip injury and hip OA. Tepper and Hochberg (1993) studied the association between hip injury and radiographic OA of the hip in 2,358 subjects aged 55 to 74 years who participated in NHANES I; of these, only 73 (3.1%) had definite OA of one or both hips. In multiple logistic regression models adjusted for age, race, and education, a history of hip injury was significantly associated with higher odds of hip OA: the odds ratio was (95% CI) 7.84 (2.11, 29.10). When the analysis was performed examining the relationship between hip injury and either unilateral or bilateral hip OA, however, the odds ratio (95% CI) for the association of hip injury with unilateral hip OA was 24.2 (3.84, 153), as compared with a bilateral hip OA odds ratio of 4.17 (0.50, 34.7). Heliovaara and colleagues (1993) studied the relation between history of lower-limb injury and clinically diagnosed hip OA in a population study in Finland. In multiple logistic regression models adjusted for age, gender, body mass index, and physical stress at work, a history of lower-limb injury was associated with OA in both sexes. As in the NHANES I dataset, the association was stronger with unilateral than with bilateral hip OA. Thus, these data suggest that hip and knee injury are an important risk factor for hip and knee OA, respectively, especially unilateral hip and knee OA.

Conclusions

This chapter has reviewed published epidemiologic studies focusing on potentially modifiable risk factors for the development of hip and knee OA. Primary prevention strategies directed toward preventing overweight through dietary instruction and regular low-intensity physical exercise, workplace modification to reduce the physical stress on lower-extremity joints, and prevention of major joint injury would be expected to reduce the incidence of hip and knee OA in the population. This would lead to reduced health care utilization (including a reduction in the need for total joint arthroplasty), reduced morbidity and disability, and reduced health care costs.

How much of an impact on the burden of OA would be expected if young persons were to adopt the preventive strategies noted above? This can be estimated not from the odds ratio, which measures the strength of the association of a risk factor with the disease, but rather from the attributable risk, or etiologic fraction, which indicates what proportion of all the cases of the disease in the population are due to that risk factor.

Several studies provide data on the estimated proportion of knee OA attributable to individual risk factors. For overweight, on the basis of data from the Framingham Osteoarthritis Study, Felson (1995) estimated that the incidence of OA of the knee could be reduced by 33 percent in women and 21.4 percent in men if those in the highest tertile of body mass index moved into the middle tertile and if those in the middle tertile moved into the lowest tertile. On the basis of data from the Baltimore Longitudinal Study of Aging, Hochberg and colleagues (1995) estimated that the proportion of knee OA attributed to overweight (being overweight was defined as being in the highest tertile with regard to the body mass index) was 31.6 percent in men and 52.4 percent in women. For occupational activity, Felson and colleagues (1991) estimated that the proportion of cases of radiographic knee OA attributable to jobs with both physical demands and knee bending was 15 percent, while Cooper and colleagues (1994a) suggested that 5 percent of cases of symptomatic knee OA might result from jobs involving repetitive knee usage. The amount of knee OA attributable to sports and joint injury and/or trauma would be expected to be lower because of the low prevalence of these exposures in the general population. Thus, for knee OA, overweight is the most important modifiable risk factor, followed by occupational activity.

The available data on which to base estimates for OA of the hip come from studies from Scandinavia (Heliovaara et al., 1993; Olsen et al., 1994). Heliovaara and colleagues (1993) examined the cumulative effect of the three modifiable risk factors for hip OA: a body mass index greater than 25 kg/m^2, physical stress at work, and a history of lower-limb injury. They found the population-attributable fraction of hip OA to be 18.6 percent if one risk factor was present, 30.8 percent if two risk factors were present, and 9.1 percent if all three risk factors were present. (The low figure of 9.1% reflects the small number of cases that had all three risk factors.) Thus, 58.5 percent of all hip OA could be attributed to these three risk factors, either alone or in combination. Olsen and colleagues (1994) calculated the etiologic fraction for physical work load, participation in sports activity, and overweight in their case-control study of patients with hip OA who underwent total joint arthroplasty. The etiologic fraction was 55 percent for sports, 40 percent for physical work load, and 15 percent for overweight; overall, approximately 80 percent of cases could be attributed to one of these three risk factors.

Thus, the majority of cases of both knee and hip OA could be prevented by adoption of the primary prevention strategies outlined above.

REFERENCES

Acheson R, Collart AB. 1975. New Haven survey of joint diseases: XVII. Relationship between some systemic characteristics and osteoarthrosis in a general population. *Ann Rheum Dis* 34:379–387.

Anderson JJ, Felson DT. 1988. Factors associated with osteoarthritis of the knee in the First National Health and Nutrition Examination Survey (HANES I): Evidence for an association with overweight, race, and physical demands of work. *Am J Epidemiol* 128:179–189.

Axmacher B, Lindberg H. 1993. Coxarthrosis in farmers. *Clin Orthop Rel Res* 287:82–86.

Bagge E, Bjelle A, Eden S, Svanborg A. 1991. Factors associated with radiographic osteoarthritis: Results from a population study 70-year-old people in Goteborg. *J Rheumatol* 18:1218–1222.

Bovenzi M, Petronio L, DiMarino F. 1980. Epidemiological survey of shipyard workers exposed to hand-arm vibration. *Int Arch Occup Environ Health* 46:251–266.

Bovenzi M, Fiorito A, Volpe C. 1987. Bone and joint disorders in the upper extremities of chipping and grinding operators. *Int Arch Occup Environ Health* 59:189–198.

Buckwalter JA. 1995. Osteoarthritis and articular cartilage use, disuse, and abuse: Experimental studies. *J Rheumatol* 22(suppl. 43):13–15.

Cooper C. 1995. Occupational activity and the risk of osteoarthritis. *J Rheumatol* 22(suppl. 43): 10–12.

Cooper C, McAlindon T, Coggon D, Egger P, Dieppe P. 1994a. Occupational activity and osteoarthritis of the knee. *Ann Rheum Dis* 53:90–93.

Cooper C, McAlindon T, Snow S, Vines K, Young P, Kirwan J, Dieppe P. 1994b. Mechanical and constitutional risk factors for symptomatic knee osteoarthritis: Differences between medial tibiofemoral and patellofemoral disease. *J Rheumatol* 21:307–313.

Copeman W. 1940. The arthritis sequelae of pneumatic drilling. *Ann Rheum Dis* 2:141–146.

Croft P, Coggon D, Cruddas M, Cooper C. 1992a. Osteoarthritis of the hip: An occupational disease in farmers. *Br Med J* 304:1269–1272.

Croft P, Cooper C, Wickham C, Coggon D. 1992b. Osteoarthritis of the hip and occupational activity. *Scand J Work Env Health* 18:59–63.

Davis MA, Ettinger WH, Neuhaus JM. 1988a. The role of metabolic factors and blood pressure in the association of obesity with osteoarthritis of the knee. *J Rheumatol* 15:1827–1832.

Davis MA, Ettinger WH, Neuhaus JM, Hauck WW. 1988b. Sex differences in osteoarthritis of the knee: The role of obesity. *Am J Epidemiol* 127:1019–1030.

Davis MA, Ettinger WH, Neuhaus JM, Cho SA, Houck WW. 1989. The association of knee injury and obesity with unilateral and bilateral osteoarthritis of the knee. *Am J Epidemiol* 130:278–288.

Davis MA, Neuhaus JM, Ettinger WH, Mueller WH. 1990. Body fat distribution and osteoarthritis. *Am J Epidemiol* 132:701–707.

Department of Rheumatology and Medical Illustration, University of Manchester. 1973. *The epidemiology of chronic rheumatism.* Vol. 2, *Atlas of standard radiographs of arthritis.* Pp. 1–15. Philadelphia: FA Davis.

Felson DT. 1988. Epidemiology of hip and knee osteoarthritis. *Epidemiol Rev* 10:1–28.

———. 1994. Do occupation-related physical factors contribute to arthritis? *Ballieres Clin Rheumatol* 8:63–77.

———. 1995. Weight and osteoarthritis. *J Rheumatol* 22(suppl. 43):7–9.

Felson DT, Anderson JJ, Naimark AA, Walker AM, Meenan RF. 1988. Obesity and knee osteoarthritis: The Framingham study. *Ann Intern Med* 109:18–24.

Felson DT, Hannan MT, Naimark A, Berkeley J, Gordon G, Wilson PWF, Anderson J. 1991. Occupational physical demands, knee bending, and knee osteoarthritis: Results from the Framingham study. *J Rheumatol* 18:1587–1592.

Felson DT, Zhang Y, Anthony JM, Naimark A, Anderson JJ. 1992. Weight loss reduces the risk for symptomatic knee osteoarthritis in women: The Framingham study. *Ann Intern Med* 116:535–539.

Genti G. 1989. Occupation and osteoarthritis. *Ballieres Clin Rheumatol* 3:193–204.

Hadler NM, Gillings DB, Imbus HR, Levitin PM, Makuk D, Utsinger PD, Yount WJ, Slusser D, Moskowitz N. 1978. Hand structure and function in an industrial setting. *Arthritis Rheum* 21: 210–220.

Hart DJ, Spector TD. 1993. The relationship of obesity, fat distribution, and osteoarthritis in women in the general population: The Chingford study. *J Rheumatol* 20:331–335.

Hartz AJ, Fischer ME, Bril G, Kelber S, Rupley D Jr., Okan B, Rimm AA. 1986. The association of obesity with joint pain and osteoarthritis in the HANES data. *J Chronic Dis* 39:311–319.

Heliovaara M, Makela M, Imprivaara O, Knekt P, Aromaa A, Sievers K. 1993. Association of overweight, trauma, and workload with coxarthrosis: A health study of 7,217 persons. *Acta Orthop Scand* 64:513–518.

Hochberg MC, Lawrence RC, Everett DF, Cornoni-Huntley J. 1989. Epidemiologic associations of pain in osteoarthritis of the knee: Data from the National Health and Nutrition Examination Survey and the National Health and Nutrition Examination—I. Epidemiologic Followup Survey. *Semin Arthritis Rheum* 18(suppl. 2):4–9.

Hochberg MC, Lethbridge-Cejku M, Scott WW Jr., Reichle R, Plato CC, Tobin JD. 1995. The association of body weight, body fatness, and body fat distribution with osteoarthritis of the knee: Data from the Baltimore Longitudinal Study of Aging. *J Rheumatol* 22:488–493.

Hunter D, McLaughlin A, Perry K. 1945. Clinical effects of the use of pneumatic tools. *Br J Ind Med* 2:10–16.

Jacobson B, Dalen N, Tjornstrand B. 1987. Coxarthrosis and labour. *Int Orthop* 11:311–313.

Kellgren JH, Lawrence JS. 1952. Rheumatism in coal miners: II. X-ray study. *Br J Ind Med* 9:197–207.

Kelsey JL, Hochberg MC. 1988. Epidemiology of chronic musculoskeletal disorders. *Annu Rev Public Health* 9:379–401.

Klunder KB, Rud B, Hansen J. 1980. Osteoarthritis of the hip and knee joint in retired football players. *Acta Orthop Scand* 51:925–927.

Konradsen L, Hansen EM, Sondegaard L. 1990. Long distance running and osteoarthritis. *Am J Sports Med* 18:379–381.

Kujala UM, Kaprio J, Sarna S. 1994. Osteoarthritis of weight bearing joints of lower limbs in former elite male athletes. *Br Med J* 308:231–234.

Kujala UM, Kettunen J, Paananen H, Aalto T, Battie MC, Impivaara O, Videman T, Sarna S. 1995. Knee osteoarthritis in former runners, soccer players, weight lifters, and shooters. *Arthritis Rheum* 38:539–546.

Lane NE, Bloch DA, Jones HH, Marshall W Jr., Wood PD, Fries JF. 1986. Long distance running, bone density, and osteoarthritis. *JAMA* 255:1147–1151.

Lane NE, Bloch DA, Hubert HB, Jones H, Simpson U, Fries JF. 1990. Running, osteoarthritis, and bone density: Initial 2-year longitudinal study. *Am J Med* 88:452–459.

Lane NE, Michel B, Bjorkengren A, Oehlert J, Shi H, Bloch DA, Fries JF. 1993. The risk of osteoarthritis with running and aging: A 5-year longitudinal study. *J Rheumatol* 20:461–468.

Lawrence JS. 1961. Rheumatism in cotton operatives. *Br J Ind Med* 18:270–276.

———. 1977. *Rheumatism in populations.* Pp. 98–155. London: William Heinemann Medical Books.

Lindberg H, Montgomery F. 1987. Heavy labor and the occurrence of gonarthrosis. *Clin Orthop Rel Res* 214:235–236.

Lindberg H, Roos H, Gardsell P. 1993. Prevalence of coxarthrosis in former soccer players: 286 players compared with matched controls. *Acta Orthop Scand* 64:165–167.

Louyot P, Savin R. 1966. La coxarthrose chez l'agriculture. *Rev Rheum Mal Osteoartic* 33:625–632.

Marti B, Knobloch M, Tschopp A, Jucker A, Howald H. 1989. Is excessive running predictive of degenerative hip disease? Controlled study of former elite athletes. *Br Med J* 299:91–93.

Martin K, Lethbridge-Cejku M, Muller D, Elahi D, Andres R, Plato C, Tobin J, Hochberg M. 1995. Risk factors for cardiovascular disease and radiographic features of knee osteoarthritis: Data from the Baltimore Longitudinal Study of Aging. *Arthritis Rheum* 38(9, suppl.):S342.

Neyret P, Donell ST, DeJour D, DeJour H. 1993. Partial meniscectomy and anterior cruciate ligament rupture in soccer players: A study with a minimum 20-year followup. *Am J Sports Med* 21:455–460.

Olsen O, Vingard E, Koster M, Alfredsson L. 1994. Etiologic fractions for physical work load, sports, and overweight in the occurrence of coxarthrosis. *Scand J Work Environ Health* 20:184–188.

Panush RS, Lane NE. 1994. Exercise and the musculoskeletal system. *Ballieres Clin Rheumatol* 8:79–102.

Panush RS, Schmidt C, Caldwell JR, Edwards NL, Longley S, Yonker R, Webster E, Nauman J, Stork J, Pettersson H. 1986. Is running associated with degenerative joint disease? *JAMA* 255:1152–1155.

Partridge REH, Duthie JJR. 1968. Rheumatism in dockers and civil servants: A comparison of heavy manual and sedentary workers. *Am Rheum Dis* 27:559–568.

Puranen J, Ala-Ketola L, Peltokallio P, Saarela J. 1975. Running and primary osteoarthritis of the hip. *Br Med J* 1:424–435.

Roach KE, Persky V, Miles T, Budiman-Mak E. 1994. Biomechanical aspects of occupation and osteoarthritis of the hip: A case-control study. *J Rheumatol* 21:2334–2340.

Roos H, Lindberg H, Gardsell P, Lohmander LS, Wingstrand H. 1994. The prevalence of gonarthrosis and its relation to meniscectomy in former soccer players. *Am J Sports Med* 22:219–222.

Saville PD, Dickson J. 1968. Age and weight in osteoarthritis of the hip. *Arthritis Rheum* 11:635–644.

Scott JC, Hochberg MC. 1987. Epidemiologic insights into the pathogenesis of hip osteoarthritis. In: *Clinical concepts in regional musculoskeletal illness*, edited by NM Hadler. Pp. 89–107. Orlando: Grune and Stratton.

Scott JC, Hochberg MC. 1993. Arthritis and musculoskeletal disorders. In: *Chronic disease epidemiology and control*, edited by RC Brownson, PL Remington, JR Davis. Pp. 285–305. Washington, D.C.: American Public Health Association.

Silman AJ, Hochberg MC. 1993. *Epidemiology of the rheumatic diseases*. Pp. 257–288. Oxford: Oxford University Press.

Sohn RS, Micheli LJ. 1985. The effect of running on the pathogenesis of osteoarthritis of the hips and knees. *Clin Orthop* 198:106–109.

Spector TD, Hart DJ, Doyle DV. 1994. Incidence and progression of osteoarthritis in women with unilateral knee disease in the general population: The effect of obesity. *Ann Rheum Dis* 53:565–568.

Tepper S, Hochberg MC. 1993. Factors associated with hip osteoarthritis: Data from the First National Health and Nutrition Examination Survey (NHANES-I). *Am J Epidemiol* 137:1081–1088.

Thelin A. 1990. Hip joint arthrosis: An occupational disorder among farmers. *Am J Ind Med* 18:339–343.

Typpo T. 1985. Osteoarthritis of the hip: Radiologic findings and etiology. *Ann Chir Gynaecol* 74 (suppl. 201):5–38.

van Saase JLCM, Vandenbroucke JP, van Romunde LKJ, Valkenburg HA. 1988. Osteoarthritis and obesity in the general population: A relationship calling for an explanation. *J Rheumatol* 15:1152–1158.

Vingard E. 1991. Overweight predisposes to coxarthrosis: Body-mass index studied in 239 males with hip arthroplasty. *Acta Orthop Scand* 62:106–109.

Vingard E, Alfredsson L, Goldie I, Hogstedt C. 1991a. Occupation and osteoarthrosis of the hip and knee: A register-based cohort study. *Int J Epidemiol* 20:1025–1031.

Vingard E, Hogstedt C, Alfredsson L, Fellenium E, Goldie I, Koster M. 1991b. Coxarthrosis and physical work load. *Scand J Work Environ Health* 17:104–109.

Vingard E, Alfredsson L, Goldie I, Hogstedt C. 1993. Sports and osteoarthrosis of the hip: An epidemiologic study. *Am J Sports Med* 21:195–200.

Wickstrom G, Haninen K, Mattsson T, Niskanen T, Riihimaki H, Waris P. 1983. Knee degeneration in concrete reinforcement workers. *Br J Ind Med* 40:216–219.

11

Skeletal and Inflammation Markers in Aging and Osteoarthritis

Implications for Early Diagnosis and
Monitoring of the Effects of Therapy

A. Robin Poole, Ph.D., D.Sc.

Osteoarthritis involves profound alterations in the metabolism, and consequently the structure, of articular cartilages and juxta-articular bone. These structural changes are accompanied by alterations in synovial metabolism and are distinct from those observed in aging. Their measurement in vivo offers the potential to distinguish pathologic alterations in osteoarthritis (OA) from the alterations associated with aging, to measure disease activity, and to assess the efficacy of therapeutic management. Available human data indicate that these pathologic changes may occur early in the disease process and precede clinical symptoms. Hence, we may be able to identify preclinical changes apart from aging and to monitor the effects of therapy.

The potential for detecting changes in the metabolism of cartilage and of joint tissues is made possible by the recent and ongoing development of new, very sensitive and specific chemical and immunochemical assays for the detection of what are often tissue-specific macromolecules, their biosynthetic products, and their degradation products in body fluids such as serum and plasma, synovial fluid, and urine (see reviews by Lohmander et al., 1992; Thonar and Glant, 1992; Poole, 1994; Poole and Dieppe, 1994).

Changes in the Metabolism and Structure of Cartilage and Bone in Osteoarthritis

Cartilage

One of the most striking anatomical features of OA is the loss of joint space as a consequence of the degeneration of articular cartilage resulting from an abnormal turnover of the extracellular matrix of cartilage and the progressive destruction of that matrix. This may be a very lengthy process lasting for decades. Not only are chondrocytes responsible for the synthesis of the extensive extracellular matrix, but current data point to these cells as playing a key role in cartilage degradation in health and OA (fig. 11.1; for reviews, see Poole, 1993; Poole et al., 1995). This latter aspect is clearly demonstrated by recent immunochemical analyses of type II collagen, the primary component of cartilage matrix. This molecule forms with type XI and type IX collagens an extensive network of fibrils in the extracellular matrix of articular cartilage. The fibrils provide the cartilage with its tensile properties (Poole, 1993). In aging, damage to these collagen fibrils develops as a result of cleavage of the triple helix of type II collagen by collagenases. This is even more pronounced in OA (Hollander et al., 1994, 1995). The weakened matrix then fibrillates as the damage develops (Hollander et al., 1995); this is first seen in the immediate pericellular matrix of chondrocytes. This process starts at the articular surface, and increasing degeneration spreads progressively deeper, eventually penetrating the entire depth. The same pattern of collagen damage is seen in aging, but the degree of damage is much less, always developing first in the immediate pericellular matrix of chondrocytes (Hollander et al., 1995).

These changes, which directly implicate the chondrocytes in the pathology, are accompanied by enhanced proteolytic cleavage of the core protein of the large proteoglycan aggrecan. This molecule, which produces the compressive stiffness of cartilage (Poole, 1993), is also progressively degraded, resulting in a loss of keratan sulfate–rich molecules (Rizkalla et al., 1992). This loss is seen particularly in more superficial sites, where type II collagen fibril damage is most pronounced in early disease (Hollander et al., 1995); often, pericellular loss of aggrecan is also noted. In more advanced disease, these damaged aggrecan molecules are replaced by larger, more intact molecules (Rizkalla et al., 1992) as a consequence of a marked increase in biosynthesis (Mankin et al., 1971; Thompson and Oegema, 1979; Poole, 1986) and extensive changes in aggrecan composition (Rizkalla et al., 1992). The biosynthesis of aggrecan can now be detected by immunoassay of a chondroitin sulfate epitope that is likely to be present pri-

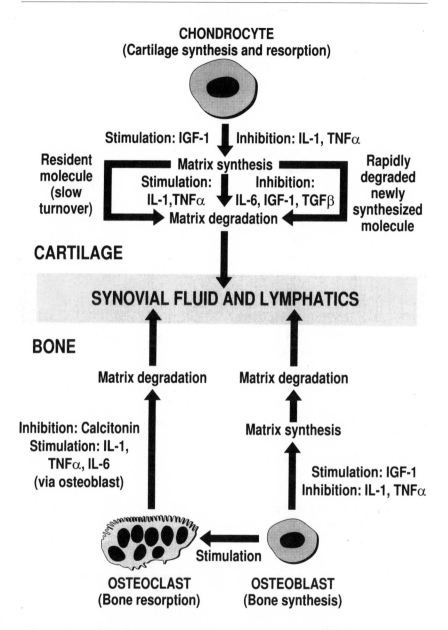

Figure 11.1. The influence of cytokines and growth factors on the synthesis and degradation of matrix molecules and their release from cartilage and bone tissues

marily on newly synthesized aggrecan molecules, or degradation products thereof, which are not normally retained in the matrix (Rizkalla et al., 1992; H. Jugessur and A. R. Poole, unpublished results, 1996). This epitope is recognized and defined by a mouse monoclonal antibody 846.

Type II procollagen synthesis is also enhanced in OA (Lippiello et al., 1977; Aigner et al., 1992, 1993). This can be detected by the immunoassay of the C-propeptide of this molecule, which is released from procollagen in the extracellular matrix when collagen fibrils form. The C-propeptide content directly correlates with the rate of type II procollagen synthesis (Nelson et al., 1994, 1996), and consequently the C-propeptide increases in osteoarthritic cartilage (Nelson et al., 1994, 1996).

The release from cartilage of a thrombospondin called cartilage oligomeric protein (COMP) is also enhanced in OA (Lohmander et al., 1994). This may result from a combination of increased synthesis and degradation.

Bone

Bone is formed from an organic extracellular matrix called osteoid, which is synthesized and secreted by osteoblasts. Like cartilage, bone contains a number of proteins that are primarily, or exclusively, found in this tissue. These molecules, which can now also be detected by immunoassay, include bone sialoprotein and osteocalcin. The primary organic component is type I collagen, which differs in its chemistry from the type II collagen of articular cartilage and, unlike type II collagen, is present in a wide variety of tissues.

In OA, the degeneration of articular cartilage is accompanied by an increase in bone density. This so-called sclerosis of bone is obvious on radiographic examination and results from enhanced synthesis of bone (see chapter 7). These changes contrast to the marked osteopenia seen in juxta-articular bone in a rheumatoid joint as a consequence of excessive bone resorption: this increased turnover of bone, which leads to both sclerosis and osteopenia, can be detected by scintigraphy using radiolabeled bone-seeking biophosphonates.

Whereas osteoblasts synthesize the organic matrix of bone, which then mineralizes, it is the osteoclasts that resorb this mineralized matrix (fig. 11.1). Their activity is physiologically coupled to that of osteoblasts by cytokines such as interleukin-6 (IL-6). Specific hormones such as calcitonin (acting upon osteoclasts) and parathyroid hormone (PTH) and PTH-related peptide (acting upon osteoblasts) can arrest and stimulate bone resorption, respectively. The resorption of bone results in the degradation of type I collagen, which is normally cross-linked after it has been present for a while in the extracellular matrix.

When the bone is resorbed, these cross-links are released into body fluids, where they escape degradation and can be detected in urine. Most of these cross-links are derived from bone.

The detection of the synthesis and degradation of these molecules within these skeletal tissues now makes it possible to study their turnover in vivo.

Reasons for Changes in Cartilage and Bone Metabolism

The biosynthetic and degradative activities of chondrocytes are, like those of osteoblasts and osteoclasts, ordinarily regulated hormonally or by cytokines and growth factors (fig. 11.1). Insulin-like growth factor I (IGF-I) is a potent stimulator of matrix synthesis by chondrocytes (for a review, see Poole, 1993) and by osteoblasts (Hock et al., 1988; Canalis et al., 1989). Cyclic compressive loading is also stimulatory for synthesis in chondrocytes, whereas passive loading can inhibit synthesis and stimulate degradation (for a review, see Sah et al., 1991; Poole, 1993). Bone and cartilage metabolism are both profoundly influenced by changes in the mechanical loading of these tissues as a result of alterations or abnormalities in the articulation of joint surfaces which arise from joint injury and joint instability (Poole, 1986); incongruity of articulating surfaces; or abnormal matrix structure, such as might result from a genetic abnormality (Poole, 1993). Unloading bone, or immobilization, can cause net resorption; increased loading produces an increase in bone mass (Cruess, 1982). Increased loading of bone must occur in OA as a consequence of the loss of articular cartilage, and is reflected by increased bone density, or sclerosis. Changes in bone density, or in the structure and mechanical properties and thickness of neighboring articular cartilage, would cause changes in loading of chondrocytes as well as osteoblasts, which could alter the metabolism of these cells. This is especially likely since bone and cartilage contact each other and are both involved in the process of load dissipation during articulation. Damage to the articular surface of cartilage could also influence the metabolism of chondrocytes deeper within the cartilage by changing the physical properties of the neighboring extracellular matrix and, hence, load transmission. Thus, a change in one tissue, or in one site, could markedly influence the metabolism of the other tissue or that of an adjacent region in the same tissue, and lead to structural changes in the adjacent site or tissue. These alterations could then "feed back" and further influence the tissue in which these changes began, thereby establishing a chain reaction of degenerative changes. That is why it is so important to study bone as well as articular cartilage in OA: the changes in these tissues and the mechanisms producing them are interlinked and are reflected by both tissues. These changes are a consequence of dynamic mechanical and biochemical interactions. In a chronic inflammatory disease, such as rheumatoid arthritis (RA), or in cases of OA with inflammatory overtones (see below), we would anticipate that the changes would be more influenced by cytokines and growth factors produced by the inflammatory process.

Cytokines, such as interleukin-1 (IL-1) and tumor necrosis factor–α (TNF-α) can inhibit the synthesis of cartilage (for a review, see Poole, 1993) and bone (Canalis, 1987; Stashenko et al., 1987) (fig. 11.1), and at higher concentrations can also stimulate cartilage matrix degradation (by up-regulation of matrix metalloproteinase synthesis and activation [Poole et al., 1995]), and bone resorption (Saklatvala, 1986; Boyce et al., 1989). In chondrocytes, the stimulation of degradation by IL-1 can be enhanced by fibroblast growth factor (FGF) or inhibited by IGF-I (Poole et al., 1995), probably through IL-1 receptor regulation. Some of these cytokines are also produced by chondrocytes (Poole et al., 1995) and by osteoblasts. The latter produce IL-6, which can potently induce bone resorption (Ishimi et al., 1990; Jilka et al., 1992). Interleukin-6 production by bone cells is normally suppressed by estradiol-17β (Jilka et al., 1992). The fact that cytokine production in these tissues can be regulated by sex hormones may help explain in part the greater incidence of OA in women. How these cytokines, growth factors, and hormones are involved in OA is unclear, yet the evidence for their fundamental effects on bone and cartilage metabolism in the pathobiology of OA is compelling, especially in more rapidly progressive joint disease.

Inflammation and Osteoarthritis

Although OA clearly involves the degeneration and remodeling of cartilage and bone, there is now clear evidence for an inflammatory component in established OA. As we will discuss later, only when this inflammation is more pronounced is there evidence to indicate that it may recognizably influence the disease process by enhancing cartilage degeneration. The potential for inflammation to influence cartilage and, to a lesser extent, bone metabolism in OA is considerable, particularly by way of cytokines generated by synovial cells and macrophages in the synovial membrane. Until recently, little attention was paid to inflammation and its involvement in the pathogenesis of OA. One school of thought was so anti-inflammation that the term *osteoarthrosis* was used instead of *osteoarthritis*.

Interleukin-6, which, as noted above, can play a fundamental role in bone resorption (fig. 11.1) and cartilage metabolism (Poole et al., 1995), is elevated in synovial fluids of patients with RA and OA (Houssiau et al., 1988) and in those with arthritis following traumatic injury (Waage et al., 1989). Levels of the soluble receptor of TNF-α, an index of the involvement of this cytokine, are elevated in synovial fluids from osteoarthritic joints and are similar to levels found in joints of patients with reactive arthritis and RA (Steiner et al., 1995). These changes all point to the presence of an active inflammatory component in patients with OA.

The metabolism of the synovium plays an essential role in normal joint function. Macrophage lining cells help ensure asepsis, and the fibroblastic lining cells secrete essential components of the synovial fluid. These lining cells produce proinflammatory cytokines and also synthesize a large glycosaminoglycan called hyaluronan (hyaluronic acid), a soft tissue boundary lubricant for joint movement (fig. 11.2). In inflammatory arthritis, the synthesis of hyaluronan is enhanced (Dahl and Husby, 1985) as a result of the known stimulation by cytokines, such as IL-1 and TNF-α (Yaron et al., 1989), and transforming growth factor β (TGF-β) (Haubeck et al., 1995), all of which are also found in increased amounts in synovial fluid from arthritic joints. The increase in hyaluronan synthesis in itself points to an active production of cytokines. In RA, this increased production of hyaluronan is reflected by a rise in serum levels of this molecule, detected by radioassays or immunoassays. These serum levels directly correlate with joint inflammation and disease progression (Engström-Laurent and Hallgren 1985, 1987; Hørslev-Petersen et al., 1988; Konttinen et al., 1990; Paimela et al., 1991) and with levels of circulating TNF-α (Manicourt et al., 1993). Therefore, hyaluronan offers the potential to detect synovitis in OA as well as in RA.

Genetic Mutations Cause Chondrodysplasias with Early Onset Osteoarthritis

Abnormalities of the COL2A1 (type II procollagen) gene result in chondrodysplasias characterized by alterations in the growth plate and abnormal cartilage matrix, which lead to premature joint degeneration and early onset OA (R. Stanescu et al., 1987; V. Stanescu et al., 1984, 1985). These genetic conditions include the Stickler syndrome (Ahmad et al., 1991; Winterpacht et al., 1993), spondyloepiphyseal dysplasia (Lee et al., 1989; Tiller et al., 1990; Ritvaniemi et al., 1995), and undefined dysplasias (Palotie et al., 1989; Ala-Kokko et al., 1990; Knowlton et al., 1990). Similarly, defects in the COL11A2 gene encoding the type XI procollagen α_2 (X1) chain can also produce the Stickler syndrome and spondyloepiphyseal dysplasia (Vikkula et al., 1995). Abnormalities in cartilage oligomeric protein structure resulting from genetic defects produce pseudo-achondroplasia and multiple epiphyseal dysplasia (Briggs et al., 1995;

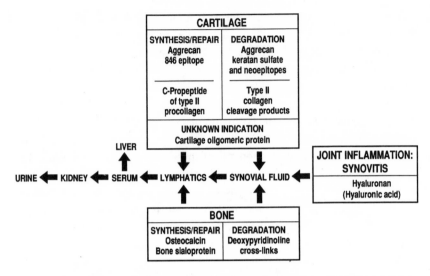

Figure 11.2.   Candidate skeletal markers for the study of matrix synthesis and degradation in cartilage and bone, and the release of these markers into body fluids. Some markers, such as aggrecan and hyaluronan, are removed by the liver, whereas others, such as osteocalcin, are mainly removed by the kidneys.

Hecht et al., 1995). In subjects with such molecular defects in a single molecule, the structure and the turnover of other cartilage matrix molecules are also altered (Bleasel et al., 1995), due to the chain of reactions and alterations at the cellular and molecular levels.

Mutations that influence cell surface receptors can cause abnormal cellular responses to growth factors and result in chondrodysplasias and early onset of OA. Achondroplasia, the most common chondrodysplasia, results from a mutation in the fibroblast growth factor receptor 3 (FGF R3) gene (Shiang et al., 1994; Bellus et al., 1995). Mutations in this receptor can also cause thanatotrophic dysplasia (types I and II) (Tavormina et al., 1995). Moreover, an abnormality in the gene encoding the receptors for parathyroid hormone and parathyroid hormone–related peptide causes Jansen-type metaphyseal chondrodysplasia (Schipani et al., 1995).

Although persons with skeletal dysplasias usually develop OA, the early onset and accompanying skeletal dysplasias set them apart from those with onset of OA later in life.

What Do Our Measurements of Cartilage and Bone Markers in Body Fluids Reflect?

If we are to be able to use biological markers to examine the metabolism of bone and cartilage in vivo, we must know what we are measuring and what these changes represent in terms of tissue turnover. Otherwise, we will be denied the opportunity to clearly interpret how our findings relate to disease pathology and activity. It is essential, therefore, that we study specific, well-defined markers of biosynthesis and of degradation in bone and cartilage. If a molecule is not known to be a specific product of either process, then experiments must be performed to ascertain what its release does, in fact, represent. Is the molecule the degradation product of a newly synthesized cartilage-specific component, such as the C-propeptide of type II procollagen? Or does the molecule represent the release, following synthesis, of an intact molecule that is not incorporated into matrix? Or is the molecule the degradation product of a molecule previously incorporated and "resident" in the extracellular matrix, such as a cross-link of collagen?

The content of a molecule, and/or its fragments, present in a body fluid may therefore reflect the rate of synthesis of that molecule or its rate of degradation, or a combination of both. Changes in degradation and synthesis may, in turn, reflect disease-related hormonal, cytokine, or growth factor activity, biomechanical alterations that influence matrix turnover, or a combination of all of these. For these reasons, if we are able to interpret our data effectively, measurements of these biological markers must be matched by equally careful studies on what these markers truly represent, both structurally and metabolically. We need to know exactly which part of the molecule we are measuring. Can we only detect intact molecules, or only degradation products, or both? What are the structures of the epitopes recognized by the antibodies we use to detect these molecules? All of this information is essential if these studies are to be successful.

Moreover, the levels of these molecules in body fluids are the product of the molecules' release and clearance (fig. 11.2), and therefore, any change in these levels may reflect modifications in one process or the other, or both. Depending on the molecule, the liver and/or the kidney are primarily responsible for its removal from blood. Usually this happens relatively quickly—in minutes rather than hours (Poole and Dieppe, 1994). Joint fluid clearance rates must also be studied in health and disease, and these too are also usually rapid (Page-Thomas et al., 1987). Clearance from synovial fluids may be influenced by inflammatory changes in the synovium—although, in the case of the proteoglycan aggrecan, there is no indication for this (Page-Thomas et al., 1987). Liver disease can lead to an accumulation of hyaluronan, since it is normally cleared by the liver (Fraser et al., 1986). Awareness of how clearance may influence the levels of these tissue and inflammation markers is obviously of great importance for their study and for data interpretation; we have much to understand about the molecules that we may choose to study and whose metabolism we wish to track in vivo.

Individual Skeletal Markers of Cartilage Metabolism in Osteoarthritis

The Proteoglycan Aggrecan

Initial studies of epitopes of keratan sulfate, a glycosaminoglycan of aggrecan, which is particularly concentrated in degradation products of resident aggrecan molecules in aging human cartilage (Webber et al., 1987), were made by Thonar et al. (1985) and Sweet et al. (1988) using an ELISA assay employing a monoclonal antibody that reacted with a highly sulfated region of keratan sulfate (Caterson et al., 1983; Mehmet et al., 1986). The assays revealed an elevation of immunoreactive keratan sulfate–containing degradation products in the sera of patients with OA. Although further investigations by these investigators confirmed this increase (Campion et al., 1991), others using the same or similar monoclonal antibodies to this glycosaminoglycan failed to confirm the earlier findings (Seibel et al., 1988; Spector et al., 1992; Poole et al., 1994b). The radioimmunoassays used by Poole et al. (1994b) employed either whole immunoglobulin G or Fab′. Previous studies of competitive radioimmunoassays had revealed that, whereas whole immunoglobulin molecules primarily detected the larger immunoreactive keratan sulfate–containing degradation products (Poole et al., 1989), the use of Fab′ fragments enabled the detection of smaller aggrecan fragments as well. These fragments proved to be more common in age- and sex-matched normal sera (Poole et al., 1994b). When either the large fragments or all the keratan sulfate–containing fragments were measured (by IgG assay or Fab′ assay, respectively), serum levels of this epitope were found to be slightly depressed in OA, certainly not elevated (Poole et al., 1994b). This was confirmed in a more recent study (Petersson et al., 1996). This reduction was also observed in sera of patients with RA, where it is was more pronounced (Poole et al., 1990, 1994b).

In patients with RA, inverse relationships between circulating immunoreactive keratan sulfate and markers of inflammation have been consistently seen. These include circulating acute phase proteins, erythrocyte sedimentation rate (Poole et al., 1990; Spector et al., 1992), and TNF-α (Manicourt et al., 1993). These relationships point to an inhibitory effect of inflammation on aggrecan release, suggesting that in sera from subjects with arthritis, these fragments may be more reflective of proteoglycan synthesis and particularly of the inhibitory effects of inflammation on aggrecan synthesis (followed by its degradation), mediated most probably systemically via cytokines, such as TNF-α and IL-1, as described above. It is unlikely, therefore, that these aggrecan molecules detected in serum are solely products of matrix degradation of resident molecules. Thus, at the present time, measurement of keratan sulfate epitopes in sera or plasma may reflect both synthesis and degradation.

In synovial fluids from joints of subjects with OA, aggrecan degradation products can also be detected (Witter et al., 1987). Here a keratan sulfate epitope has shown some interesting disease-related changes in cross-sectional studies of chronic large-joint OA and RA (Poole et al., 1994b). In *synovial fluid* of patients with OA as in *peripheral blood* of patients with RA, there are inverse relationships between keratan sulfate epitope concentration and synovial fluid inflammation markers, namely, eosinophil cationic protein, myeloperoxidase, and neutrophil count (Poole et al., 1994b). This suggests that (as observed systemically in RA) within the osteoarthritic joint, low-level inflammation impairs aggrecan synthesis rather than stimulates degradation. This is in contrast to rheumatoid joints, where inflammation is much more pronounced and is associated with an increase in keratan sulfate epitope content (Poole et al., 1994b). These disease-related differences are likely due to different cytokine concentrations and/or profiles. Thus, the study of immunoreactive keratan sulfate–rich fragments in serum and in synovial fluid from osteoarthritic joints has not been shown to provide a definitive marker of aggrecan cleavage, a finding more likely to occur in synovial fluids from patients with RA (Poole et al., 1994b). Systemically, therefore, keratan sulfate epitopes appear to reflect the degradation products of newly synthesized molecules, the turnover of which is more influenced by inflammation at the level of biosynthesis than at the level of degradation. But when the inflammation is more pronounced, as in a rheumatoid joint, keratan sulfate epitopes are more reflective of degradation.

More specific antibodies to study aggrecan degradation are, however, now available. Recently, antibodies have been produced to the amino- and carboxy-terminal neoepitopes that are produced when link protein (Hughes et al., 1992) and aggrecan core protein (Hughes et al., 1995; Lark et al., 1995; Singer et al., 1995) (fig. 11.2) are cleaved by tissue proteases. Although immunoassays of body fluids have not yet been reported, it is almost certainly only a matter of time before the use of these new antibodies will provide direct indications of the degradation of these molecules. Whether the molecules are resident or newly synthesized may be more difficult to determine. Then it will be possible to compare data obtained with these new assays with data obtained from assays based on keratan sulfate epitopes.

Whereas in our analysis the content of the keratan sulfate epitope in synovial fluid shows little increase over serum levels in OA and RA (the mean increase is about 2-fold), the 846 epitope found on the most intact, fully functional, and newly synthesized aggrecan molecules (Rizkalla et al., 1992; H. Jugessur and A. R. Poole, unpublished results, 1996) is usually elevated in osteoarthritic cartilage (Rizkalla et al., 1992), and is often strikingly so in synovial fluid of patients with OA (on average, 38-fold) (Poole et al., 1994b). The synovial fluid content was found to be highest in patients with greater joint space narrowing and in those with longer duration of disease and cartilage damage. When the 846 epitope content was analyzed relative to the keratan sulfate content in synovial fluids from osteoarthritic joints, a clear inverse relationship was observed by Spearman rank analyses ($r = -0.510$; $p = 0.0004$; $n = 49$) (Poole et al., 1994b). This was also noted in RA but was less pronounced (Poole et al., 1994b). With increased duration of OA, ratios of 846 to keratan sulfate epitopes were also increased in synovial fluid. These studies suggest that these epitopes are indicative of different processes and are present on different molecules and fragments. Thus, the keratan sulfate epitope in *synovial fluid* is probably never reflective of synthesis alone, even in OA. However, in *peripheral blood* from normal subjects and from persons with OA, there are direct correlations between these two epitopes (Poole et al., 1994b), suggesting that serum keratan sulfate epitope is more reflective of synthesis. In contrast, in RA, the serum keratan sulfate content was significantly directly correlated with synovial fluid 846 content, although 846 or keratan sulfate correlations were not observed for either marker alone between joint fluids and sera of individual patients. Therefore, circulating keratan sulfate epitope may be derived from joints of patients with RA and may more directly reflect the synthesis of aggrecan in diseased joints rather than systemic synthesis by all cartilages. That serum keratan sulfate epitope is also indirectly correlated to joint myeloperoxidase levels and joint damage (Poole et al., 1994b) also supports a direct link between serum keratan sulfate epitope content and joint inflammation and damage.

Elevations of serum 846 epitope have also been noted in about 20 percent of patients with chronic OA—a proportion much less than the almost 60 percent of subjects with RA with chronic inflammatory disease who showed marked elevations (Poole et al., 1994b). It remains to be seen whether these subjects with OA are indicative of a subgroup with a better prognosis (increased matrix synthesis) or have an underlying inflammatory component that produces this increase. In a separate general survey of patients with OA compared with a much smaller normal group, the 846 epitope was found to be reduced compared to normal levels (Otterness et al., 1995). Patients with RA who have early rapid erosive joint disease with a poor prognosis normally have serum levels at the lower end or below the normal range, suggesting impairment of biosynthesis by the acute inflammation (Månsson et al., 1995). The elevation of the 846 epitope in serum is thus indicative of slower disease progression and a better prognosis in RA. The same may therefore also apply in OA.

In a majority of subjects with chronic RA, longitudinal studies have revealed some interesting inverse relationships between serum levels of 846, the number of inflamed joints, and serum keratan sulfate content (Poole et al., 1994a). This suggests that the effects of inflammation on synthesis within the joint are reflected systemically by markers of aggrecan synthesis and degradation. Thus, serum levels of 846 epitope are inversely related to the number of inflamed joints, whereas serum levels of immunoreactive keratan sulfate are directly related. Whether such relationships will be evident in patients with OA remains to be established.

Studies of both aggrecan core protein epitopes (Lohmander et al., 1989; Dahlberg et al., 1992) and other aggrecan chondroitin sulfate epitopes (Hazell et al., 1995) have revealed that these are both rapidly elevated in synovial fluids within days or weeks after traumatic knee injury. Later these elevations are reduced but do not return to normal. Joint injuries, such as cruciate ligament rupture or meniscal tears, are known to predispose the injured joints to the development of OA. Hence it is interesting that these apparently permanent changes in cartilage metabolism can precede onset of clinical OA and are detectable so soon after injury. These epitope elevations may also be a consequence of inflammatory changes, since following joint injury there are corresponding increases in synovial fluid levels of the metalloproteinases collagenase and stromelysin, as well as the tissue inhibitor of metalloproteinases (TIMP) (Lohmander et al., 1993). It remains to be established whether the changes in these proteinases and inhibitor reflect synovitis, which could result in cytokine production that alters cartilage and bone metabolism. But experimental studies of canine OA induced surgically have revealed increases in synovial cell hyaluronan synthesis (Myers and Brandt, 1987), as well as elevations in serum hyaluronan that were not seen in sham operated controls (Manicourt et al., 1995). Thus, it may be that the development of synovitis alters cartilage metabolism and is additive to changes in loading produced by destabilization following injury. Whether altered synovial metabolism may be involved in development of OA and its progression in humans remains to be seen, but there are indications that this may be the case, as will be discussed below.

Do the changes in the joint fluid detected so early reflect the development of OA, and is it possible to identify persons at risk for disease progression using aggrecan markers? We do not yet know. Cross-sectional studies of healthy individuals have revealed that, in individual cases, serum keratan sulfate epitope may be elevated (Thonar and Glant, 1992). Ordinarily, levels of this epitope are constant for each individual (Block et al., 1989; Poole et al., 1990). The significance of this elevation is not yet known, but it may, like the synovial fluid measurements, be of prognostic value once longitudinal clinical data are available.

In contrast to others with OA, those patients with a familial OA resulting from a mutation in the COL2A1 gene exhibit elevations of a keratan sulfate epitope (Bleasel et al., 1995). So in these cases, earlier identification of abnormalities during growth which may predispose toward the development of arthritis may be possible.

The levels of a keratan sulfate epitope are generally higher in runners than in soccer players (Roos et al., 1995). This is probably a reflection of increased matrix turnover, but the long-term significance remains to be established. Animals exposed to excessive treadmill exercise exhibit abnormal changes in cartilage collagen and aggrecan content and structure, which are indicative of early OA (Säämämen et al., 1994). Serum analyses should be done in these animals to determine whether changes in keratan sulfate and other epitopes are observed.

Differences in metabolism have been found between the sexes. Levels of keratan sulfate are higher in males than in females (Poole et al., 1990; Campion et al., 1991; Roos et al., 1995), a difference that was not originally noted (Thonar et al., 1985). Again, is this elevation in males of significance, since the incidence of OA is higher in women?

Cartilage Oligomeric Protein

There have been fewer studies of cartilage oligomeric protein, which has been cloned and its structure elucidated (Hedbom et al., 1992; Oldberg et al., 1992). We know little about its turnover, about its half life in the extracellular matrix, and about whether its release is reflective of synthesis and/or degradation. Yet some recent reports have shown interesting relationships between COMP content in sera and disease progression in arthritis. In one study, serum COMP levels increased significantly above baseline during the first year of the study in those persons with progression of OA, as defined by loss of more than 2 mm in joint space on x-ray, or a requirement for knee surgery within a 5-year period (Sharif et al., 1995c). A high proportion of those with positive scintig-raphy scans after several years (associated with increased bone turnover) also showed elevated levels of serum COMP. In another study, increased serum COMP levels were observed in persons with progressive manifestations of joint OA but were not observed in those persons with only joint pain (Petersson et al., 1996). In a general survey comparing subjects without OA and those with OA, levels of COMP served to discriminate the former from the latter (Otter-ness et al., 1995).

Patients with early RA presenting with rapid erosive joint destruction also show elevations of serum COMP, together with elevations of erythrocyte sedimentation rate and serum acute phase protein content (Forslind et al., 1992; Månsson et al., 1995). Thus, COMP measurements may have prognostic value in determining disease outcome in both types of arthritis. Moreover, they point to links between the metabolism of cartilage and underlying changes in bone turnover in OA.

Like aggrecan, synovial fluid COMP shows a persistent increase follow-ing traumatic joint injury, a change that is also seen in patients with OA (Loh-mander et al., 1994). Moreover, abnormal cartilage turnover in patients with familial OA, reflected by elevated keratan sulfate epitope in serum, is also accom-panied by elevations in serum COMP (Bleasel et al., 1995).

C-Propeptide of Type II Procollagen

Newly synthesized type II procollagen contains amino and carboxy pro-peptides, just like type I and type III procollagens. These propeptides are re-quired for the fibril formation that occurs following secretion when the pro-peptides are removed by amino and carboxy proteinases. Immunoassays have been used to detect the C-propeptide (Månsson et al., 1995) and hence the syn-thesis of type II procollagen. The content of the C-propeptide in cartilage is directly proportional to the rate of type II procollagen synthesis measured by incorporation of proline into hydroxyproline (Nelson et al., 1994). The C-propeptide can also be detected in synovial fluids of patients with arthritis (Shinmei et al., 1993), in sera of normal individuals (Månsson et al., 1995; Roos et al., 1995), and in sera of patients with RA (Månsson et al., 1995) and OA (A. R. Poole, M. Ionescu, A. Swan, and P. Dieppe, manuscript in preparation).

In athletes the serum level is reduced by comparison with that of a nonathletic reference group. This is in contrast to a keratan sulfate epitope that is elevated (Roos et al., 1995). These changes in the C-propeptide must point to differences in the synthesis of type II procollagen compared to aggrecan turnover as reflected by the glycosaminoglycan epitope. The significance of this for long-term cartilage metabolism and structural integrity remains to be established. Such differences are also seen in patients with early RA with rapid erosive disease. Here the serum C-propeptide is frequently elevated, whereas aggrecan 846 epitope is markedly reduced. This contrasts to less rapid erosive early disease (Månsson et al., 1995) and chronic disease, in which both C-propeptide and 846 epitope levels may be elevated (Poole et al., 1994b; A. R. Poole, M. Ionescu, A. Swan, and P. Dieppe, manuscript in preparation). Similar elevations in serum C-propeptide are seen in OA, but only in about 20 percent of patients with chronic large joint involvement (A. R. Poole, M. Ionescu, A. Swan, and P. Dieppe, manuscript in preparation). Other basic studies revealed that an increase in the C-propeptide content in articular cartilage occurs in parallel with the increased synthesis of this molecule (Lippiello et al., 1977; Aigner et al., 1992, 1993; Nelson et al., 1994, 1996) which is observed in OA. The increased C-propeptide content of articular cartilage also correlates with higher synovial fluid content (Nelson et al., 1996). These systemic elevations may reflect increased type II procollagen synthesis in diseased articular cartilage.

Type II Collagen Degradation Products

It is not yet possible to identify cartilage-specific collagen cross-links in body fluids as is reflected in bone turnover. However, it is possible to detect collagenase cleavage products of the cartilage-specific type II collagen owing to the recent development of immunoassays for type II collagen α chain neo-epitopes produced by collagenase cleavage (C. Billinghurst, M. Ionescu, and A. R. Poole, unpublished results, 1996). These epitopes are currently being studied in synovial fluids and urine from individuals with arthritis, and reflect the cleavage of cartilage type II collagen in disease.

Individual Skeletal Markers of Bone Metabolism in Osteoarthritis

Collagen Cross-Links and α-Chain Degradation Products

There are two types of collagen cross-links, designated as deoxypyridinoline (or lysylpyridinoline) and pyridinoline (or hydroxylyslpyridinoline) cross-links (Eyre et al., 1984); they are also known as pyridinium and hydroxypyridinium cross-links, respectively. The cross-links found in type I collagen of human adult bone are both pyridinoline and deoxypyridinoline cross-links and are approximately present in a ratio of about 3.5:1, respectively. Mature human cartilage contains the same cross-links, but these are predominantly pyridino-line cross-links in a ratio of about 10:1 (Eyre et al., 1988). Thus, the bulk of the deoxypyridinoline cross-links are thought to arise from bone. These mature cross-links take a while to form in the extracellular matrix and are absent from newly synthesized molecules. Only resident molecules contain them. Elevations in their concentration in urine correlate closely with enhanced bone resorption, which can result in the development of osteoporosis. These bone resorption products are only detectable in urine by either HPLC or immunoassays for the N-telopeptide to helix cross-link (Hanson et al., 1992), the pyridinoline and deoxypyridinoline cross-links (Seyedin et al., 1993), free deoxypyridinoline (Robins et al., 1994), and the C-telopeptide pyridinoline cross-link (Bonde et al., 1994).

Because of the involvement of bone changes in arthritis, it is not surprising that the measurement of alterations in cross-link content in urine is proving to be of value in studies of subjects with arthritis, as well as those with clinical osteoporosis. Measurements are made relative to creatinine excretion to account for any changes in kidney function. Although values are generally higher in the morning than in the evening, no consistent diurnal changes have been seen in healthy controls and in those with OA (McLaren et al., 1993). The observation that pyridinoline is significantly increased in OA was made by immunoassay (Robins et al., 1986; Seibel et al., 1989). The increase of cross-link excretion is most pronounced in RA, in which it is directly related to disease activity (Gough et al., 1994). In OA, increased cross-link excretion is related to narrowing of the knee joint space (Thompson et al., 1992). Whether the increases in pyridinoline may also reflect the degradation of cartilage collagens remains to be established.

Noncollagenous Bone Proteins

Despite the fact that little work has been done on noncollagenous bone proteins in OA, some interesting findings have emerged. Serum osteocalcin is increased in patients with longstanding OA, whereas there is a general lack of any increase in RA (A. R. Poole, M. Ionescu, A. Swan, and P. Dieppe, unpublished results, 1996). Again, this corresponds to the increase in bone turnover leading to the increase in density seen in juxta-articular bone in OA. The changes further suggest that there is also a systemic component and not only juxta-articular change, as discussed in chapter 7. These results are in contrast to an earlier study in which serum osteocalcin was reduced in nondestructive OA but tended to be more elevated in those with destructive OA (Campion et al.,

1989). The discrepancies may be due to the use of widely different assays for osteocalcin, which can give quite different results depending on the molecule or fragments that are detected. Better-defined assays for osteocalcin are now available and should prove more interpretable. Synovial fluid osteocalcin is significantly elevated in osteoarthritic joints with abnormal scintigraphic scans (Sharif et al., 1995a), reflecting local juxta-articular changes.

Bone-specific bone sialoprotein can also be detected in serum. In OA, sialoprotein is increased with time in patients showing disease progression over a 3-year period (Petersson et al., 1996). In patients with RA, this protein is increased in serum, irrespective of the severity of joint disease (Månsson et al., 1995). Sialoprotein is therefore another candidate worth studying in OA. Whether its presence in body fluids truly reflects synthesis of bone remains to be clarified.

Hyaluronan and Other Markers of Inflammation in Osteoarthritis

As indicated earlier, relatively little is known of the relationships between joint inflammation and disease activity in OA, although we know that the inflammation may ultimately prove to be of pivotal importance in the pathology of OA, as it is in RA (Poole et al., 1995). Cartilage and bone markers combined with scintigraphic imaging now provide some insights into changes in bone and cartilage turnover and joint space narrowing in OA. Evidence for joint inflammation may be reflected, as in RA, by the content of hyaluronan in serum. In the presence of normal liver function, measurements of serum hyaluronan can provide valuable information in RA about synovitis as a reflection of joint inflammation. Interestingly, similar elevations of hyaluronan have been observed in patients with OA (Goldberg et al., 1991; A. R. Poole, M. Ionescu, A. Swan, and P. Dieppe, unpublished results, 1996). The increases are less marked than those observed in RA, but as in the case of the collagen cross-links, they are clearly recognizable. That patients with knee OA with more rapid disease progression are characterized by more elevated serum hyaluronan at baseline and after 5 years of continuing disease (Sharif et al., 1995b) may reflect an underlying persistent synovitis that contributes to the accelerated pathologic change.

Recent preliminary studies of the acute phase reactant C-reactive protein, and of tumor necrosis factor receptor type II, have revealed their potential value to distinguish between persons with knee OA and those without OA (Otterness et al., 1995). The elevations of these molecules in OA raise important questions about the role that inflammation may play in the pathogenesis of this condition.

Table 11.1 summarizes the skeletal and inflammation markers that have been studied in OA, and the differences that have been observed between subjects with OA and nonarthritic "normal" subjects with regard to the content of these markers in body fluids.

Conclusions: Future Strategies and Issues in the Development and Use of Skeletal Markers

Much of what we know today has resulted from studies of individual markers, with most of the emphasis being placed on patients with RA, in whom disease activity is more definable and measurable. In the future we must ensure that we do careful comparative studies of these different markers by analyzing the same types of body fluid samples. Such collaborative studies have already started, as exemplified by the work of Manicourt et al. (1993), Månsson et al. (1995), and Roos et al. (1995). Longitudinal analyses of cartilage and bone markers in relation to disease activity, measured both clinically and by using markers of inflammation, are urgently required. Undoubtedly, the best way of performing such analyses is by implementing studies of these integrated markers as part of clinical trials. In this way we can promote the participation of different investigators obtaining data on various markers in relationship to established clinical measurements. Furthermore, the value of these markers can be critically assessed and promising candidates identified with respect to their prognostic value for measuring disease outcome and their diagnostic value for interpreting disease activity and evolving joint pathology. The proven value of the markers in clinical trials would permit changes in disease activity produced by a therapeutic intervention to be detected and evaluated even before clinical changes became apparent. This would obviously be of great value for the pharmaceutical industry (see chapter 13).

To more fully interpret our data from human studies, we need to know much more about the pathology in the osteoarthritic joint so that we can understand how changes in these markers reflect disease onset and progression. Studies on humans must be accompanied by investigations using animal and human tissues in vitro, and animals in vivo. Since comprehensive animal studies are often not affordable for most investigators in academia, the collaboration of multiple investigators in conjunction with the pharmaceutical industry in such studies is again strongly urged.

Table 11.1. Summary of Changes in Skeletal and Inflammation Markers in Osteoarthritis

Marker	Synovial Fluid	Reference	Serum	Reference
Aggrecan keratan sulfate epitope	not markedly increased over serum	Poole et al., 1994b	elevated	Thonar et al., 1985 Sweet et al., 1988 Campion et al., 1991
	inversely related to inflammation	Poole et al., 1994b	decreased or unchanged	Seibel et al., 1988 Spector et al., 1992 Poole et al., 1994b
Aggrecan chondroitin sulfate 846 epitope	markedly elevated over serum, particularly in advanced disease; inversely related to keratan sulfate epitope ($r = 0.510$, $p = 0.0004$, $n = 49$)	Poole et al., 1994b	directly correlated with keratan sulfate epitope; elevated in about 20% of patients with chronic disease	Poole et al.,. 1994b
Cartilage oligomeric protein (COMP)	elevated	Lohmander et al., 1994	increased with time in patients exhibiting disease progression	Sharif et al., 1995c Petersson et al., 1996
C-propeptide of type II procollagen of cartilage	elevated over serum levels	Poole, Dieppe et al., unpublished results, 1996	elevated in about 20% of patients	Poole, Dieppe et al., unpublished results
Deoxypyridinoline and pyridinoline cross-links of cartilage (pyridinoline only) and bone	not detectable		not detectable in urine both are elevated in urine, related to joint degeneration	Robins et al., 1986 Seibel et al., 1989 Thompson et al., 1992

Table 11.1—*Continued*

Marker	Synovial Fluid	Reference	Serum	Reference
Osteocalcin	elevated in patients with positive scintigraphic scans	Sharif et al., 1995a	elevated	Poole, Dieppe et al., unpublished results
			elevated in those with destructive disease	Campion et al., 1989
Bone sialoprotein	not studied		increased in patients during early disease progression	Petersson et al., 1996
Hyaluronan	not studied		elevated and associated with more rapid joint destruction	Goldberg et al., 1991 Sharif et al., 1995b

The search for new and precise markers of cartilage and bone matrix synthesis and degradation must also continue. New assays are needed to detect the degradation of cartilage or bone collagen. New markers are necessary to study inflammatory changes in OA. Fortunately, as we have seen, some of these are already available and are now being used for the first time in human studies. *Serum* assays for clinical studies need to be more sensitive: that is, to include assays for collagen cross-links, which at present can usually only be analyzed in urine. However, the use of urine to study markers other than cross-links should also be explored. Priority should be given to definitive assays that measure cartilage degradation (aggrecan and type II collagen neoepitopes representing cleavage products), bone resorption (deoxypyridinoline cross-links), synthesis of cartilage (846 epitope), and bone proteins (osteocalcin and bone sialoprotein) (fig. 11.2). If we proceed in this way, it is likely that in the future the use of these assays will prove to be very valuable in the diagnosis and management of OA.

Finally, do these analyses provide us with any convincing evidence to support the hypothesis that OA is an accelerated process of aging? At present, the data do not provide evidence to support this hypothesis, particularly in view of the pronounced changes that we observe in terms of bone remodeling favoring sclerosis (see chapter 7), and the notable alterations in markers associated with the progression of joint damage. There is, as yet, no evidence to show where OA as a "disease" may part from or represent a continuum with aging. Much more needs to be done to study the "natural history" of aging populations to better address the evolution of OA.

ACKNOWLEDGMENTS

My recent studies were funded by the Medical Research Council of Canada, Pharmacia Upjohn Diagnostics, and the Shriners of North America. Jane Wishart assisted in the preparation of the figures. Audrey Wheeler processed the manuscript.

REFERENCES

Ahmad NN, Ala-Kokko L, Knowlton RG, Jiminez SH, Weaver EJ, Maguire JI, Tasman W, Prockop DJ. 1991. Stop codon in the procollagen II gene (COL2A1) in a family with the Stickler syndrome (arthro-opthalmopathy). *Proc Natl Acad Sci USA* 88:6624–6627.

Aigner T, Stäss H, Wesoloh G, Zeiler G, von der Mark K. 1992. Activation of collagen II expression in osteoarthritic and rheumatoid cartilage. *Virchows Archiv B: Cell Pathol* 62:337–345.

Aigner T, Bertling W, Stöss H, Weseloh G, von der Mark K. 1993. Independent expression of fibril forming collagens I, II, and III in chondrocytes of human osteoarthritic cartilage. *J Clin Invest* 91:829–837.

Ala-Kokko L, Baldwin CT, Moskowitz RW, Prockop DJ. 1990. Single base mutation in the type II procollagen gene (COL2A1) as a cause of primary osteoarthritis associated with a mild chondrodysplasia. *Proc Natl Acad Sci USA* 87:6565–6568.

Bellus GA, Hefferon TW, Ortiz de Luna RI, Hecht JT, Horton WA, Machado M, Kaitila I, McIntosh I, Francomano CA. 1995. Achondroplasia is defined by recurrent G380R mutations of FGF R3. *Am J Hum Genet* 56:368–373.

Bleasel JF, Poole AR, Heinegard D, Saxne T, Ionescu M, Moskowitz RW. 1995. Serum cartilage markers define osteoarthritis pathophysiologic mechanisms in families with type II collagen gene mutations. *Trans Orthop Res Soc* 20:249.

Block JA, Schnitzer TJ, Anderson GBJ, Lenz ME, Jeffery R, McNeill TW, Thonar EJ-MA. 1989. The effect of chemonucleolysis on serum keratan sulfate levels in humans. *Arthritis Rheum* 32:100–104.

Bonde M, Qvist P, Fledelius C, Riis BJ, Christiansen C. 1994. Evaluation of an immunoassay (Cross-Laps™ ELISA) for quantitation of type I collagen degradation products in urine. *Clin Chem* 40: 2022–2025.

Boyce BF, Aufdemorte TF, Garrett IR, Yates AJP, Mundy GR. 1989. Effects of interleukin-1 on bone turnover in normal mice. *Endocrinology* 125:1142–1150.

Briggs MD, Hoffmann SMG, King LM, Olsen AS, Mohrenweiser H, Leroy JG, Mortier GR, Rimoin DL, Lachman RS, Gaines ES, Cekleniak JA, Knowlton RG, Cohn DH. 1995. Pseudoachondroplasia and multiple epiphyseal dysplasia due to mutations in the cartilage oligomeric matrix protein gene. *Nature Genet* 10:330–336.

Campion GV, Delmas PD, Dieppe PA. 1989. Serum and synovial fluid osteocalcin (bone GLA protein) levels in joint disease. *Br J Rheumatol* 28:393–398.

Campion GV, McCrae F, Schnitzer TJ, Lenz ME, Dieppe PA, Thonar EJ-MA. 1991. Levels of keratan sulfate in the serum and synovial fluid of patients with osteoarthritis of the knee. *Arthritis Rheum* 34:1254–1259.

Canalis E. 1987. Effects of tumor necrosis factor on bone formation *in vitro*. *Endocrinology* 121:1596–1604.

Canalis E, Centrella M, Burch W, McCarthy TL. 1989. Insulin-like growth factor 1 mediates selective anabolic effects of parathyroid hormone in bone cultures. *J Clin Invest* 83:60–65.

Caterson B, Christner JE, Baker JR. 1983. Identification of a monoclonal antibody that specifically recognizes corneal and skeletal keratan sulfate. *J Biol Chem* 258:8848–8854.

Cruess RL. 1982. Physiology of bone formation and resorption. In: *The musculoskeletal system: Embryology, biochemistry, and physiology,* edited by RL Cruess. Pp. 219–252. New York: Churchill Livingstone.

Dahl IMS, Husby G. 1985. Hyaluronic acid production *in vitro* by synovial lining cells from normal and rheumatoid joints. *Ann Rheum Dis* 44:647–657.

Dahlberg L, Ryd L, Heinegård D, Lohmander LS. 1992. Proteoglycan fragments in joint fluid: Influence of arthrosis and inflammation. *Acta Orthop Scand* 63:417–423.

Engström-Laurent A, Hällgren R. 1985. Circulating hyaluronate in rheumatoid arthritis: Relationship to inflammatory activity and the effect of corticosteroid therapy. *Ann Rheum Dis* 44:83–88.

Engström-Laurent A, Hällgren R. 1987. Circulating hyaluronic acid levels vary with physical activity in healthy subjects and in rheumatoid arthritis patients: Relationship to synovitis mass and morning stiffness. *Arthritis Rheum* 30:1333–1338.

Eyre DR, Paz MA, Gallop PM. 1984. Cross-linking in collagen and elastin. *Annu Rev Biochem* 53:717–748.

Eyre DR, Dickson IR, van Ness K. 1988. Collagen cross-linking in human bone and articular cartilage: Age-related changes in the content of mature hydroxypyridinium residues. *Biochem J* 252:495–500.

Forslind K, Eberhardt K, Jonsson A, Saxne T. 1992. Increased serum concentrations of cartilage oligomeric matrix protein: A prognostic marker in early rheumatoid arthritis. *Br J Rheumatol* 31:593–598.

Fraser JRE, Engström-Laurent A, Nyberg A, Laurent TC. 1986. Removal of hyaluronic acid from the circulation in rheumatoid disease and primary biliary cirrhosis. *J Lab Clin Med* 107:79–85.

Goldberg RL, Huff JP, Lenz ME, Glickman P, Katz R, Thonar EJ-MA. 1991. Elevated plasma levels of hyaluronate in patients with osteoarthritis and rheumatoid arthritis. *Arthritis Rheum* 34:799–807.

Gough AKS, Peel NFA, Eastell R, Holder RL, Lilley J, Emery P. 1994. Excretion of pyridinium cross-links correlates with disease activity and appendicular bone loss in early rheumatoid arthritis. *Ann Rheum Dis* 53:14–17.

Hanson DA, Weis MA, Bollen A-M, Maslan SL, Singer FR, Eyre DR. 1992. A specific immunoassay for monitoring human bone resorption: Quantitation of type I collagen cross-linked N-telopeptides in urine. *J Bone Miner Res* 7:1251–1258.

Haubeck H-D, Kock R, Fischer D-C, van de Leur E, Hoffmeister K, Greiling H. 1995. Transforming growth factor β_1, a major stimulator of hyaluronan synthesis in human synovial lining cells. *Arthritis Rheum* 38:669–677.

Hazell PK, Dent C, Fairclough JA, Bayliss MT, Hardingham TE. 1995. Changes in glycosaminoglycan epitope levels in knee joint fluid following injury. *Arthritis Rheum* 38:953–959.

Hecht JT, Nelson LD, Crowder E, Wang Y, Elder FFB, Harrison WR, Francomano CA, Prange CK, Lennon GG, Deere M, Lawler J. 1995. Mutations in exon 17B of cartilage oligomeric matrix protein (COMP) cause pseudoachondroplasia. *Nature Genet* 10:325–329.

Hedbom E, Antonsson P, Hjerpe A, Aeschlimann D, Paulsson M, Rosa-Pimentel E, Sommarin Y, Wendel M, Oldberg A, Heinegård D. 1992. Cartilage matrix proteins: An acidic oligomeric protein (COMP) detected only in cartilage. *J Biol Chem* 267:6132–6136.

Hock JM, Centrella M, Canalis E. 1988. Insulin-like growth factor 1 has independent effects on bone matrix formation and cell replication. *Endocrinology* 122:254–260.

Hollander AP, Heathfield TF, Webber C, Iwata Y, Bourne R, Rorabeck C, Poole AR. 1994. Increased damage to type II collagen in osteoarthritic articular cartilage detected by a new immunoassay. *J Clin Invest* 93:1722–1732.

Hollander AH, Pidoux I, Reiner A, Rorabeck C, Bourne R, Poole AR. 1995. Damage to type II collagen in aging and osteoarthritis starts at the articular surface, originates around chondrocytes, and extends into the cartilage with progressive degeneration. *J Clin Invest* 96:2859–2869.

Hørslev-Petersen K, Bentsen KD, Engström-Laurent A, Junker P, Halberg P, Lorenzen I. 1988. Serum amino terminal type III procollagen peptide and serum hyaluronan in rheumatoid arthritis: Relation to clinical and serologic parameters of inflammation during 8 and 24 months treatment with levamisole, penicillamine, or azathioprine. *Ann Rheum Dis* 47:116–126.

Houssiau FA, Devogelaer J-P, van Damme J, Nagant de Deuxchaisnes C, van Snick J. 1988. Interleukin-6 in synovial fluid and serum of patients with rheumatoid arthritis and other inflammatory arthritides. *Arthritis Rheum* 31:784–788.

Hughes CE, Caterson B, White RJ, Roughley PJ, Mort JS. 1992. Monoclonal antibodies recognizing protease-generated neoepitopes from cartilage proteoglycan degradation. *J Biol Chem* 267:16011–16014.

Hughes CE, Caterson B, Fosang AJ, Roughley PJ, Mort JS. 1995. Monoclonal antibodies that specifically recognize neoepitope sequences generated by "aggrecanase" and matrix metalloproteinase cleavage of aggrecan: Application to catabolism *in situ* and *in vitro*. *Biochem J* 305:799–804.

Ishimi Y, Miyawa C, Jin CH, Akatsu T, Abe E, Nakamura Y, Yamaguchi A, Yoshiki S, Matsuda T, Hirano T, Kishimoto T, Suda T. 1990. IL-6 is produced by osteoblasts and induces bone resorption. *J Immunol* 145:3297–3303.

Jilka R, Hangoc G, Girasole G, Passeri G, Williams DC, Abrams JS, Boyce B, Broxmeyer H, Manolagas SC. 1992. Increased osteoclast development after estrogen loss: Mediation by interleukin-6. *Science* 257:88–91.

Knowlton RG, Katzenstein PL, Moskowitz RW, Weaver EJ, Malemud CJ, Pathria MN, Jiminez SA, Prockop DJ. 1990. Genetic linkage of a polymorphism in the type II procollagen gene (COL2A1) to primary osteoarthritis associated with a mild chondrodysplasia. *N Engl J Med* 322:526–530.

Konttinen YT, Saari H, Honkaanen VEA, Szocsik K, Mussalo-Rauhamaa H, Tulensalo R, Friman C. 1990. Serum baseline hyaluronate and disease activity in rheumatoid arthritis. *Clin Chim Acta* 193:39–48.

Lark MW, Williams H, Hoerrner LA, Weidner J, Ayala JM, Harper CF, Christen A, Olszewski J, Konteatis Z, Webber R, Mumford RA. 1995. Quantification of a metalloproteinases-generated aggrecan G1 fragment using monospecific anti-peptide serum. *Biochem J* 307:245–252.

Lee B, Vissing H, Ramirez F, Rogers D, Rimoin D. 1989. Identification of the molecular defect in a family with spondyloepiphyseal dysplasia. *Science* 244:978–980.

Lippiello L, Hall D, Mankin HJ. 1977. Collagen synthesis in normal and osteoarthritic human cartilage. *J Clin Invest* 59:593–600.

Lippiello L, Kaye C, Neumata T, Mankin HJ. 1985. In vitro metabolic response of articular cartilage segments. *Connect Tissue Res* 13:99–107.

Lohmander LS, Dahlberg L, Ryd L, Heinegård D. 1989. Increased levels of proteoglycan fragments in knee joint fluid after injury. *Arthritis Rheum* 32:1434–1442.

Lohmander LS, Lark MW, Dahlberg ML, Walakovits LA, Roos H. 1992. Cartilage matrix metabolism in osteoarthritis: Markers in synovial fluid, serum, and urine. *Clin Biochem* 25:167–174.

Lohmander LS, Hoerrner LA, Lark MW. 1993. Metalloproteinases, tissue inhibitor, and proteoglycan fragments in knee synovial fluid in human osteoarthritis. *Arthritis Rheum* 36:181–189.

Lohmander LS, Saxne T, Heinegård D. 1994. Release of cartilage oligomeric matrix protein (COMP) into joint fluid after knee injury and in osteoarthritis. *Ann Rheum Dis* 53:8–13.

Manicourt D-H, Triki R, Fukuda K, Devogelaer J-P, Nagant de Deuxchaisnes C, Thonar EJ-MA. 1993. Levels of circulating tumor necrosis factor a and interleukin-6 in patients with rheumatoid arthritis: Relationship to serum levels of hyaluronan and antigen in keratan sulfate. *Arthritis Rheum* 36:490–499.

Manicourt D-H, Cornu O, Lenz ME, Druetz–Van Egeren A, Thonar EJ-MA. 1995. Rapid and sustained rise in the serum levels of hyaluronan after anterior cruciate ligament transection in the dog knee joint. *J Rheumatol* 22:262–269.

Mankin HJ, Dorfman H, Lippiello L, Zarins A. 1971. Biochemical and metabolic abnormalities in articular cartilage from osteo-arthritic human hips: II. Correlation of morphology with biochemical and metabolic data. *J Bone Joint Surg* 53A:523–537.

Månsson B, Carey D, Alini M, Ionescu M, Rosenberg LC, Poole AR, Heinegård D, Saxne T. 1995. Cartilage and bone metabolism in rheumatoid arthritis: Differences between rapid and slow progression of disease identified by serum markers of cartilage metabolism. *J Clin Invest* 95:1071–1077.

McLaren AM, Isdale AH, Whiting PH, Bird HA, Robins SP. 1993. Physiological variations in the urinary excretion of pyridinium crosslinks of collagen. *Br J Rheumatol* 32:307–312.

Mehmet H, Scudder P, Tang PW, Hounsell EF, Caterson B, Feizi T. 1986. The antigenic determinants recognized by three monoclonal antibodies to keratan sulphate involve sulphated hepta- or larger oligosaccharides of the poly (N-acetyllactosamine) series. *Eur J Biochem* 157:385–391.

Myers SL, Brandt KD. 1987. Studies of synovial hyaluronic acid synthesis in canine osteoarthritis. *J Rheumatol* 14:1150–1155.

Nelson F, Reiner A, Ionescu M, Brooks E, Bogoch E, Poole AR. 1994. The content of the C-propeptide of type II collagen in articular cartilage is an index of synthesis of this molecule which is increased in osteoarthritis. *Trans Orthop Res Soc* 19:216.

Nelson F, Dahlberg L, Reiner A, Pidoux I, Fraser G, Brooks E, Tanzer M, Bogoch E, Rosenberg LC, Poole AR. 1996. The content of C-propeptide of type II procollagen in cartilage reflects the synthesis of this molecule which is marked by an increase in osteoarthritis. Submitted.

Oldberg A, Antonsson P, Lindblom K, Heinegård D. 1992. COMP (cartilage oligomeric matrix protein) is structurally related to the thrombospondins. *J Biol Chem* 267:22346–22350.

Otterness IG, Zimmerer RO, Swindell AC, Poole AR, Saxne T, Heinegård D, Ionescu M, Weiner E. 1995. An examination of some molecular markers in blood and urine for discriminating patients with osteoarthritis from healthy individuals. *Acta Orthop Scand* 66(suppl. 266):148–150.

Page-Thomas DP, Bard D, King B, Dingle JT. 1987. Clearance of proteoglycan from joint cavities. *Ann Rheum Dis* 46:934–937.

Paimela L, Heiskanen A, Kurki P, Helve T, Leirisalo-Repo M. 1991. Serum hyaluronate levels as a predictor of radiologic progression in early rheumatoid arthritis. *Arthritis Rheum* 34:815–821.

Palotie A, Väisänen P, Ott J, Ryhänen L, Elima K, Vikkula M, Cheah K, Vuorio E, Peltonen L. 1989. Predisposition to familial osteoarthritis linked to type II collagen gene. *Lancet* 1:924–927.

Petersson IF, Boegård T, Svensson B, Heinegård D, Poole AR, Ionescu M, Saxne T. 1996. Differences in cartilage and bone metabolism identified by serum markers in early development of osteoarthritis of the knee. Submitted.

Poole AR. 1986. Changes in the collagen and proteoglycan of articular cartilage in arthritis. *Rheumatology* 10:316–371.

———. 1993. Cartilage in health and disease. In: *Arthritis and allied conditions: A textbook of rheumatology,* edited by D McCarty, W Koopman. 12th ed. Pp. 279–233. Philadelphia: Lea and Febiger.

———. 1994. Immunochemical markers of joint inflammation, skeletal damage and repair: Where are we now? *Ann Rheum Dis* 53:3–5.

Poole AR, Dieppe P. 1994. Biological markers in rheumatoid arthritis. *Semin Arthritis Rheum* 23(suppl. 2, June):17–31.

Poole AR, Webber C, Reiner A, Roughley PJ. 1989. Studies of a monoclonal antibody to skeletal keratan sulphate: Importance of antibody valency. *Biochem J* 260:849–856.

Poole AR, Witter J, Roberts N, Piccolo F, Brandt R, Paquin J, Baron M. 1990. Inflammation and cartilage metabolism in rheumatoid arthritis: Studies of the blood markers hyaluronic acid, orosomucoid, and keratan sulfate. *Arthritis Rheum* 33:790–799.

Poole AR, Ionescu M, Fitzcharles MA. 1994a. The relationship of the turnover of the cartilage proteoglycan aggrecan to disease activity in patients with rheumatoid arthritis. *Arthritis Rheum* 37:S363.

Poole AR, Ionescu M, Swan A, Dieppe P. 1994b. Changes in cartilage metabolism in arthritis are reflected by altered serum and synovial fluid levels of the cartilage proteoglycan aggrecan: Implications for pathogenesis. *J Clin Invest* 94:25–33.

Poole AR, Alini M, Hollander AP. 1995. Cellular biology of cartilage degradation. In: *Mechanisms and models in rheumatoid arthritis,* edited by B Henderson, R Pettifer, J Edwards. Pp. 163–204. London: Academic Press.

Ritvaniemi P, Körkko J, Bonaventure J, Vikkula M, Hyland J, Paassilta P, Kaitila I, Käärianen H, Sokolov BP, Hakala M, Mannismäki P, Meerson EM, Klemola T, Williams C, Peltonen L, Kivirikko KI, Prockop DJ, Ala-Kokko L. 1995. Identification of COL2A1 gene mutations in patients with chondrodysplasias and familial osteoarthritis. *Arthritis Rheum* 33:999–1004.

Rizkalla G, Reiner A, Bogoch E, Poole AR. 1992. Studies of the articular cartilage proteoglycan aggrecan in health and osteoarthritis: Evidence for molecular heterogeneity and extensive molecular changes in disease. *J Clin Invest* 90:2268–2277.

Robins SP, Stewart P, Astbury C, Bird HA. 1986. Measurement of the cross-linking compound pyridinoline in urine as an index of collagen degradation in joint disease. *Ann Rheum Dis* 45: 969–973.

Robins SP, Woitge H, Hesley R, Ju J, Seyedin S, Seibel MJ. 1994. Direct, enzyme-linked immunoassay for urinary deoxypyridinoline as a specific marker for measuring bone resorption. *J Bone Miner Res* 9:1643–1649.

Roos H, Dahlberg L, Hoerrner LA, Lark MW, Thonar EJ-MA, Shinmei M, Lindqvist U, Lohmander

LS. 1995. Markers of cartilage matrix metabolism in human joint fluid and serum: The effect of exercise. *Osteoarthritis Cartilage* 3:7–14.

Säämämen A-M, Kiviranta I, Jurvelin J, Helminen H, Tammi M. 1994. Proteoglycan and collagen alterations in canine knee articular cartilage following 20 km daily running exercise for 15 weeks. *Connect Tiss Res* 30:191–201.

Sah RL-Y, Doong J-YH, Grodzinsky AJ. 1991. Effects of compression on the loss of newly synthesized proteoglycans and proteins from cartilage explants. *Arch Biochem Biophys* 286:20–29.

Saklatvala J. 1986. Tumour necrosis factor a stimulates resorption and inhibits synthesis of proteoglycan in cartilage. *Nature* 322:547–549.

Schipani E, Kruse K, Jappner H. 1995. A constitutively active mutant PTH-PTHrP receptor in Jansentype metaphyseal chondrodysplasia. *Science* 268:98–100.

Seibel MJ, Towbin H, Braun DG, Kiefer B, Müller W, Paulsson M. 1988. Serum keratan sulphate in rheumatoid arthritis and different clinical subsets of osteoarthritis. In: *Keratan sulphate: Chemistry, biology, chemical pathology*, edited by H Greiling, JE Scott. Pp. 191–198. Biochemical Society Symposia. London.

Seibel MJ, Duncan A, Robins SP. 1989. Urinary hydroxy-pyridinium crosslinks provide indices of cartilage and bone involvement in arthritic diseases. *J Rheumatol* 16:964–970.

Seyedin SM, Kung VT, Daniloff YN, Hesley RP, Gomez B, Nielsen LA, Rosen HN, Zuk RF. 1993. Immunoassay for urinary pyridinoline: The new marker for bone resorption. *J Bone Miner Res* 8:635–641.

Sharif M, George E, Dieppe PA. 1995a. Correlation between synovial fluid markers of cartilage and bone turnover and scintigraphic scan abnormalities in osteoarthritis of the knee. *Arthritis Rheum* 38:78–81.

Sharif M, George E, Shepstone L, Knudson W, Thonar EJ-MA, Cushnaghan J, Dieppe P. 1995b. Serum hyaluronic acid level as a predictor of disease progression in osteoarthritis of the knee. *Arthritis Rheum* 38:760–767.

Sharif M, Saxne T, Shepstone L, Kirwan JR, Elson CJ, Heinegård D, Dieppe PA. 1995c. Relationship between serum cartilage oligomeric matrix protein levels and disease progression in osteoarthritis of the knee joint. *Br J Rheumatol* 34:306–310.

Shiang R, Thompson LM, Zhu YZ, Church DM, Fielder TJ, Bocian M, Winokur ST, Wasmuth JJ. 1994. Mutations in the transmembrane domain of FGF R3 cause the most common genetic form of dwarfism, achondroplasia. *Cell* 78:335–342.

Shinmei M, Ito K, Matsuyama S, Yoshihara Y, Matsuzawa K. 1993. Joint fluid carboxy-terminal type II procollagen peptide as a marker of cartilage collagen biosynthesis. *Osteoarthritis Cartilage* 1:121–128.

Singer II, Kawka DW, Bayne EK, Donatelli SA, Weider JR, Williams HR, Ayala JM, Mumford RA, Lark MW, Glant TT, Nabozny GH, David CS. 1995. VDIPEN, a metalloproteinase-generated neoepitope, is induced and immunolocalized in articular cartilage during inflammatory arthritis. *J Clin Invest* 95:2178–2186.

Spector TD, Woodward L, Hall GM, Hammond A, Williams A, Butler MG, James IT, Hart DJ, Thompson PW, Scott DL. 1992. Keratan sulphate in rheumatoid arthritis, osteoarthritis, and inflammatory diseases. *Ann Rheum Dis* 51:1134–1137.

Stanescu R, Stanescu V, Bordat C, Maroteaux P. 1987. Pathologic features of the femoral heads in a patient aged 14 1/2 years with spondyloepiphyseal dysplasia with osteoarthritis. *J Rheumatol* 14:1061–1067.

Stanescu V, Stanescu R, Maroteaux P. 1984. Pathogenic mechanisms in osteochondrodysplasias. *J Bone Joint Surg* 66A:817–836.

Stanescu V, Stanescu R, Maroteaux P. 1985. Articular degeneration as a sequela of osteochondrodysplasias. *Clin Rheum Dis* 11:239–270.

Stashenko P, Dewhirst FD, Rooney ML, Desjardins LA, Heeley JD. 1987. Interleukin-1b is a potent inhibitor of bone formation *in vitro. J Bone Miner Res* 2:559–565.

Steiner G, Studnicka-Benke A, Witzmann G, Höfler E, Smolen J. 1995. Soluble receptors for tumor necrosis factor and interleukin-2 in serum and synovial fluid of patients with rheumatoid arthritis, reactive arthritis, and osteoarthritis. *J Rheumatol* 22:406–412.

Sweet MBE, Coelho A, Schnitzler CM, Schnitzer TJ, Lenz ME, Jakim I, Kuettner KE, Thonar EJ-MA. 1988. Serum keratan sulfate levels in osteoarthritis patients. *Arthritis Rheum* 31:648–652.

Tavormina PL, Shiang R, Thompson LM, Zhu Y-Z, Wilkins DJ, Lachman RS, Wilcox WR, Rimoin DL, Cohn DH, Wasmuth JJ. 1995. Thanatotrophic dysplasia (types I and II) caused by distinct mutations in fibroblast growth factor receptor 3. *Nature Genet* 9:321–328.

Thompson PW, Spector TD, James IT, Henderson E, Hart DJ. 1992. Urinary collagen crosslinks reflect the radiographic severity of knee osteoarthritis. *Br J Rheumatol* 31:759–761.

Thompson RC, Oegema TR. 1979. Metabolic activity of articular cartilage in osteoarthritis: An *in vitro* study. *J Bone Joint Surg* 61A:407–416.

Thonar EJ-MA, Glant T. 1992. Serum keratan sulfate—a marker of predisposition to polyarticular osteoarthritis. *Clin Biochem* 25:175–180.

Thonar EJ-MA, Lenz ME, Klintworth GK, Caterson B, Pachman LM, Glickman P, Katz R, Huff J, Kuettner KE. 1985. Quantification of keratan sulfate in blood as a marker of cartilage catabolism. *Arthritis Rheum* 28:1367–1376.

Tiller GE, Rimoin DL, Murray LW, Cohn DH. 1990. Tandem duplication within a type II collagen gene (COL2A1) exon in an individual with spondyloepiphyseal dysplasia. *Proc Natl Acad Sci USA* 87:3889–3893.

Vikkula M, Mariman ECM, Lui VCH, Zhidkova NI, Tiller GE, Goldring MB, van Beersum SEC, de Waal Malefijt MC, van den Hoogen FHJ, Ropers H-H, Mayne R, Cheah KSE, Olsen BR, Warman ML, Brunner HG. 1995. Autosomal dominant and recessive osteochondrodysplasias associated with the COL11A2 locus. *Cell* 80:431–437.

Waage A, Kaufmann C, Espevik T, Husby G. 1989. Interleukin-6 in synovial fluid from patients with arthritis. *Clin Immunol Immunopathol* 50:394–398.

Webber C, Glant TT, Roughley PJ, Poole AR. 1987. The identification and characterization of two populations of aggregating proteoglycans of high buoyant density isolated from post-natal human articular cartilages of different ages. *Biochem J* 248:735–740.

Winterpacht A, Hilbert M, Schwarze U, Mundlos S, Spranger J, Zabel BU. 1993. Kniest and Sticklers dysplasia phenotypes caused by collagen II gene (COL2A1) defect. *Nature Genet* 3:323–326.

Witter J, Roughley PJ, Webber C, Roberts N, Keystone E, Poole AR. 1987. The immunological detection and characterization of cartilage proteoglycan degradation products in synovial fluids of patients with arthritis. *Arthritis Rheum* 30:519–529.

Yaron I, Meyer FA, Dayer J-M, Bleiberg I, Yaron M. 1989. Some recombinant human cytokines stimulate glycosaminoglycan synthesis in human synovial fibroblast cultures and inhibit it in human articular cartilage cultures. *Arthritis Rheum* 32:173–180.

12

Magnetic Resonance Imaging and the Progression of Osteoarthritis, Osteoporosis, and Aging

Laurance D. Hall, Ph.D., Paul J. Watson, Ph.D., and Jenny A. Tyler, D.Phil.

It is becoming increasingly accepted that magnetic resonance imaging (MRI) is uniquely capable of visualizing the human articular joint as a complete organ (Crues, 1991). Thus, besides providing direct visualization of all of the major soft tissues (synovial fluid, cartilage, synovial membrane, ligaments, tendons, discs, and menisci) within the joint capsule, as well as the surrounding musculature, it also gives an outline for the cortical, and sometimes the trabecular, bone. The fact that those structures can all be imaged by a single noninvasive MRI scan in two dimensions within a scan time of 0.1 second to 12 minutes (depending on the spatial resolution and the required image contrast), or in three dimensions in 1–15 minutes, is a further inducement to use MRI in preference to other imaging methods such as plane-film x-ray. Although at present its major clinical uses in orthopedics and rheumatology are in the diagnosis of knee trauma and in spinal column examinations, the literature describes clinical results—including the effects of osteoarthritis (OA) (Karvonen et al., 1994; Hall and Tyler, 1995) and, recently, of osteoporosis (OP) (Jara et al., 1993)—for all other articular joints.

We shall compare the current use of MRI, both in clinical practice and in research into OA and OP, and the application of MRI to studies of aging. At present, few MRI data are available to demonstrate quantitative measurement of temporal progression for OA and OP. Consequently, the focus of this chapter will be directed to the basic MRI methodology, along with an outline of the approaches actively under way which are designed to quantitate time-progression of OA damage and of natural aging. Since the latter studies must include cadres of young subjects (aged 10–30 years), ethical considerations require that the measurement method used be noninvasive, and it is principally for that reason that we have largely excluded from this discussion both x-ray studies (Buckland-Wright and MacFarlane, 1995; Lequesne, 1995) and those that used nuclear medicine techniques.

The discussion will start with an introduction to MRI of the articular joint, along with a description of representative pathologic damage that can be directly visualized; some such studies have been in progress for 10 years, and they can be discussed definitively. This will be followed by a summary of the methods now becoming available for the quantitative measurements that will, in the future, be used to monitor longitudinal progression; given that some of those methods were developed only recently, relatively few comparative data are as yet available. In light of the above, this chapter will inevitably differ from the others in this book: whereas the discussions of the methodology are *firm*, in the absence of the necessary body of clinical data the speculations about following progression by MRI are necessarily *tentative*.

Magnetic Resonance Imaging

MRI depends on the fact that the hydrogen nuclei of water and fat are weakly magnetic (Morris, 1986). Consequently, when an articular joint is placed at the center of a powerful magnet, those "nuclear-magnets" tend to become aligned by the field, like a magnetic compass needle in the earth's field. If the tissues are then bathed with radio waves of the appropriate frequency, the orientation of those nuclear magnets is changed and can be detected as a magnetic resonance image. The intensity of the signal in each part of the image depends both on the imaging protocol used and on the type of tissue involved. In practice, each imaging protocol is optimized to heighten the contrast between the tissue of interest and those that surround it, and to select the orientation of the image plane (slice).

The two-dimensional (2D) slice image of the distal interphalangeal joint of a 31-year-old male which is shown in figure 12.1 is one of five parallel slice images obtained in 24 minutes total acquisition time (Hall and Tyler, 1995; Hodgson et al., 1995). It clearly demonstrates that a single protocol can distinguish all of the main structural entities of this articular joint; visualization of the fingerprint indicates the high spatial resolution achieved. It is important to

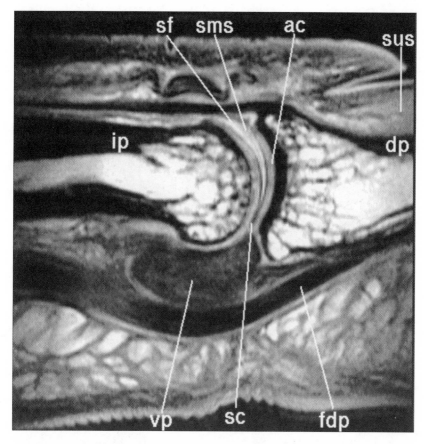

Figure 12.1. Sagittal magnetic resonance image of the distal interphalangeal (DIP) joint of a male (31 years old) measured using a spin-echo sequence (SE 1500/40) lasting 24 minutes. In plane-resolution 0.075 mm × 0.15 mm, slice thickness, 1 mm. *Sf,* synovial fluid; *sms,* synovial membrane sac; *ac,* articular cartilage; *sus,* subungual space; *ip,* intermediate phalanx; *dp,* distal phalanx; *vp,* volar plate; *sc,* superficial cartilage; *fdp,* flexor digitorum profundus.

note that the image contrast can be controlled by selecting an appropriate MRI protocol. In the case of an articular joint, it is important to distinguish between cartilage and synovial fluid. Fortunately, this can be achieved by use of magnetization transfer (MT) contrast (Wolff and Balaban, 1989), as illustrated in figure 12.2. Thus, in the upper right image, MT contrast has been used to suppress the signal from cartilage and thereby clearly identifies the high signal intensity from the synovial fluid.

From the standpoint of aging, it is important to draw attention to the

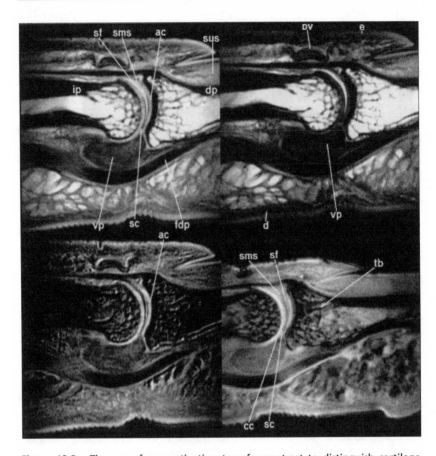

Figure 12.2. The use of magnetization transfer contrast to distinguish cartilage from synovial fluid. *Top left,* same image as figure 12.1. *Top right,* identical slice, but with signal intensity from cartilage suppressed by magnetization transfer. *Lower left,* subtraction between those two images, now showing cartilage as high signal intensity. *Lower right,* MR image of another DIP joint acquired using a different sequence (CHESS 1500/40) in 12 minutes. *Cc,* central cartilage; *tb,* trabecular bone; *e,* epidermis, *d,* dermis.

sharp line of low signal intensity which defines the entire surface of the two layers of cartilage in figure 12.1, regardless of whether they are in close contact or separated by synovial fluid. Loss of this line from a finger MRI scan is almost certainly the first measurable indication for an intact joint that the cartilage surface has lost some of its integrity.

Although simultaneous acquisition of several parallel slice images results in efficient use of scanner time, the disadvantage of that approach for studying the longitudinal development of joint changes is that incorrect slice alignment can lead to substantial difficulties in comparing a sequential series of images. Consequently, whenever scanning time permits, it is advantageous to acquire a complete three-dimensional (3D) data set. Thereafter, any slice of any arbitrary orientation can be visualized after completion of the scan. This can now be achieved for a human knee in 8–15 minutes scan time with a spatial resolution of 0.5 × 0.5 × 1.0 mm. As for the distal interphalangeal (DIP) joint, a protocol can show both the cartilage-bone boundaries; however, that spatial resolution is not sufficient in the knee to delineate between the two surfaces when they are in contact.

Given that the image in figure 12.1 is representative of all typical articular joints, it is now appropriate to turn to the visualization of joint damage. The images shown in figure 12.3 are from the DIP joints of four separate subjects and illustrate the various appearances of cartilage in different states, ranging from normalcy to end-stage disease. It is important to note that these images also demonstrate the ease with which MRI can visualize osteophytes and cysts; this sensitivity to the status of bone is an unexpected bonus and clearly extends the diagnostic scope of the method. However, those images have even greater strategic implications for studies of aging, in that it is now possible within clinical ethics to study joints that are clinically silent but may have early pathologic lesions in the cartilage and/or bone. Thus, it may now be possible to establish studies to distinguish between the early onset of OA pathology and the damage associated with a lifetime of minor trauma and overuse. It is clear that selection of age-matched subjects for any OA clinical drug trial would be significantly aided by MRI selection of articular joints that, although clinically asymptomatic, nevertheless have defined pathology.

The use of MRI to detect damage to trabecular bone structure of either the hip or spine due to osteoporosis is at present confined largely to research studies. For example, Jara and co-workers (1993) developed an MRI protocol in which the image intensity depends on the extent of disruption of the trabecular bone. The images shown in figure 12.4, which are from a cadaveric proximal interphalangeal (PIP) joint, show what can be achieved under idealized conditions insofar as they delineate the complete array of trabecular architecture for both bones. It is improbable that spatial resolution adequate to allow such images to be obtained for patients known to be affected by OP will ever be achieved; however, it may be possible to sensitize other forms of MRI protocol to changes in trabecular architecture (Jara et al., 1993).

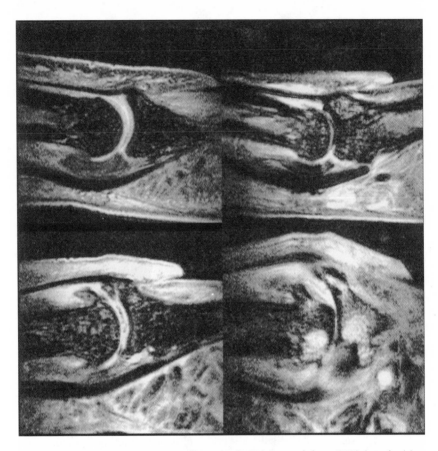

Figure 12.3.   Sagittal MRI images of a normal DIP joint and three DIP joints showing different stages of osteoarthritis. *Top left,* asymptomatic joint; *top right,* joint with loss of cartilage on the distal-phalanx; *lower left,* focal loss of cartilage, and large osteophyte; *lower right,* extensive joint degeneration, with major osteophyte formation and cystic lesions, and almost complete loss of cartilage.

Quantitative MRI Measurements of Cartilage Dimensions and Composition

Although the pronounced anatomical and pathologic features discussed thus far can be visually scored on the basis of their size, this is time consuming, and it is difficult to achieve a sufficiently high level of accuracy from such measurements to follow the progression of early pathologic damage (Hall and Tyler, 1995). Consequently, even for following substantial pathologic changes, it is desirable to have objective accurate measurements; for those more subtle features associated with aging, such measurements are mandatory. In this section we draw attention to the possibilities for fully automated quantitative measurements of cartilage dimensions and also of the various MRI parameters of water in cartilage, which reflects cartilage quality. It is encouraging that the basic methodology is now available. Furthermore, the feasibility of using MRI to follow progression has been demonstrated in a longitudinal study of the natural progression of damage to the guinea pig knee.

A number of groups have independently reported quantitative measurements of cartilage dimensions. For the human knee, Peterfy et al. (1994) used software to abstract the total volume of human knee cartilage from 3D MRI

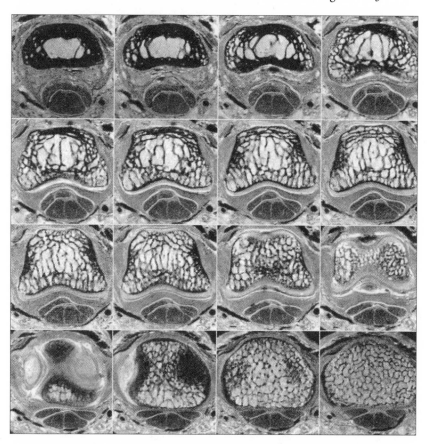

Figure 12.4. Representative axial MRI scans of a cadaveric proximal interphalangeal (PIP) joint showing the variations in trabecular bone structure along the length of the two phalanxes. A spin-echo (1500/20) sequence was used to give a 3D data set, resolution 0.075 × 0.075 × 0.075 mm, total scan time 26 hours.

University of Cambridge School of Clinical Medicine
Herchel Smith Laboratory for Medicinal Chemistry

Automated MRI DIP analyser output, version 1.1

File name (GRASS): fing9221.cmr   SNR: 38.5275
File name (MTC): fing9222.cmr   SNR: 16.8491

Mean total cartilage thickness for central slices 0.75 s.d. 0.03 mm

Slice No.	Cartilage Thickness (s.d.) mm	Fluid ?
0	0.860 (0.041)	×
1	0.787 (0.026)	×
2	0.705 (0.054)	√
3	0.748 (0.057)	√
4	0.895 (0.037)	√

Figure 12.5.   Report from automated measurement of cartilage thickness for a DIP joint. The images on the *right* record the fact that the MRI scans were successful, as was the edge-detection. The graphs on the *left* demonstrate the statistical analysis of the edge-detected regions.

scans optimized for cartilage; they validated their measurements by physically removing the cartilage. Other studies of cadaveric human knees have compared MRI cartilage thickness with the cartilage thickness revealed by sectioning the knee with a band saw (Eckstein et al., 1995). In an important knee study, Karvonen et al. (1994) presented data for 52 patients with idiopathic OA plus 40 reference subjects, and concluded that although age accounted for a significant decrease in the thickness of femoral cartilage in both the lateral and medial compartments, variations elsewhere were not significant. A similar conclusion was made for the right knee, whereas for the left knee only the lateral compartment showed significant changes.

To the best of our knowledge, the only fully automated procedure for quantitation of the thickness of living human articular cartilage is from the Herchel Smith Laboratory for Medicinal Chemistry at Cambridge University. Originally developed for the DIP joint (Robson et al., 1995), that technique has since been extended to the knee. Appropriate MRI scans are obtained which delineate the cartilage-bone interface and the cartilage–synovial fluid (or cartilage-cartilage) surface. Software written at the Herchel Smith Laboratory then automatically identifies the surfaces of the cartilage, and the space between them corresponds to its thickness. The data are printed as a report of thickness for each slice imaged, plus the mean-deviations; the method can be applied to 2D slice images directly, or to images abstracted from a 3D volume data set. A typical example of the former is shown in figure 12.5, with the measured thickness and an indication of whether or not synovial fluid has been detected in the scan.

The image of the cartilage for each of the central three slice images is shown along the right side of the report; these images demonstrate that the automated measurements have worked properly. Given below each of those images is the edge detection for the cartilage-bone and cartilage–synovial fluid boundaries, which show that the data-processing stage has also worked. Finally, for each of those three slices the plots of cartilage thickness are given at the left of the report. If there is no synovial fluid (as in the upper trace), then the measurement gives the total cartilage thickness; if there is, then each of the two cartilage layers is measured separately and their total is given as the mean value at the top of the report.

As shown in figure 12.6, a histogram plot of DIP-joint cartilage thickness, the most significant findings of the preliminary measurements made thus far are as follows: first, the range of thickness for cartilage in the DIP joints of patients clinically diagnosed as having established OA is larger than that for those with early OA or for their age-matched controls; second, the mean thickness values for each of those three groups are not significantly different. Since

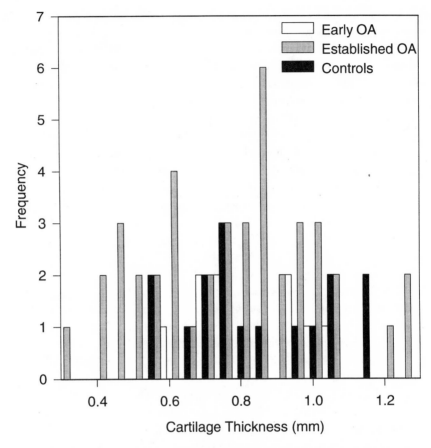

Figure 12.6.   Histogram plot of DIP-joint cartilage thickness for three groups of subjects: early osteoarthritis, established osteoarthritis, age-matched controls.

equivalent sets of data are not available for other age ranges, it is not yet possible to detect any age-related dependence. In addition to those evaluations it will also be necessary to study dependencies on the gender or the size of each individual. For such measurements it would be helpful to measure simultaneously three DIP joints plus three PIP joints, for each hand. Besides providing interjoint comparisons for joints having varying degrees of OA damage, it may be possible to assess OA patients by using the cartilage dimensions of the uninvolved PIP joints as a thickness reference, thereby eliminating the need to use age-matched control subjects.

Now that such approaches provide a noninvasive measure of the "quantity" of cartilage in a joint, it is clearly desirable also to assess its "quality." In principle, it should be possible to obtain that from the MRI parameters of water in cartilage, such as the spin-lattice (T_1-value) and the spin-spin (T_2-value) relaxation time, the water concentration (M_0-value), the magnetization transfer rates (T_{1sat}), the MT-saturation level (M_{sat}/M_0), and the self-diffusion coefficient (ADC-value). Several laboratory studies (Bernstein et al., 1993; Xia et al., 1994; Tyler et al., 1995) have demonstrated the gravimetric dependencies between those parameters and the concentration of water, proteoglycan, and collagen. The problem is to invent MRI protocols that are fast enough for clinical use yet accurate enough to detect small changes associated with early damage to human cartilage. Such detection would provide a quantitative measure of cartilage quantity which, because it is noninvasive, could be used to study aging as well as the evolution of OA.

This has now been achieved at the Herchel Smith Laboratory for the DIP joint, using a protocol that measures, for all the pixels in a single MRI slice image in 40 minutes scan time, the values for M_0, T_1, T_2, MT, and M_{sat}/M_0. Like the cartilage thickness measurements, this protocol is also automated. A typical report is shown in figure 12.7; the mean values for all the parameters and their standard deviations are shown at the top. Importantly, the histogram plots show the distribution for each parameter; if the values for damaged cartilage are sufficiently different from those for normal cartilage, those plots should show a wider distribution of values for damaged cartilage than they should show if all the cartilage of the joint is "normal" for that individual. Table 12.1 clearly demonstrates that the above expectations are supported by the data currently available. In particular, the mean T_2-values for cartilage of OA patients are not only approximately 30 percent larger on average than those for control subjects, but their standard deviation is 600 percent broader, suggesting that there is a wider range of cartilage composition. Although insufficient data are available to calculate the sensitivity statistics, the variations observed are nevertheless very encouraging. While the above data require further experimental confirmation based on data from a broader range of subjects, at present they are unique for human cartilage, and confirm the substantial potential of quantitative MRI.

Conclusions: Prospects for Future MRI Studies of Age-Associated Changes in Joints

Given the noninvasive nature of MRI and its proven capability for visualizing many forms of damage to human osteoarthritic articular joints, it is clear that MRI is also ideally suited for studies of clinically asymptomatic joints.

University of Cambridge School of Clinical Medicine
Herchel Smith Laboratory for Medicinal Chemistry

Quantitative MRI DIP analyser, version 1.0

File name: finq0003.cmr	SNR: 67.3296	File name: finq0006.cmr	SNR: 64.5952
File name: finq0004.cmr	SNR: 58.117	File name: finq0007.cmr.shift	SNR: 68.1248
File name: finq0005.cmr	SNR: 30.66	File name: finq0008.cmr.shift	SNR: 65.949

Parameter	Value	(s.e.)
T1	911	35
T2	26.8	0.7
Msat/M0	0.159	0.008
T1sat	109	5

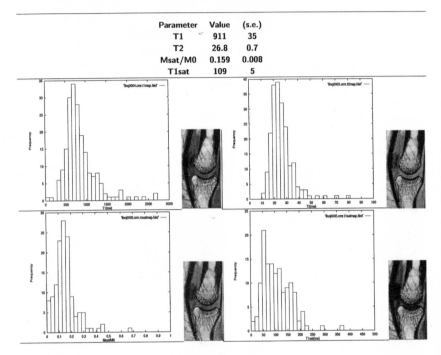

Figure 12.7. Report from an automated measurement of the MRI parameters for the water in the cartilage of a DIP joint of a 45-year-old female. The images demonstrate that each measurement module has worked. The histogram plots show the distribution of each of the four parameters.

That few such studies have been reported so far is largely a reflection of the fact that the technologies for making quantitative MRI measurements with adequate sensitivity and accuracy have not previously been available clinically, and is also partly due to the high cost and potentially long duration that such studies might involve. In the section that follows we address in turn each of those points in terms of the strategic planning that must precede such studies.

Future MRI studies of the effects of aging in individuals should include as many articular joints as possible but should place special emphasis on those that are known to be susceptible to degeneration and/or to OA or OP. According to the existing evidence from clinical evaluation (Dieppe, 1995) and x-ray studies (Buckland-Wright and MacFarlane, 1995; Lequesne, 1995), those joints include—in addition to the DIP and PIP joints of the hand—the knee, the hip, and the spine; both the hip and spine are also particularly susceptible to trabecular bone degeneration associated with OP in postmenopausal women. Although it is not easy to justify taking additional x-ray scans of clinically asymptomatic joints, all available information should be used to help define any clinical problem at entry. It is also clear that studies of aging must be made of joints that are free from overt pathology, and it is in that context that the noninvasive nature of MRI creates an ethically acceptable opportunity.

On entry of each patient to a study, the joints should each be imaged using a 3D volume protocol so that the entire joint can be viewed by appropriate clinicians and pathologists. By suitable choice of protocol, that same 3D data set can also be used for automated calculation of cartilage thickness and for estimation of trabecular bone degeneration. A protocol for quantitating all the MR parameters of the cartilage water should then be used; since it will have limited spatial coverage in terms of the total joint cartilage, it is important to position that slice to include the locations known to be most susceptible to the particular pathology. There may be some potential conflict between a study intended solely to delineate osteoarthritic changes and one that has to distinguish those from the effects of natural aging. Clearly, the former must focus the MRI scans on the regions already known to be most susceptible to OA, whereas the latter needs to include regions that are likely to be relatively uninfluenced by that pathology. For the hand, the solution is to study as many fingers per scan session as is feasible, and at the Herchel Smith Laboratory a single protocol is available that can now be applied simultaneously to all DIP and PIP joints of fingers 2, 3, and 4. This ensures that as many data as possible are obtained from clinically asymptomatic joints, which can then be compared with the data from

Table 12.1. Preliminary Data for the MRI Parameters for Cartilage Water for Three Groups of Subjects

Parameter	Early OA ($n = 10$)		Established OA ($n = 24$)		Control ($n = 8$)	
T_1 (ms)	1032	(379)[a]	1054	(202)	1017	(114)
T_2 (ms)	32.9	(15.5)	33.1	(18.1)	26	(2.7)
M_{sat}/M_0	0.27	(0.16)	0.31	(0.13)	.0.21	(0.03)
T_{1sat} (ms)	70.5	(14.8)	64.7	(18.1)	69.5	(9.2)

[a]Numbers in parentheses are standard deviations.

the clinically involved joints. It is a big advantage that the PIP joints have a prevalence for RA while the DIP joints tend to be more susceptible to OA.

For other human articular joints, there are two options. In all instances it is advantageous to ensure that the imaging slices that pass through the pathology also encompass tissues less likely to be clinically involved. For those joints that are bilateral (knee, hip, ankle, shoulder), it may also be possible to examine the uninvolved joint as a control; clearly this doubles the scan time, and hence the cost, of the study; it may also reduce patient compliance (which is clearly of great importance), as many elderly subjects, who may have other disabilities, do not always welcome additional, time-consuming exposure to high technology.

Although at present relatively few MRI centers have a capacity for, or a commitment to, the quantitative MRI approaches recommended here, the methods discussed in this chapter can now be applied to many clinical problems. Furthermore, the extent of interest by researchers in OA is growing rapidly, in part because of the need of the pharmaceutical industry to have an accurate measure of disease severity with which to demonstrate to regulatory agencies, such as the FDA, the clinical efficacy of new chondroprotective agents (see chapter 13). A similar pharmaceutical interest has previously motivated studies of trabecular bone degeneration and its treatment, and it is clear that interest in MRI will grow if it can provide information not only about bone density but also about trabecular bone morphology and the connectivity of the trabecular spurs. Taken in conjunction with the need to study skeletal and joint disorders of the ever-increasing aged population of developed countries, it seems highly desirable that MRI studies of aging and arthritic articular joints should be given increased attention.

ACKNOWLEDGMENTS

The collaborative research upon which this chapter is based would not have been possible without a generous benefaction from Dr. Herchel Smith (to Laurance D. Hall) and a Senior Research Fellowship from the Arthritis and Rheumatism Council (for Jenny A. Tyler).

REFERENCES

Bernstein D, Gray ML, Hartman AL, Gipe R, Foy BD. 1993. Diffusion of small solutes in cartilage as measured by nuclear magnetic resonance (NMR) spectroscopy and imaging. *J Orthop Res* 11: 456–478.
Buckland-Wright JC, MacFarlane DG. 1995. Radioanatomic assessment of therapeutic outcome in osteoarthritis. In: *Osteoarthritic disorders,* edited by KE Kuettner, VM Goldberg. Pp. 51–65. Rosemont, Ill.: American Academy of Orthopedic Surgeons.
Crues JV III, ed. 1991. *MRI of the musculoskeletal system.* New York: Raven Press.

Dieppe PA. 1995. The classification and diagnosis of osteoarthritis. In: *Osteoarthritic disorders,* edited by KE Kuettner, VM Goldberg. Pp. 5–12. Rosemont, Ill.: American Academy of Orthopedic Surgeons.

Eckstein F, Sittek H, Milz S, Schulte E, Kiefer B, Reiser M, Putz M. 1995. The potential of magnetic resonance imaging (MRI) for quantifying articular cartilage thickness: A methodological study. *Clin Biomech* 10:434–440.

Hall LD, Tyler JA. 1995. Can quantitative magnetic resonance imaging detect and monitor the progression of early osteoarthritis? In: *Osteoarthritic disorders,* edited by KE Kuettner, VM Goldberg. Pp. 67–84. Rosemont, Ill.: American Academy of Orthopedic Surgeons.

Hodgson RJ, Barry MA, Carpenter TA, Hall LD, Hazleman BL, Tyler JA. 1995. MRI protocol optimization for evaluation of hyaline cartilage in the interphalangeal joint of fingers. *Invest Radiology* 30:522–531.

Jara H, Wehrli FW, Chung H, Ford JC. 1993. High resolution variable flip angle 3D MR imaging of trabecular microstructure in vivo. *Magn Reson Med* 29:528–539.

Karvonen RL, Negendank WG, Tietge RA, Reed AH, Miller PR, Fernandez-Madrid F. 1994. Factors affecting articular cartilage thickness in osteoarthritis and aging. *J Rheumatol* 21:1310–1318.

Lequesne M. 1995. Quantitative measurements of joint space during progression of osteoarthritis: Chondrometry. In: *Osteoarthritic disorders,* edited by KE Kuettner, VM Goldberg. Pp. 427–444. Rosemont, Ill.: American Academy of Orthopedic Surgeons.

Morris PG, ed. 1986. *Nuclear magnetic resonance imaging in medicine and biology.* Oxford: Clarendon Press.

Peterfy CG, van Dijke SV, Janzen EL, Gluer CC, Namba R, Majumdar S, Lang P, Genant HK. 1994. Quantification of articular cartilage in the knee with pulsed saturation transfer subtraction and fast-suppressed MR imaging: Optimisation and validation. *Radiology* 192:485–491.

Robson MD, Hodgson RJ, Herrod NJ, Tyler JA, Hall LD. 1995. A combined analysis and magnetic resonance imaging technique for computerized automatic measurement of cartilage thickness in the distal interphalangeal joint. *Magn Reson Imag* 13:709–718.

Tyler JA, Watson PJ, Koh H-L, Herrod NJ, Robson MD, Hall LD. 1995. Detection and monitoring of progressive degeneration of osteoarthritic cartilage by MRI. *Acta Orthop Scand* 66(suppl. 266): 130–138.

Wolff SD, Balaban RS. 1989. Magnetization transfer contrast (MTC) and tissue water proton relaxation in-vivo. *Magn Reson Med* 10:135–144.

Xia Y, Farquhar T, Burton-Wurster N, Ray E, Jelinski LW. 1994. Diffusion and relaxation mapping of cartilage-bone plugs and excised disks using microscopic magnetic resonance imaging. *Magn Reson Med* 31:273–282.

13

The Pharmaceutical Industry and Therapeutic Approaches to Osteoarthritis in the Next Decade

Helmut Fenner, Ph.D.

No major progress has been made in recent decades in improving the management of osteoarthritis (OA). Obviously, research on and development of new therapeutic modalities in OA have been neglected by the pharmaceutical industry, although the medical need for novel agents and the enormous marketing opportunity presented by such drugs have been appreciated. Paradoxically, major resources have been dedicated in recent years to research programs dealing with issues arising from the use of currently available agents—for example, demonstrating marginal in vitro differences among nonsteroidal anti-inflammatory drugs (NSAIDs) with respect to cartilage damage—instead of addressing the more relevant basic and clinical questions that might have provided answers for progress in drug discovery programs. In general, there was no lack of interest in drug research on OA within the pharmaceutical industry; however, for several reasons, rheumatoid arthritis (RA) has been a more attractive target. Despite the huge impact of OA on the quality of life of millions of elderly persons, the perception of OA as a degenerative disorder with less dramatic signs and symptoms and a slower progression of joint damage than occurs in RA may have contributed to the fact that improvement of therapeutic interventions in OA is still only a vision.

Until recently, the molecular targets for a mechanism-based search for interventional strategies could not be defined clearly enough to provide a rationale for drug discovery programs. This situation has now changed, since significant progress has been made in understanding the mechanisms underlying inflammatory and destructive processes in RA and OA. Much of the complex system of soluble factors and direct cell-cell interactions involved in the initiation, manifestations, and perpetuation of articular inflammation and structural damage has been unraveled, and the time has come to define and explore a number of molecular targets utilizing the advanced technologies of drug discovery programs, including recombinant DNA techniques.

Among other more speculative interventional strategies, two major research avenues are currently followed and will provide novel treatment modalities for OA:

1. Novel types of anti-inflammatory and antinociceptive agents with an improved safety profile will be available in the near future (Vane, 1994). Selective inhibitors for the cyclooxygenase pathway (COX-2) that generates proinflammatory and nociceptive prostanoids have been shown to have no effect on the formation of regulatory prostanoids in the gut mucosa and the kidney (COX-1-derived prostanoids). As a consequence of the discovery of COX-1 and COX-2, the two distinct isoforms of cyclooxygenase, the separation of the targets for therapeutic intervention presented an opportunity to develop a new generation of anti-inflammatory drugs challenging the existing concepts of NSAID use. Since the functional roles of COX-1 and COX-2 are separated in tissue compartments, anti-COX-1 activity is reflected by tissue exposure to the circulating drug levels, whereas anti-COX-2 activity is exerted in the synovial system. This new generation of drugs will replace the currently used class of NSAIDs in the treatment of osteoarthritic pain and inflammation.

2. While well-tolerated novel NSAIDs are used to control the symptoms of OA, the destructive process will be addressed by inhibition of the matrix metalloproteinases (MMPs) involved in osteoarthritic articular cartilage matrix degradation, mainly collagenase and stromelysin. Orally active metalloproteinase inhibitors are expected to prevent erosive changes, or at least to decrease the rate of progression of articular matrix damage and to support cartilage repair mechanisms. Several MMP inhibitors with a promising profile in animal models are candidates for clinical development. This will be a time-consuming process and demands significant investments in new clinical research tools, thus presenting a major challenge to the pharmaceutical industry in the next decade.

The Inflammatory Process in Osteoarthritis

OA presents in a variety of clinical manifestations probably deriving from a common inflammatory disease process, initiated and maintained in many patients for many years without major signs and symptoms, although structural joint damage may ultimately be detected by radiographic assessment. Most of the early biochemical events involved in triggering the imbalance in matrix remodeling pathways and the failure of cartilage "healing" are not well understood at present. This is also true for the role of biomechanical effects, including trauma, and for the predisposing genetic and environmental factors associated with the initiation and the manifestation of disease.

However, basic and clinical research in OA has made progress in providing understanding of many of the molecular mechanisms that contribute to articular matrix damage and disease progression. There is now clear evidence for the existence, in OA and in RA, of qualitatively similar cascades of effector mechanisms of synovitis, which resemble each other with regard to the role of pro-inflammatory cytokines in the formation of effector molecules of inflammation and matrix degradation (see also chapter 11):

— Pro-inflammatory cytokines (tumor necrosis factor–α [TNF-α] and interleukin-1 [IL-1]) can be detected by immunohistochemistry in tissue derived from osteoarthritic joints (Miller et al., 1993).
— In response to elevated synovial cytokine levels, physiologic cytokine inhibitors (soluble receptors, IL-1 receptor antagonist) are up-regulated. Patients with RA, patients with OA, and healthy subjects can be differentiated by measuring their circulating levels of soluble TNF receptors (Dayer and Fenner, 1992; Otterness et al., 1995).
— This local response may contribute to regulatory control of disease manifestations and progression in some patients. If the amount of inhibitors produced in response to elevated ligand concentrations is not sufficient to restore cytokine homeostasis, cytokine-mediated effector mechanisms will be initiated (Dayer and Fenner, 1992).
— TNF-α and IL-1 induce or up-regulate gene expression of the phospholipase A2–activating protein (PLAP), subsequently activating biochemical pathways leading to the formation of pro-inflammatory and nociceptive prostanoids and leukotrienes (Bomalski and Clark, 1993).
— The cytokine-induced expression of COX-2 in the synovial system seems to be the predominant source of mediators of synovial inflammation in RA and OA (McCarthy and Crofford, 1995).

Novel Anti-inflammatory Therapies for the Treatment of Osteoarthritis

A number of targets can be defined for intervention against the inflammatory cascade in the synovitis within the osteoarthritic joint, including phospholipase A2 (PLA2) activation and function and initiation of the cyclooxygenase and lipoxygenase pathways. Drug discovery programs have addressed most of these targets in recent years. Although lipoxygenase inhibitors or receptor antagonists for individual leukotrienes have shown interesting profiles in animal models of inflammation, thus far a promising benefit/risk ratio has not been demonstrated for any of these agents in early clinical trials. In theory, PLA2 inhibitors would have great potential as anti-inflammatory agents, but no promising drug candidates have been well characterized so far.

Whereas many novel approaches to therapeutic intervention need to be explored carefully in the future, drug discovery and development have made considerable progress on the basis of new insights into basic mechanisms in two areas: anticytokine therapy, and selective intervention with the synovial generation of pro-inflammatory prostanoids mediated by cyclooxygenase 2 (COX-2).

Interventions Aimed at Controlling Inflammatory Mechanisms: Cytokine Inhibitors

The dominant role of pro-inflammatory cytokines in initiating and perpetuating synovial inflammation suggests that intervention against TNF and/or IL-1 formation or function by anticytokine therapies in immunoinflammatory disease states would represent a promising therapeutic approach. At present, TNF inhibitors (monoclonal antibodies to TNF and soluble TNF receptor fusion proteins) and IL-1 inhibitors (human recombinant IL-1 receptor antagonist and soluble IL-1 receptors) are under clinical investigation in RA and have shown dramatic and long-lasting effects on clinical and laboratory parameters of inflammatory synovitis. Although anticytokines are expected to have beneficial effects also in OA, systemic administration of these biological agents in a disease with local manifestations of inflammation will be difficult to justify for many reasons, including safety concerns and cost-benefit considerations.

Nevertheless, for the purpose of "proof of concept," the effects of anti-TNF or anti-IL-1 therapies in severe progressive OA should be explored by serial intra-articular injection of these biological agents. Persistent cytokine inhibitor levels are expected to control the inflammatory response for several weeks. Measurement of various synovial and systemically circulating immunochemical markers, including those reflecting articular matrix remodeling, could generate further evidence for the role of cytokine-mediated events in different disease stages of OA.

In the near future, small molecules will be available from drug discovery programs utilizing the information on structure and function of ligands and receptors for molecular modeling of agents with anticytokine activity. These drugs will be explored in various immuno-inflammatory disease states. Although they may have a potential as anti-inflammatory agents in OA, their systemic use will be restricted to autoimmune diseases, since the risk of affecting TNF-associated host-defense mechanisms cannot be taken in patients with OA.

Novel Cyclooxygenase Inhibitors

Nonsteroidal anti-inflammatory drugs are widely used in OA to control pain and symptoms of inflammation. For the currently used NSAIDs, two major drawbacks have to be considered: toxicity for the gut and the kidney, and the risk of a detrimental effect on cartilage and bone metabolism. Although numerous animal studies and in vitro experiments have compared the potential risk that NSAIDs will interfere with proteoglycan metabolism and chondrocyte function (many of the results of such studies have been used heavily in marketing campaigns by certain drug companies), the clinical significance of these findings has never been demonstrated in properly designed prospective clinical studies.

Recent work on the structure and function of cyclooxygenase has presented evidence for the existence of two different forms of cyclooxygenases (COX-1 and COX-2), which have a different functional role and represent distinct tissue-specific targets for COX inhibitors: COX-1, the constitutive enzyme, is expressed under physiologic stimuli in endothelial cells, in the gastrointestinal (GI) mucosa, in the kidney, and in many other tissues, including synoviocytes and chondrocytes of synovial membrane and cartilage, respectively. COX-1-derived prostanoids have a role in maintaining or restoring tissue integrity ("housekeeping" functions). COX-2, the inducible enzyme, is expressed during an inflammatory response in synovial cells and chondrocytes and is undetectable in other tissues (fig. 13.1). Studies on the expression and regulation of COX-1 and COX-2 in the synovial system have shown that both isoforms of COX are present under basal conditions and are up-regulated differently by pro-inflammatory cytokines: COX-1 is expressed 2- to 4-fold, whereas COX-2 is expressed 10- to 80-fold.

The predominant source of pro-inflammatory mediators derived from the COX pathway is cytokine-induced COX-2 expression, which thus is the target for intervention in inflammatory synovitis. In contrast, preferential or simultaneous inhibition of COX-1 is expected to present a risk to articular matrix components, since COX-1-derived prostaglandins are involved in the homeostatic regulation of the synovial mediator network (McCarthy and Crofford, 1995). Taken together, it cannot be excluded that in vivo effects on human car-

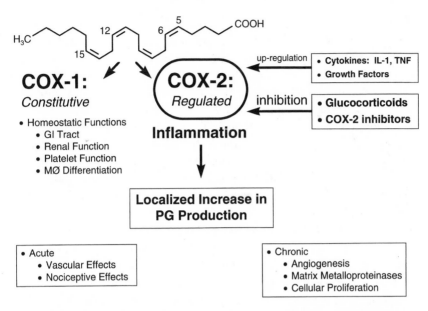

Figure 13.1.   Two different forms of cyclooxygenases (*COX-1,* cyclooxygenase 1; and *COX-2,* cyclooxygenase 2) have different functional roles and represent distinct tissue-specific targets for COX inhibitors. COX-1, the constitutive enzyme, is expressed under physiologic stimuli in endothelial cells, in the GI mucosa, the kidney, and many other tissues, including synoviocytes and chondrocytes. COX-1-derived prostanoids have a role in maintaining or restoring tissue integrity ("housekeeping" functions). COX-2, the inducible enzyme, is expressed during an inflammatory response in synovial cells and chondrocytes and is undetectable in other tissue. *MØ* = macrophage; *PG* = prostaglandin.

tilage function, and probably on cartilage repair mechanisms, due to chronic inhibition of the COX-1 pathway may translate into a risk for patients with OA during long-term use of these agents. Most of the data suggest evidence for differences among widely used NSAIDs which might be attributed to their differential COX-1 and COX-2 inhibition. This may explain why indomethacin, a preferential COX-1 inhibitor, exerts significant effects on cartilage proteoglycan and synovial prostaglandin metabolism (Rainsford et al., 1992), whereas no effect on proteoglycan metabolism could be demonstrated for meloxicam, a preferential COX-2 inhibitor (Rainsford et al., 1994).

The difference in the dose-response curves for COX-1 and COX-2 inhibition by indomethacin and meloxicam, established in a cell line expressing human COX-1 and COX-2, clearly indicates that meloxicam is a potent inhibitor of COX-2 at concentrations that do not affect COX-1, whereas indomethacin inhibits COX-1 at drug concentrations lower than the concentrations at which it inhibits COX-2 (Churchill et al., 1995; and fig. 13.2).

The future concept of anti-inflammatory intervention in OA is based on treatment modalities reflecting new insights into the role of pro-inflammatory cytokines in up-regulating pathways of osteoarthritic inflammation. Such intervention will include interventions with cytokine inhibitors, in the form of intra-articular administration of anti-TNF and anti-IL-1 therapies; however, this will be restricted to joints with severe manifestations of progressive OA.

Selective or preferential inhibitors of COX-2 will also be included. They will replace the currently used class of NSAIDs, which have an unfavorable benefit/risk ratio for use in OA due to COX-1 inhibitory effects on the gut, on the kidney, and probably on cartilage metabolism. The first representative of the new class of anti-inflammatory agents which will be available in the near future and will have the therapeutic advantage of selective or preferential inhibition of COX-2 in patients with OA will be meloxicam (Boehringer Ingelheim). In a daily dosage of 7.5–15 mg, meloxicam has been shown to be equivalent to standard NSAID treatment schedules in anti-inflammatory and anti-nociceptive activity, whereas, as compared to conventional NSAIDs, it has significantly lower GI toxicity, the major concern in prescribing NSAIDs (Hosie et al., 1996; Linden et al., 1996). The frequency of severe GI-adverse events (1.7% in both meloxicam treatment groups) was closer to the level seen with placebo than to the level seen with any of the comparators used in the trial: (piroxicam: 4.9%; naproxen: 7.8%; diclofenac sodium: 4.9%) (Distel et al., 1996).

Future Strategies in Therapeutic Intervention for Cartilage Degradation in Osteoarthritis

A number of studies have demonstrated that matrix metalloproteinases are expressed by synovial cells obtained from patients with RA (Dayer et al., 1976; Woolley et al., 1977). MMP expression is up-regulated by pro-inflammatory cytokines and the synovium in OA (Firestein et al., 1991). The role of expression of synovial tissue inhibitor of metalloproteinases (TIMP) in controlling MMP activity also must be considered. The relative local levels of collagenase or stromelysin, the presence of TIMP, and the complexes formed by MMPs and TIMP control the degradative potential at the level of the articular cartilage matrix (Walakovits et al., 1992).

A linear relationship between synovial levels of TNF-α and the latent forms of the matrix metalloproteinases MMP-1 (collagenase) and MMP-3

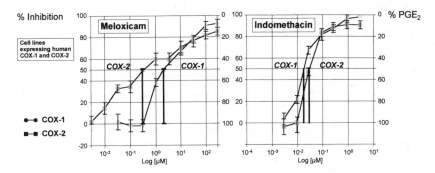

Figure 13.2.   Difference in the dose-response curves for COX-1 and COX-2 inhibition by indomethacin and meloxicam in a cell line expressing human COX-1 and COX-2 (Churchill et al., 1995). Meloxicam is a potent inhibitor of COX-2 at concentrations not affecting COX-1, whereas indomethacin inhibits COX-1 at drug concentrations lower than those at which it inhibits COX-2. PGE_2 = prostaglandin E_2.

(stromelysin) has recently been shown in synovial fluid from patients with RA (Fenner et al., 1995). The prominent role of TNF-α in MMP gene up-regulation is further confirmed by recent results from clinical trials with TNF inhibitors: a significant decrease in pro-MMP release is seen after synovial TNF-α trapping following the infusion of anti-TNF therapies. Simultaneous assessment of immunochemical serum markers for articular matrix turnover (type II collagen C-propeptide, cartilage aggrecan chondroitin sulfate epitope 846, and keratan sulfate, as discussed in chapter 11), indicates that matrix remodeling responds to TNF inhibition and MMP down-regulation (Fenner et al., 1995).

Disease-Controlling Therapy with Cytokine Inhibitors

Recent results from clinical studies with anti-TNF therapies suggest that long-term administration of TNF inhibitors represents an interventional strategy capable of decreasing radiographic disease progression in RA, thus meeting the criteria for a "disease-controlling anti-rheumatic therapy" (DC-ART) which have recently been proposed (Edmonds et al., 1993). As discussed, systemic administration of TNF inhibitors will not be a therapeutic option in OA; however, serial intra-articular injection of these proteins may represent a promising interventional strategy in severe progressive OA when the safety profile of these novel agents has been clearly defined in clinical studies.

Disease-Controlling Therapy with Orally Active Metalloproteinase Inhibitors

A number of pharmaceutical companies (e.g., Syntex, Searle, Merck, Wellcome, Stuart Pharmaceuticals, and Roche) have been involved for many years in drug discovery programs for inhibitors of cartilage breakdown. At the same time, basic research on the structure and function of metalloproteinases and their physiologic inhibitors has made considerable progress, and the most important MMPs are now available thanks to recombinant DNA technologies. Drug design by molecular modeling has been successfully used to make advance compounds available for in vitro and in vivo testing. Further programs have generated large numbers of compounds to establish the structure-activity relationship for MMP inhibitors, and the mode of action of these pseudo-peptidic agents is well understood.

A number of orally active MMP inhibitors have been synthesized in sufficient quantities and tested for specific inhibitory activities for collagenase (MMP-1), stromelysin (MMP-3), and gelatinase A (MMP-2). Several in vitro and animal models have been established for MMP inhibitor testing: inhibition of IL-1-induced degradation of bovine nasal cartilage, prevention of IL-1-induced glycosaminoglycan loss by femoral head cartilage, a rat sponge/cartilage implant model, and a rat model of *Propionibacterium acnes*–induced arthritis (Johnson et al., 1987; Nixon et al., 1991; Seed et al., 1993). However, the problems we are facing have been clearly addressed recently: "Using inhibitors of metalloproteinases to treat arthritis. Easier said than done" (Vincenti et al., 1994, p. 1115).

Concepts and Strategies for the Clinical Development of MMP Inhibitors

The clinical development of MMP inhibitors is challenging, as it presents a number of methodological issues which have never been addressed before in anti-arthritic drug development. A close cooperation has to be established between scientists who understand the biology of this intervention, clinical pharmacologists familiar with the specific pharmacology of antirheumatic agents, and clinical trial specialists experienced in difficult long-term drug trials. And, most important, new clinical research tools have to be established and validated which are sensitive to change in osteoarthritic joint damage and can be used for monitoring drug effects and defining clinical endpoints.

Points to Consider in Clinical Research and Development of MMP Inhibitors

Matrix metalloproteinase inhibitors for use in arthritis have to be active orally and show sufficient bioavailability. For compliance reasons they should not be given more frequently than twice a day.

MMPs are synthesized by various cells in the synovial system and are released from there in their latent forms (pro-MMPs) to be activated and enzymatically active in the extracellular milieu. An important issue in early clinical development, therefore, is pharmacokinetic/pharmacodymamic modeling to gain information on a dose-response relationship. An essential requirement for MMP inhibitors acting on target enzymes located in the synovial system is sufficient synovial fluid concentrations of the inhibitors to have access to the target tissue. Only if MMP-inhibitory drug levels are built up, persist over time, and are presented to the pericellular environment of synoviocytes and chondrocytes can trapping of the active form of the target MMP result in down-regulation of MMP-mediated cartilage breakdown. Information on the actual drug concentrations having access to the site of the MMP inhibitor–MMP interaction should be correlated to in vitro IC_{50} data in order to predict the locally active fraction of the total systemic drug level by measuring simultaneously systemic and synovial fluid concentrations after the administration of different dose levels in different intervals. Ideally, data should be generated defining the synovial area-under-the-curve (AUC) of the drug in relation to the systemic AUC to be able to correlate preclinical information on inhibitory drug levels with data on drug disposition in patients.

This is important information for defining a rationale for dose selection in early dose-finding trials. If a dose range theoretically capable of achieving inhibitory target tissue concentrations of the agent can be determined in early clinical pharmacology studies, the number of dose levels introduced in dose-finding studies for pharmacodynamic reasons can be limited dramatically, which will save development time and resources.

It is known from other therapeutic enzyme inhibitors that the pharmacokinetic profile of the agent may not reflect its therapeutic effects. The kinetics of enzyme inhibition are defined by equilibrium constants of the enzyme-substrate interaction. Information on the off-rates of these complexes provides an important contribution to pharmacokinetic and pharmacodynamic models of drug activity.

When evaluating systemic exposure to therapeutic agents with the potential to affect matrix remodeling, one has to consider not only the diseased tissue that represents the target of intervention but also the physiologic remodeling process in connective tissues other than articular matrix, or in unaffected joints.

Several MMP inhibitors have been tested in animal models to determine whether they prevent or significantly decrease the rate of progression of structural damage. For some agents, in vitro MMP inhibition and inhibitory activity at the level of the target tissue, resulting in a lower rate of degradation, has been demonstrated by histologic assessment of cartilage damage in animal models (Johnson et al., 1987; Nixon et al., 1991).

Radiographic Assessment of Disease Progression: Sample Size for Comparative Clinical Drug Trials

For comparative clinical drug trials in patients with RA, a sample size of more than 150 patients per treatment group has been estimated (Sharp et al., 1993) "to assure 90 percent power for detecting a 50 percent slowing of radiological progression at a significance of 0.05" (p. 332). Such cohorts of patients with a diagnosis of RA might be recruitable if the test drug promises some short-term or mid-term benefit for the patient. In this case the drop-out rate over 1 year may be not much higher than 20 percent, and 180 patients per treatment group have to be enrolled in such trials.

Because radiographic disease progression is much slower and much more variable in patients with OA than in those with RA, the mean progression rate in OA treatment groups will be much lower. For that reason, the sample to be recruited for trials for anti-osteoarthritic agents has to be a multiple of the sample size estimated for RA patients, and in order to demonstrate intertreatment differences OA trials must be much longer than RA trials. Furthermore, the sample size calculation has to consider a much higher drop-out rate because the study duration has to cover an active treatment period of 2–3 years on top of the recruitment time. Since patients are not expected to have any short-term or midterm subjective benefit from participating in such trials, their compliance will be difficult to maintain.

Dose-finding studies with novel anti-osteoarthritic agents claiming to be disease-controlling anti-osteoarthritic therapies have to cover a wide range of dose levels in order to identify a few doses with a probability of showing efficacy in larger phase III trials. Basing the success of the clinical dose-finding program on the use of conventional radiographic assessment procedures will consume several years and enormous resources and will have a limited chance of producing clear-cut results.

Imaging and Absorptiometry Techniques for Clinical Trials

Rapid progress in novel imaging techniques in recent years has provided more sensitive and more specific assessment procedures, which are currently used for basic and clinical research. Magnetic resonance imaging (MRI) has the potential to detect early changes in the structure of matrix components and may also be useful to monitor disease progression in OA. This methodology should be applied in future studies in which conventional outcome measures, other new imaging techniques, and immunochemical serum markers for articular cartilage turnover are assessed simultaneously (see chapters 11 and 12).

Automated MRI measurement represents the only technology available to detect minor changes in cartilage thickness and quality and to determine whether a treatment is capable of producing repair mechanisms (Tyler et al., 1995). However, owing to the magnitude of investment costs and logistic issues during drug trials, MRI is not expected to be established as a standard assessment procedure for use as a clinical development tool, since it is difficult to imagine that MRI use will be feasible and affordable in clinical dose-finding trials monitoring hundreds of patients spread over a huge geographical area.

Advanced technologies using dual-energy x-ray absorptiometry (DEXA) have the potential to quantify minor changes in bone density and cartilage thickness of the metacarpophalangeal (MCP) joints, to measure joint space width, and to measure total bone density alterations resulting from erosive or remodeling processes. If these DEXA methods could be validated for the purpose of monitoring disease progression in OA by computerized grading procedures, they would have a chance to qualify as important clinical development tools for novel drugs affecting matrix turnover and repair. Serial assessment of patients is less expensive with DEXA than with MRI, the assessment time is short, and longitudinal data analysis can be fully computerized.

These technologies would also be valuable research tools for use in addressing safety issues during the clinical development program in longitudinal studies with whole-body scans.

Serum Markers for Proteoglycan and Collagen Turnover as Clinical Drug Development Tools

A recent conference on molecular markers for joint and skeletal diseases has defined the status of immunochemical markers in basic and clinical research and addressed the issues related to their use as future tools in drug development for OA and RA (Heinegård et al., 1995). A number of promising marker candidates have been established and explored in smaller studies in patients with these disorders. None of the existing reagents, however, has gone through a validation procedure, which is a prerequisite for the use of a reagent as a clinical development tool in trials with drugs that have the potential to interfere with the synthesis and degradation of proteoglycans and collagens. Serum markers reflecting cartilage and bone metabolism and degradation are the most valuable novel research tool for future drug development in OA (see chapter 11).

In considering the directions that future improvement of therapeutic modalities in OA will take, answers will be needed to many open questions, including the following:

— Do immunochemical serum markers support the diagnosis of OA before x-ray changes are apparent?
— Does the use of serum markers in longitudinal studies provide information on disease manifestation, disease activity, and disease progression?
— Do certain immunochemical markers reflect repair of cartilage and bone?
— Do serum markers have the potential to discriminate between certain subpopulations of OA that are distinguished by genetic and environmental factors?
— Which are the most sensitive and specific markers for structural damage in OA? (These might not be the same as the markers that are most sensitive and specific for bone loss in osteoporosis, and rheumatoid joint destruction.)
— Do certain serum markers indicate drug-induced effects on extra-articular connective tissue or on healthy articular cartilage matrix?
— Finally, who is prepared to support financially the collaboration between basic scientists, clinicians, statisticians, and molecular biologists capable of solving the technical problems related to the large-scale production of reagents necessary for their clinical validation?

Conclusions: Perspectives for the Next Decade

A number of promising drug candidates are available for clinical testing to qualify as disease-controlling anti-osteoarthritic therapies. It is, however, difficult to speculate how long it will take to translate the progress in drug discovery into improving OA treatment by providing novel agents for patients. One of the reasons for this uncertainty is the lack of appropriate drug development technologies. Because up to the present time basic research in OA has been widely neglected, no major efforts have been made by the pharmaceutical industry to establish the clinical research methodology needed in this area and to prepare for trials with novel agents for OA. As demonstrated several times in the past, the driving force in improving the drug-specific methodology of clinical testing has evolved from needs recognized during clinical programs sponsored by the pharmaceutical industry. Without novel surrogate markers for articular matrix turnover, more sensitive imaging techniques validated for use in clinical trials, and the development and clinical testing of agents that interfere with inflammation and matrix degradation in OA, it is unlikely that novel therapies will reach the market within the next 10–15 years. Well-tolerated drugs for OA not only acting on symptoms but also decreasing the rate of progression of structural damage would be a reality much earlier if the appropriate combined efforts of academic and industry research could be initiated as soon as possible. The results would be appreciated by an increasing number of patients—and would present a major marketing opportunity for those pharmaceutical companies who commit themselves to this interesting and important field.

REFERENCES

Bomalski JS, Clark MA. 1993. Phospholipase A2 and arthritis. *Arthritis Rheum* 36:190–198.

Churchill L, Graham A, Farina P, Grob P. 1995. Inhibition of human cyclooxygenase 2 (COX-2) by meloxicam. *Rheumatol Eur* 24(suppl. 3):272.

Dayer J-M, Fenner H. 1992. The role of cytokines and their inhibitors in arthritis. In: *Ballieres Clin Rheumatol* 6:485–516.

Dayer J-M, Krane SM, Russell RGG, Robinson DR. 1976. Production of collagenase and prostaglandins by isolated adherent rheumatoid synovial cells. *Proc Natl Acad Sci USA* 730:945–949.

Distel M, Mueller C, Bluhmki E, Fries J. 1996. Global analysis of safety of a new NSAID, meloxicam. *Br J Rheumatol* 35(suppl. 1):68–77.

Edmonds JP, Paulus HE, Scott DL, Furst DE, Brooks P. 1993. Antirheumatic drugs: A proposed new classification. *Arthritis Rheum* 36:336–339.

Fenner H, Taylor D, Folkers G, Zueger S. 1995. The TNF-MMP-matrix network and serum markers for cartilage synthesis and degradation. *Acta Orthop Scand* 66(suppl. 266):156–157.

Firestein GS, Paine MM, Littman BH. 1991. Gene expression in rheumatoid arthritis and osteoarthritis synovium. *Arthritis Rheum* 34:1094–1105.

Heinegård D, Lohmander S, Saxne T. 1995. Molecular markers for joint and skeletal diseases. *Acta Orthop Scand* 66(suppl. 266):i.

Hosie J, Distel M, Bluhmki E. 1996. Meloxicam in osteoarthritis: A 6-month, double-blind comparison with diclofenac sodium. *Br J Rheumatol* 35(suppl. 1):39–43.

Johnson WH, Roberts NA, Borkakoti N. 1987. Collagenase inhibitors: Their design and potential therapeutic use. *J Enz Inhib* 2:1–18.

Linden B, Distel M, Bluhmki E. 1996. A double-blind study to compare the efficacy of safety of meloxicam 15 mg with piroxicam 20 mg in patients with osteoarthritis of the hip. *Br J Rheumatol* 35(suppl. 1):35–38.

McCarthy CJ, Crofford LJ. 1995. Interleukin 1 reduces expression of prostaglandin E subtype 2 receptors in rheumatoid synoviocytes. *Arthritis Rheum* 38:S273.

Miller VE, Rogers K, Muirden KD. 1993. Detection of tumor necrosis factor alpha and interleukin 1β in the rheumatoid arthritic cartilage pannus junction by immunohistochemical methods. *Rheumatol Int* 13:77–82.

Nixon JS, Bottomley KMK, Broadhurst MJ, Brown PA, Johnson WH, Lawton G, Marley J, Sedgwick AD, Wilkinson E. 1991. Potent collagenase inhibitors prevent IL-1 induced cartilage degradation in vitro. *Int J Tissue React* 13:237–241.

Otterness IG, Zimmerer RO, Swindell AC, Poole AR, Saxne T, Heinegard D, Ionescu M, Weiner E.

1995. An examination of some molecular markers in blood and urine for discriminating patients with osteoarthritis from healthy individuals. *Acta Orthop Scand* 66(suppl. 266):148–150.

Rainsford KD, Rashad SY, Revell PA. 1992. Effects of NSAIDs on cartilage proteoglycan metabolism. In: *Rheumatology, state of the art,* edited by G Balint, L Gömor, L Hodinka. Pp. 177–183. Amsterdam: Elsevier.

Rainsford KD, Ying C, Smith F. 1994. Comparative effects of meloxicam on cartilage-synovial components of joint injury in vitro. *Osteoarthritis Cartilage* 2(suppl. 1):58.

Seed MP, Ismaiel S, Cheung CY, Thomson TA, Gardner CR, Atkins RM, Elson CJ. 1993. Inhibition of interleukin 1β induced rat and human cartilage degradation in vitro by the metalloproteinase inhibitor U27391. *Ann Rheum Dis* 52:37–43.

Sharp JT, Wolfe F, Corbett M, Isomaki H, Mitchell DM, Furst DE, Sibley J, Shipley M. 1993. Radiological progression in rheumatoid arthritis: How many patients are required in a treatment trial to test disease modification? *Ann Rheum Dis* 52:332–337.

Tyler JA, Watson PJ, Koh H-L, Herrod NJ, Rabson M, Hall LD. 1995. Detection and monitoring of progressive degeneration of osteoarthritic cartilage by MRI. *Acta Orthop Scand* 66(suppl. 266):130–138.

Vane JR. 1994. Towards a better aspirin. *Nature* 367:215–216.

Vincenti PM, Clark IM, Brickerhoff CE. 1994. Using inhibitors of metalloproteinases to treat arthritis: Easier said than done? *Arthritis Rheum* 37:1115–1126.

Walakovits LA, Moore VL, Bhardwaj N, Gallick GS, Lark MW. 1992. Detection of stromelysin and collagenase in synovial fluid from patients with rheumatoid arthritis and posttraumatic knee injury. *Arthritis Rheum* 35:35–42.

Woolley DE, Crossley MJ, Evanson JM. 1977. Collagenase at sites of cartilage erosion in the rheumatoid joint. *Arthritis Rheum* 20:1231–1239.

Index

Library of Congress Cataloging-in-Publication Data

Osteoarthritis : public health implications for an aging population /
edited by David Hamerman.
    p.   cm.
    Includes index.
    ISBN 0-8018-5561-6 (alk. paper)
    1. Osteoarthritis.   2. Aging.   3. Aged—Diseases.   I. Hamerman,
David.
    [DNLM: 1. Osteoarthritis.   2. Aging. WE 348 O849 1997]
RA645.O74O85   1997
362.1'967223—dc21
DNLM/DLC
for Library of Congress   96-45259
                                                 CIP